AF668355

A Practical Guide to **Oxygen Therapy**

A Practical Guide to **Oxygen Therapy**

Previously known as Oxygen Therapy

Third Edition

SK Jindal MD FAMS FCCP
Emeritus Professor
Postgraduate Institute of
Medical Education and Research, Chandigarh, India
Medical Director, Jindal Clinics, Chandigarh, India

Ritesh Agarwal MD DM
Professor, Department of Pulmonary Medicine
Postgraduate Institute of Medical Education and Research
Chandigarh, India

Foreword
Randeep Guleria

JAYPEE BROTHERS MEDICAL PUBLISHERS
The Health Sciences Publisher
New Delhi | London

Jaypee Brothers Medical Publishers (P) Ltd

Headquarters
EMCA House
23/23-B, Ansari Road, Daryaganj
New Delhi 110 002, India
Landline: +91-11-23272143, +91-11-23272703
+91-11-23282021, +91-11-23245672
E-mail: jaypee@jaypeebrothers.com

Overseas Office
J.P. Medical Ltd.
83, Victoria Street, London
SW1H 0HW (UK)
Phone: +44-20 3170 8910
E-mail: info@jpmedpub.com

Corporate Office
4838/24, Ansari Road, Daryaganj
New Delhi 110 002, India
Phone: +91-11-43574357
Fax: +91-11-43574314
E-mail: jaypee@jaypeebrothers.com

EU GPSR Authorised Representative
Logos Europe, 9 rue Nicolas Poussin
17000, La Rochelle, France
Phone: +33 (0) 6 67 93 73 78
E-mail: contact@logoseurope.eu

Website: www.jaypeebrothers.com
Website: www.jaypeedigital.com

© 2022, Jaypee Brothers Medical Publishers

The views and opinions expressed in this book are solely those of the original contributor(s)/author(s) and do not necessarily represent those of editor(s) and publisher of the book.

All rights reserved. No part of this publication may be reproduced, stored or transmitted in any form or by any means, electronic, mechanical, photocopying, recording or otherwise, without the prior permission in writing of the publishers.

All brand names and product names used in this book are trade names, service marks, trademarks or registered trademarks of their respective owners. The publisher is not associated with any product or vendor mentioned in this book.

Medical knowledge and practice change constantly. This book is designed to provide accurate, authoritative information about the subject matter in question. However, readers are advised to check the most current information available on procedures included and check information from the manufacturer of each product to be administered, to verify the recommended dose, formula, method and duration of administration, adverse effects and contraindications. It is the responsibility of the practitioner to take all appropriate safety precautions. Neither the publisher nor the author(s)/editor(s) assume any liability for any injury and/or damage to persons or property arising from or related to use of material in this book.

This book is sold on the understanding that the publisher is not engaged in providing professional medical services. If such advice or services are required, the services of a competent medical professional should be sought.

Every effort has been made where necessary to contact holders of copyright to obtain permission to reproduce copyright material. If any have been inadvertently overlooked, the publisher will be pleased to make the necessary arrangements at the first opportunity.

Inquiries for bulk sales may be solicited at: jaypee@jaypeebrothers.com

A Practical Guide to Oxygen Therapy

First Edition: 1998

Second Edition: 2009

Third Edition: **2022**

Reprint: 2026

ISBN: 978-93-5465-580-7

Printed at Replika Press Pvt. Ltd.

Contributors

Ritesh Agarwal MD DM
Professor
Department of Pulmonary Medicine
Postgraduate Institute of Medical Education and Research
Chandigarh, India

AN Aggarwal MD DM
Professor and Head
Department of Pulmonary Medicine
Postgraduate Institute of Medical Education and Research
Chandigarh, India

Pankaj Arora MBBS MHA DNB
Associate Professor
Department of Hospital Administration
Postgraduate Institute of Medical Education and Research
Chandigarh, India

Paramez Ayyappath MD IDCCM
Head and Senior Consultant
Department of Pulmonary and Critical Care Medicine
Lissie Hospital, Ernakulam
Kerala, India

Balamugesh T MD DM
Professor
Department of Pulmonary Medicine
Christian Medical College
Vellore, Tamil Nadu, India

Poonam Chaudhary PhD
Department of Biochemistry
All India Institute of Medical Sciences
Bhopal, Madhya Pradesh, India

Ravindran Chetambath MD FRCP
Professor and Head
Department of Pulmonary Medicine
DM Wayanad Institute of Medical Sciences, Wayanad, Kerala, India

Uma Devaraj MD
Professor
Department of Pulmonary Medicine
St. Johns National Academy of Health Sciences
Bengaluru, Karnataka, India

Navneet Dhaliwal MBBS
Associate Professor
Department of Hospital Administration
Postgraduate Institute Medical Education and Research
Chandigarh, India

Sahajal Dhooria MD DM
Assistant Professor
Department of Pulmonary Medicine
Postgraduate Institute of Medical Education and Research
Chandigarh, India

Abhishek Goyal MD DM
Professor
Department of Pulmonary Medicine
All India Institute of Medical Sciences
Bhopal, Madhya Pradesh, India

Vijay Hadda MD FCCP FISCCM
Associate Professor
Pulmonary, Critical Care and Sleep Medicine
All India Institute of Medical Sciences
New Delhi, India

Ajay Handa MD DNB DM
Senior Consultant and
Interventional Pulmonologist
Sakra World Hospital and Visiting
Senior Consultant
Pulmonologist and Professor of
Internal Medicine, Baptist Hospital
Bengaluru, Karnataka, India

Hariharan Iyyer MD DM
Senior Research Associate
Pulmonary, Critical Care and
Sleep Medicine
All India Institute of Medical Sciences
New Delhi, India

Aditya Jindal MD DM
Senior Medical Consultant and
Intervention Pulmonologist
Director, Jindal Clinics
Chandigarh, India

SK Jindal MD FAMS FCCP
Emeritus Professor
Postgraduate Institute of Medical
Education and Research
Chandigarh, India
Medical Director
Jindal Clinics
Chandigarh, India

VK Jindal PhD
Formerly Professor of Physics and
Coordinator Nanoscience and
Nanotechnology
Panjab University, Chandigarh and
CSIR Emeritus Scientist
Honorary Professor in Biotechnology
and Nanotechnology
Guru Jambheshwar University of
Science and Technology
Hisar, Haryana, India

Parvaiz A Koul MD
Professor and Head
Pulmonary Medicine, SKIMS
Srinagar, Jammu and Kashmir, India

Jesin Kumar C MD
Assistant Professor
Department of Pulmonary Medicine
DM Wayanad Institute of Medical
Sciences, Wayanad, Kerala, India

Karan Madan MD DM
Department of Pulmonary,
Critical Care and Sleep Medicine
All India Institute of Medical Sciences
New Delhi, India

Uma Maheshwari K
MD DM FCCP
Professor and Head
Department of Pulmonary Medicine
St. Johns National Academy
of Health Sciences
Bengaluru, Karnataka, India

Venkata Nagarjuna Maturu
MD DM
Consultant
Department of Pulmonary Medicine
Yashoda Superspeciality Hospitals
Somajiguda, Hyderabad, Telangana,
India

Nazia Mehfooz MD
Assistant Professor
Pulmonary Medicine, SKIMS
Srinagar, Jammu and Kashmir, India

Saurabh Mittal MD
Department of Pulmonary,
Critical Care, and Sleep Medicine
All India Institute of Medical Sciences
New Delhi, India

Anant Mohan MD PhD
Professor and Head
Department of Pulmonary,
Critical Care and Sleep Medicine
All India Institute of Medical Sciences
New Delhi, India

Valliappan Muthu MD DM
Assistant Professor
Department of Pulmonary Medicine
Postgraduate Institute of Medical
Education and Research
Chandigarh, India

Anil Narang MD
Former Professor and Head
Department of Paediatrics
Postgraduate Institute of Medical
Education and Research
Chandigarh, India

Sourabh Pahuja MD
Department of Pulmonary,
Critical Care, and Sleep Medicine
All India Institute of Medical Sciences
New Delhi, India

Virender Pratibh Prasad MD
Associate Consultant
Department of Pulmonary Medicine
Yashoda Superspeciality Hospitals
Somajiguda, Hyderabad
Telangana, India

Priya N MD
Assistant Professor
Department of Pulmonary Medicine
Christian Medical College
Vellore, Tamil Nadu, India

Srinivas Rajagopala MD DM
Senior Consultant Pulmonologist
Director, Transplant Pulmonology
Medical Director, ECMO Unit and
Transplant Critical Care
Yashoda Hospitals
Secunderabad, Telangana, India

Puneet Saxena MD
Classified Specialist
Department of Pulmonary Medicine
Army Hospital (Research and Referral)
New Delhi, India

Inderpaul Singh Sehgal MD DM
Assistant Professor
Department of Pulmonary Medicine
Postgraduate Institute of Medical
Education and Research
Chandigarh, India

Manvi Singh MD
Assistant Professor
Advanced Pediatrics Centre
Postgraduate Institute of Medical
Education and Research
Chandigarh, India

Meenu Singh MD
Professor
Advanced Pediatrics Centre and
In-Charge, Telemedicine
Postgraduate Institute of Medical
Education and Research
Chandigarh, India

Ruchi Singh MD
Department of Physiology
Pulmonary Medicine
All India Institute of Medical Sciences
Bhopal, Madhya Pradesh, India

Tejas M Suri MD DM
Senior Resident
Department of Pulmonary,
Critical Care and Sleep Medicine
All India Institute of Medical Sciences
New Delhi, India

PS Tampi MD DM FCCP
Senior Consultant, Pulmonologist and Physician, Bombay Hospital and Medical Research Center
Mumbai, Maharashtra, India
(Former Honorary Faculty and Unit Head, Department of Medicine, Grant Medical College and Sir JJ Group of Hospitals
Former Professor of Medicine and Respiratory Diseases
Indian Navy and Armed Forces
Mumbai, Maharashtra, India

Rohit Vadala MD
Senior Resident
Pulmonary, Critical Care and Sleep Medicine
All India Institute of Medical Sciences
New Delhi, India

S Venkatseshan MD
Ex-Senior Resident
Advanced Pediatrics Centre
Postgraduate Institute of Medical Education and Research
Chandigarh, India

Foreword

Oxygen is essential for life and is a critical requirement for all living beings even though the medical use of oxygen became popular only in the modern times. The recent COVID-19 pandemic, however, has made it almost a house-hold commodity. Nonetheless, oxygen use for a disease state requires immense caution and care. It is like a prescription-drug which should be used under strict supervision for the maximum benefit and safety.

The healthcare system uses oxygen at all levels including wards, surgeries, trauma, intensive care units and maternal and child care. Oxygen is also given for long-term use at home in patients with chronic lung diseases. Oxygen should be considered a pharmacological agent with standard indications, side effects, prescribing information and auditing. The ongoing pandemic has emphasized the need to evaluate oxygen therapy critically and in a scientific manner. Often, oxygen delivery to patients is taken in a casual manner and left to untrained professionals. There is a need to understand the physiology behind oxygen uptake in the lungs, its transport in the blood and tissue oxygenation. There is also a need to understand the different ways in which oxygen is produced and supplied to a healthcare facility and the challenges in seeing that the supply chain, storage and production are well maintained and regularly monitored for optimum delivery. For clinicians working in both pulmonary and non-pulmonary areas understanding the various oxygen delivery systems becomes very important. The issues need and ways to give high flow or low flow oxygen to a patient need to be well understood. Moreover, the monitoring parameters while delivering oxygen and the goals of oxygen therapy are important.

There are certain circumstances where oxygen therapy becomes more specialized. This includes air travel (fitness to fly and other issues), oxygen at high altitude, oxygen therapy in diving, hyperbaric oxygen, etc. Detailed understanding of the pathophysiology of the underlying process is needed to be able to deliver oxygen in these special circumstances. Also, like any drug oxygen therapy also has side effects. Oxygen toxicity is a well-known entity but in day-to-day clinical practice it is often ignored.

There are many misgivings and misconceptions regarding the use of oxygen among not only the lay patients but also the doctors. The issue is rarely discussed at clinical rounds and bed-side discussions in the medical colleges. Students are left to gather information from scattered sources. They frequently find themselves stuck in the quagmire of internet and articles in different journals.

I am glad to write this foreword for a book which attempts to provide concise and comprehensive information for doctors of all categories. It bridges the requirements on importance and use of oxygen across multiple specialties. In this multi-authored book, various aspects of oxygen have been covered by experienced teachers and physicians who provide reliable scientific information for students, teachers and physicians of all hues. The mere fact that this is the 3rd edition of the book proves its popularity in the medical fraternity.

I am sure that the readers will find the book useful in their day-to-day clinical practice in all settings. It will greatly add to the knowledge spectrum of students and other readers. I do hope that it becomes a value addition to the existing medical literature.

Randeep Guleria MD DM FAMS
Director
All India Institute of Medical Sciences, New Delhi

Preface

No other event seems to prove the preciousness of Oxygen than the second wave of the pandemic COVID-19 during the year 2021. The sheer number of patients requiring oxygen coupled with the widespread panic created an acute shortage of this life-saving gas. There was almost round the clock media coverage creating ripples in the international circle. There had been a lot of misinformation affecting clinical judgment of physicians and administrative decisions. This prompted us to revise our book on the subject which had been published twice in the past during normal times. The third edition in any case was due after a gap of over ten years. We thought it prudent to tell about the updated information on different aspects of oxygen and its administration to medical students and health personnel of different hues.

In this edition, we have added the term 'A Practical Guide' to the earlier nomenclature of 'Oxygen Therapy' to stress upon the basic and introductory character of the book meant for medical students, teachers and practicing clinicians. All the chapters in this book are written and revised by distinguished pulmonary and critical care physicians who are actively engaged with administration of oxygen for their patients. Besides the pulmonary and intensive care physicians, the book is useful for internists and general physicians, anesthesiologists, cardiologists, pediatricians and all others who are required to prescribe oxygen for their patients.

For the purpose of cohesiveness and scientific understanding of students, the book includes the first few chapters on general introductory issues related to the history, physics of gases, respiratory physiology and tissue oxygenation. Thereafter we have discussed issues of indications and administration in different clinical disorders. Oxygen therapy for intensive care and long-term domiciliary use of oxygen find special mention. Some of the relatively uncommon issues seen in routine clinical practice such as the high altitude problems, air travel and oxygen therapy, oxygen use in diving medicine and hyperbaric oxygen therapy have been discussed in separate chapters. Considerations for neonates and children have been also added for the purpose of wider coverage. Besides the general principles, indications and use, we have also added oxygen therapy for COVID-19 infection and 'high flow oxygen nasal cannula system' in view of the recent crisis and interest in the subject. Finally, there is general introduction to the delivery devices, storage and supply.

We have attempted to compose this book as a day-to-day reference document on medical oxygen. It is meant for internists, general physicians, pulmonologists, intensive care physicians and postgraduate students of medical and pediatric specialties. It provides short but concise information on different aspects of oxygen meant as a therapeutic agent. It not only lays the scientific foundations of oxygen therapy, but also lays stress on a rational and well regulated use of oxygen as a core drug than a mere 'add on tonic'. We are hopeful that the readers will enjoy the reading and find it useful for their day-to-day practice of medicine.

SK Jindal
R Agarwal

Acknowledgments

We are grateful to our patients especially during this COVID-19 pandemic who made it critical to revise the various aspects of oxygen therapy to serve as a practical guide for the physicians. The book reflects the joint effort of the faculty and the alumni of the Department of Pulmonary Medicine, Postgraduate Institute of Medical Education and Research, Chandigarh and some other senior pulmonologists of India. We thankfully acknowledge their contributions.

Contents

Part A: General Introduction

Part B: Physiological Considerations

Part C: Clinical Considerations

Part A General Introduction

Chapter Outline

Chapter 1

Historical Aspects

SK Jindal

INTRODUCTION

Oxygen, constituting almost half of the earth's crust, is crucial for the living process. Its evolution had long preceded the appearance of life on earth. Subsequently, it has supported the survival of all living beings—man, animals, and plants. The history of the evolution of atmospheric oxygen is a matter of intense investigation for anthropologists, geophysicists, and chemists. Oxygen reflects the story of life for an ordinary man. Oxygen for treating medical diseases was discovered only in the last few centuries. Sadly, the story of this discovery is also laced with tragic happenings. Lavoisier, the man who first used the term oxygen, was guillotined during the French Revolution without any recognition of his immense contributions.

EVOLUTION OF ATMOSPHERIC OXYGEN

It is believed that the earth was practically devoid of oxygen, only about one-thousandth of the present level when it was formed some 4.6 billion years ago. Water itself had appeared much later after the earth had cooled down. Oxygen was produced by photo-dissociation of water by the ultraviolet light from the sun. There was plenty of water on earth and the ultraviolet light from the sun. Why was then the concentration of oxygen negligible? One single oxygen atom (or radical) is unstable and does not exist in the natural form. The oxygen molecule (O_2), which we need and breathe, is formed of two oxygen radicals. Whenever there is an excess of oxygen radicals, they formed ozone (O_3), cutting out the ultraviolet light from the sun. This would decrease further photo-dissociation and the production of oxygen.

There are two very puzzling facts about the relationship of origin of life and oxygen—one, life could initially develop only in an oxygen-free atmosphere. Two, it was the presence of living organisms that resulted in an increase in oxygen in the atmosphere. The explanation for the development of life in an oxygen-free atmosphere is attributed to the formation of organic compounds, which are essential components in the structure of all living things, both plants and animals. The compounds could form from water, carbon dioxide, and ammonia only in oxygen-free surroundings. Oxygen would have oxidized and destroyed the compounds. In the absence of oxygen, the organic compounds could accumulate and result in the formation of life. The presence of primitive cellular life encouraged an increase in oxygen concentration by permitting an increase in photo-dissociation of water.

Almost half the duration of the existence of earth had passed when primitive life had surfaced in the form of a single-celled organism. It is interesting to know that the living organisms themselves were responsible for the increase in the concentration of oxygen in the atmosphere. They started consuming oxygen for respiration and thereby encouraging further photo-dissociation and production of oxygen. Algae, the most primitive form of life, appeared around a billion years after forming organic compounds. Algae are photosynthetic in its function, i.e., it synthesizes energy in the presence of sunlight. At this stage, there was a marked increase in oxygen, about ten times the previous concentration. This concentration remained constant for the next two billion years by process of stabilization known as the Pasteur effect. An increase in oxygen encouraged respiration, which in turn reduced the available oxygen. This caused a reversal to fermentation and dissociation to produce more oxygen. This cycle went on for the next two billion years when there was a dramatic increase in oxygen concentration and the development of multi-cellular organisms. This was perhaps a major milestone in the evolution of life. Even though the atmospheric oxygen got established at the same levels as of now some 100 million years ago, it was less than 2 million years when the primitive man appeared. It has been explicitly illustrated with a simple example of a time clock. If the total time of the earth's formation is reduced to 24 hours, man had surfaced on the earth in the last half-minute.

Talking of oxygen, it is only about 100 million years since when we have concentrations like those of today. This is attributed to the formation of the ozone layer above the earth's atmosphere. The ozone layer formed from excess oxygen, could screen the dangerous ultraviolet light from the sun and other stars of the universe. Ozone acts like a canopy (or a tent) under which life could evolve without the danger of death from extraterrestrial rays.

It is difficult to know when the importance of oxygen in the sustenance of life was realized. Although the scientific references to its role were not available until the medieval period, the ancient Egyptian and Greek physicians did refer to the need for respiration and the requirement of air for sustenance of life. Most of the beliefs on the essential role of air were based on philosophical ideas than physiological evidence. The views were somewhat like those of other cultures. But oxygen as an independent component of air was neither known nor firmly conceived.

ANCIENT GREEK CONCEPTS

The purpose of breathing had remained enigmatic in the pre-Biblical periods. More than 2500 years ago, the Greek philosophers believed that air or some essential component of air distributed a vital need to the body. Even the role of lungs in breathing was not known during the Hippocratic period. Empedocles and Plato believed in the movement of air through the pores of the skin. This belief was later refuted by Aristotle, who, in the 4th century BC, identified a few essential elements, including earth, air, fire, and water. The need for 'air' remained well recognized, although its role was not identifiable. Aristotle believed that the role of breathing was to cool the body. Perhaps in the 3rd century BC, Erasistatus, a medical teacher at Alexandria in Egypt, recognized the interplay between air and blood as an essential function for life. It took four more centuries to postulate a theoretical concept of life based on knowledge from multiple sources. Galen, in the 1st-2nd century AD made several conclusions, one of whom related to air exchange. He laid down a schema that involved two-way traffic of inspired air and effluent waste vapors.

ANCIENT HINDU CONCEPT OF OXYGEN

The presence of lungs had been recognized in ancient Hindu medicine. Both Charaka and Sushruta, the two famous physicians/ surgeons of the Vedic period (500 BC), recognized a 'prana vayu,' i.e., life-air. Charaka mentions the head, the chest, the ears, the tongue, the mouth, and the nose as the seat of the 'pran vayu'. Sushruta (1000 BC) spoke of 'prana vayu' as flowing in the mouth. What else than oxygen can this 'prana vayu' be identified with? It was Sarangadhara, a 13th century physician, who explicitly described the concept of respiration:

नाभिस्थ : प्राणपवन : स्पृष्ट्वा हृत्कभलान्तरम् ।।
कण्ठाद्बहिर्विनिर्याति पातुं विष्णुपदामृतम्।
पीत्वा चाम्बरपीयूषं पुनरायति वेगतः ।।
प्रीणयन्देहमखिलं जीवयश्रुठरालनम् ।

In summary, it implied that the 'vayu' located in the 'hrdaya' (Chest) goes out, and after drinking the 'Ambarapiyush' (nectar), it goes back very quickly. It touches the interior of 'hrdaya', promotes the 'Jatharanatha' (life), and nourishes the entire body.

Sarangadhara had described the sequences leading to the inhalation of ambrosia, the food of gods, or nectar-like substance vital to life, from the outside air, its circulation through the heart to the brain and all other parts of the body. This 'nectar like substance' is likely to be what we now known as oxygen.

MODERN HISTORY OF OXYGEN

Paracelsus, a Swiss alchemist, had suggested in 1541 that air contained a life-sustaining substance. But the more precise basis of physiology was laid by William Harvey, who discovered the circulation of blood, although nothing much was talked of breathing. The credit of the work on the role of breathing goes to the four famous Oxford physiologists of 17th century. The physiologists clearly demonstrated that air was necessary for life and could keep an animal alive even when breathing movements were arrested. It was also shown that the dark venous blood became bright red when it passed through the lungs. This color change was attributed to the uptake of "nitro-aerial particles" from the air insufflated into the lungs. In the 17th century, John Mayow had suggested that only a portion of air was necessary for life. Still, his work was not acknowledged during his lifetime. More than a century later, this was to be labeled as oxygen when the gas was discovered and produced in the laboratory.

Medieval Europe from the 14th century onwards had gone through a period of renaissance which saw changes in innumerable scientific concepts. The mid-eighteenth century was the discovery of gases such as hydrogen, nitrogen, and carbon dioxide. Oxygen was isolated by Joseph Priestley in 1772 and prepared in a pure form by heating mercuric oxide. He had also demonstrated that the gas supported life of a mouse better than the air. He commented: *"It might be salutary to the lungs in certain cases when the common air would not be sufficient to carry off the phlogistic putrid effluvium fast enough".* Priestley, a clergyman, teacher, and librarian, was the son of a weaver and a farmer's daughter. Priestley also discovered that the gas obtained on fermenting grain (now known as CO_2) produces the drink known as seltzer when dissolved in water. He fell seriously ill from tuberculosis but got well to die at the age of seventy-one in 1801.

Interestingly, oxygen was independently discovered a year before Priestley by Scheele, who had named oxygen as 'fire-air'. Most of the gases were being actively investigated for their role in burning, which had remained a significant concern for the survival of man since the very inception of life. Different materials on burning (i.e., oxidation) were supposed to lose a substance called phlogiston as per Stahl's belief; Priestley, therefore, called oxygen as the dephlogisticated air.

It was later when the dephlogisticated air was labeled as "oxygen" (means "acid begetting" in Greek) by Antoine Laurent Lavoisier. He compared respiration with the process of combustion. He demonstrated that animal respiration involved the absorption of oxygen by the lungs from the inhaled air and elimination of carbon dioxide and water. Lavoisier also showed the essential nature of oxygen for human life that oxygen consumption increased with increased body activity. Lavoisier was executed during the French Revolution in 1789 since he was an aristocrat by birth.

One important development that significantly advanced our knowledge on clinical applications of oxygen related to assessing oxygen and carbon dioxide in the blood. Blood was first described to be slightly alkaline by Des Plantes in 1776. Oxygen and carbon dioxide were detected by Davy in 1799. Robert Boyle extracted "air" from blood. Magnus, in 1837, used the vacuum extraction technique to measure the content of these gases in the whole blood. Several other methods were employed in the first half of this century by Van Slyke, Scholander, and others, including the manometric or volumetric methods that were slow, elaborate, and required precision. Further refinements led to the development of highly accurate and fast response analyzers.

Tissue respiration was described in 1870 by Pfluger and others who identified the locus of respiration in the cells. In the 19th century, there was considerable debate between Ludwig, Pfluger, and others about theories of gas exchange. The argument further encouraged the discovery of methods for precise blood gas assessment.

Several other discoveries ran almost parallel, such as the role of hemoglobin in the transport of oxygen by the blood by Hoppe-Seyler during the 1860s. Dalton came up with his atomic theory of respiratory gases, while Paul Bert with his oxygen-dissociation curve in the early 1870s. The curve was depicted as 'hyperbolic,' which was changed to the sigmoid shape later by Bohr. The 'Bohr' effect and the 'Haldane effect' were reported later in the early 20th century.

Oxygen deficiency was perhaps first established as "anoxemia of high altitude" in 1878 by Bert, who attributed altitude sickness and death to lack of oxygen. Even earlier, Joseph Ch. Hamel, a Russian physician, had believed that the lack of oxygen was responsible for muscular weakness at altitude. On an ascent to Mont Blanc in 1820, he had planned to study the oxygen content of air and blood at the summit and the effects of oxygen administration. Unfortunately, an avalanche that killed three of his guides shortly before the summit stopped the expedition. It was almost half a century later that the term "anoxia" was used by Barcroft and Van Slyke. Uptake of oxygen was another issue that remained controversial between Bohr and his former assistant August Krogh and wife, Marie Krogh. While Bohr supported the theory of secretion of oxygen, the Krogh team showed diffusion of gases in the lungs to explain oxygen uptake. It was Joseph Barcroft who finally demonstrated that diffusion alone was the mechanism for gas exchange.

OXYGEN THERAPY

Thomas Beddoes used oxygen for the first time in the early 1800s for treating medical disorders. He built a pneumatic piston with help from James Watt, the inventor of a steam-engine for storing and delivering oxygen. Soon after, oxygen became a therapeutic panacea for many illnesses. It was used for diseases such as cholera, infertility, hysteria, and glycosuria. It was considered a 'cure-all' medicine until the early 20th century. Cunningham, a famous US physician, treated his patients of arthritis, anemia, syphilis, glaucoma, diabetes, and cancers, with high pressures of oxygen. He reported the recovery of his patients but did not find any scientific support from others. As expected, no consistent benefit could be found for most patients, and soon oxygen use became unpopular and achieved a kind of notoriety. This got compounded by the reports on toxic effects of excessive oxygen use. William Osler, who recognized "imperfectly oxidized" blood in pneumonia, was also more fearful of its toxicity than benefits. The use of oxygen for treating pneumonia was reported first in 1885 by George Holtzapple to benefit average country practitioners.

Meanwhile, there were other developments in respiratory physiology, which helped re-establish the role of oxygen therapy. In the 1920s, it was established that oxygen deficiency resulted in severe physiological disturbances which could be corrected with supplemental oxygen. These observations were supported by firm clinical and experimental evidence. Oxygen therapy now achieved a prime role in the treatments of cardiac and respiratory diseases. Oxygen was commercially produced for the first time in 1895 by Carl von Linde using fractional distillation of liquid air.

John Haldane used oxygen to treat chlorine poisoning during World War I. He had stated that 'hypoxia not only stops the machine but wrecks the machinery.' He had also advocated the use of oxygen for the treatment of other respiratory illnesses. During this period in 1921, Meakins used oxygen therapy to manage lobar pneumonia. He reported that oxygen therapy was perhaps the most important factor in the treatment apart from the specific cure of infection. This was probably the major landmark in oxygen therapy in modern medicine after its initial use and subsequent disrepute. Its use became widespread in the following years.

Parallel to the discovery of oxygen use were the developments concerning its toxicity. Its toxic effects were suspected by Von Liebig, Pasteur, and Bent. Terms such as 'oxygen toxicity lung' and 'respirator lung' were used to describe respiratory failure caused by excessive oxygen use or 'oxygen-free radicals.' Devison compared the oxygen molecule to a grenade which could cause tremendous damage once the safety pin was pulled out.

The history of respiratory failure is relatively more recent. The terms 'anoxia' and subsequently 'hypoxia' were used in the 3rd and 4th decades of the twentieth century. The concept of 'pulmonary insufficiency' was introduced in 1940 by Cournand and Richards.

More precise and meaningful terms have been used thereafter. The definition continues to be debated and refined. But the fact that respiratory failure was directly linked to oxygen deficiency and its treatment with oxygen administration were clearly established.

The methods and devices used for oxygen administration have also undergone a sea change. Many kinds of pipes had been used in the past. Gas pipes were popular treatment devices in the late nineteenth and early twentieth centuries. Different types of masks, oxygen tents, and cannulae were developed during the world wars. Closed-circuit oxygen equipment was commonly employed in the 1930s and 1950s, for example, during mountaineering. Tom Bourdillon and Charles Evans, who had climbed to within 90 m of Mt. Everest in 1953, two days before the summit was finally conquered, had to abandon their effort because of the circuit's malfunction.

HYPERBARIC OXYGEN

The development of hyperbaric oxygen therapy is another long story that saw quite a few upheavals. Some of these developments have been discussed in the chapter on hyperbaric oxygen. Hyperbaric air chambers to treat different ailments have been used since 1662 in one or the other form with varying degrees of enthusiasm and antagonism. It was in the early 20th century when hyperbaric oxygen was first used to treat decompression sickness. Later, the scope of therapy was extended to cover several other clinical indications.

DOMICILIARY OXYGEN

Alvan Barach used oxygen for the reversal of hypoxemia in the 1920s, and recognized the need for continuous use of oxygen in patients with chronic obstructive lung disease. The ambulatory use of oxygen to improve exercise tolerance was tried by Cotes in 1956 in U.K. and Barach in North America in 1959. Rapid progress was made in the next few years. Chamberlain showed the reversal of polycythemia by oxygen administration. The first two studies on domiciliary use made by Levine et al. (1967) and Abraham et al. (1969) also showed improvements in polycythemia and pulmonary hypertension in patients of chronic obstructive lung disease.

Once the domiciliary use was found effective, refinements were introduced into the design and modes of administration. Low flow oxygen delivery with the help of nasal cannulae was shown to be effective and safe. The previously held belief that intermittent oxygen could cause greater CO_2 retention and aggravate hypoxemia was dispelled. A significant improvement in overall survival was shown by Neff and Petty in 1970. Studies by the Medical Research Council (MRC) and the National Institute of Health (NIH) in 1980-81 are considered landmark studies in the use of domiciliary oxygen. Further improvements in oxygen therapy continue to occur after that. But the role of oxygen as a maintenance drug was settled.

Domiciliary oxygen was initially introduced for patients with chronic obstructive pulmonary disease and hypoxemia, for which there is definitive clinical evidence. The indications soon expanded to include several other chronic lung diseases associated with hypoxemia or breathlessness, even though the evidence for several of these uses has not been established. Some such common conditions include kyphoscoliosis, extensive bronchiectasis, interstitial lung diseases, and pulmonary fibrosis. In some cases, the indications also include patients with chronic congestive heart failure, malignancies, and other non-respiratory illnesses. Factually, oxygen use at home has now assumed the role of a maintenance drug for many debilitating diseases.

SUGGESTED READING

1. Astrup P, Severinghaus JW. The History of Blood Gases. Acids and Bases. Copenhagen, Munksgaard International Publishers 1986.
2. Barach AL. Thetherapeutic Use of Oxygen. JAMA. 1922;79:693–98.
3. Campbell EJM. Oxygen and hypoxia. Seminar Respir Med. 1981;3:59.
4. Cotes JE, Gilson JC. Effect of oxygen on exercise ability in chronic respiratory insufficiency. Lancet. 1956;1:872.
5. Cournand A. Air and blood. In: Fishman AP, Richards DW (Eds) Circulation of the Blood, Men and Ideas. Bethesda, MD, American Physiological Society. 1982, pp. 3–70.
6. Devison DM. The distribution and use of oxygen in tissues. In: Cumming G, Scadding G (Eds). Scientific Foundations of Respiratory Medicine. London: Heineman Medical. 1981, pp. 221–37.
7. Dickerson RE. Chemical Evolution and the Origin of Life. Scientific American. 1978;239:70–86.
8. Dwarkanath C. The Development of Indian Medicine - Sarangadhara's Contribution: Central Council for Research in Ayurveda and Sidha Ministry of Health and Family Welfare, Govt. of India, New Delhi, 1991.

9. Fitting J-W. From breathing to respiration. Respiration. 2015;89:82–87
10. Flenley DC. Long-term home oxygen therapy. Chest 1985; 87:99–103.
11. Franklin KJ. A Short History of Physiology, 2nd edn. London, Staples, 1949.
12. Gerschman R. Historical Introduction to the 'Free Radical Theory' of Oxygen Toxicity. In: Gilbert DL (Ed). Oxygen and Living Processes: An Interdisciplinary Approach. New York, Springer-Verlag. 1981, pp. 44–7.
13. Grainge C. Breath of life: The evolution of oxygen therapy. J Royal Society of Medicine. 2004; 97:489–93.
14. Levine BF, Bigelow DB, Hamstra RD, et al. The role of long-term continuous oxygen administration in patients with chronic airway obstruction with hypoxaemia. Ann Intern Med. 1967;66:639.
15. McKie D. Antoine Lavoissier: Scientist, Economist, Social Reformer. New York, Schuman, 1952.
16. Meakins J. Observations on the gases in human arterial blood in certain pathological pulmonary conditions and their treatment with oxygen. J Pathol Microbiol. 1921;24:79–90.
17. Medical Research Council Working Party. Long-term domiciliary oxygen Therapy in chronic hypoxic cor pulmonale complicating chronic bronchitis and emphysema. Lancet. 1981;1:681.
18. Neff TA, Petty TL. Long-term continuous oxygen therapy in chronic airway obstruction: Mortality in relationship to cor pulmonale, hypoxia and hypercapnia. Ann Intern Med. 1970;28:784.
19. Nocturnal Oxygen Therapy Trial Group. Continuous or nocturnal oxygen therapy in hypoxaemic chronic obstructive lung disease: A clinical trial. Ann Intern Med. 1980; 93:391.
20. Perkins JF Jr. Historical development of respiratory physiology, in Fenn WO, Rahn H (Eds). Handbook of Physiology, Section 3: Respiration. Vol. 1, Bethesda, MD, American Physiological Society. 1964, pp.1–62.
21. Petty TL. Historical highlights of long-term oxygen therapy. Respir Care. 2000; 45:29–36.
22. Priestley J. Experiments and observations on different kinds of air (1775). Alembic Club Reprints. Chicago, University of Chicago Press, 1906: 1(7).
23. Rutten MG. The History of Atmospheric Oxygen. Space Life Sci. 1970; 2:5–17.
24. Sarangadharacharya P. The Sarangadhara Samhita. Nirnaya-Sagar Press, Mumbai, 1920.
25. Shultz SM, Hartmann PM. George E Holtzapple (1862-1946) and oxygen therapy for lobar pneumonia: The first reported case (1997) and a review of the contemporary literature to 1899. J Med Biogr. 2005; 13:201–6.
26. Simons E, Oelz O. Mont Blanc with Oxygen: The First Rotters. High Alt Med Biol. 2001; 2:545–9.
27. Sternbach GL, Varon J. The discovery and rediscovery of oxygen. J Emerg Med. 2005; 28:221–4.

28. Sullivan-Fowler M. The giver of oxygen: Hercules Sanche and the oxydonor. J Med Humanit. 1996; 17:31–43.
29. Warren CP. The Introduction of oxygen for pneumonia as seen through the writings of two McGill University Professors, William Osler and Gonatham Meakins. Can Respir J. 2005; 12:81–5.
30. Windson JS, Rodway GW, Dick J. The Use of Closed-circuit oxygen in the Himalayas. High Alt Med Biol. 2005; 6:263–9.
31. Wollman H, Dripps RD, Goodman LS, Gilman A. The Pharmacological Basis of Therapeutics. New York, Macmilan, 1965, p. 902.

Chapter 2

Applied Physics of Gases

VK Jindal, SK Jindal

Knowledge of physical principles governing the movement of gases in and out of the respiratory system is important for students of respiratory medicine not only for a better understanding of normal physiology of respiration and pathophysiology of diseases but also for their diagnosis and management. The air we normally breathe is a mixture of gases of which oxygen (O_2) and nitrogen (N) constitute the main bulk. Oxygen remains the most important gas in medicine. Carbon dioxide (CO_2) produced during metabolism and exhaled out of the lungs is another important gas. Breathing of additional or supplemental gases is required in abnormal situations. While the role of anesthetic gases required for brief periods, has greatly diminished, helium is another gas which has found an expanded role in emergency clinical practice. The physical properties of these gases influence the mechanics of normal breathing as well as the therapeutic strategies. Nitric oxide or nitrogen monoxide (NO), a pulmonary vasodilator is another important gas in our use. The 1998 Nobel Prize in Physiology or Medicine was awarded for discovering nitric oxide's role as a cardiovascular signaling molecule. Some of the other oxides of nitrogen (nitric dioxide or the brown gas, nitrous oxide used as an anesthetic), sulphur di-oixide and ozone are important air pollutants.

STATE OF MATTER

Matter can exist in three classically different forms in nature—solid, liquid or gas. Plasma, a fourth state of matter has also been identified under extremes of temperature and pressure. Matter is either an element made from similar atoms, e.g., iron or compound made from two or more types of atoms, e.g., water (H_2O) in nature. An element is a basic unit of matter which retains the same properties on subdivisions by chemical or mechanical means. Oxygen and other gases such as hydrogen, helium, chlorine and nitrogen are elements in nature. Oxygen (O) is an element with atomic number 8. It is highly reactive non-metal element that readily forms oxides with most elements and compounds.

Atom and Element

An atom, is the smallest part of an element which acts like its 'building block.' On further subdivision of an atom, the elemental properties are lost and therefore, sub-atomic constituents of all atoms are identical. Atoms of certain elements (e.g., hydrogen, helium) can exist in free stage (H, He) and there is no difference between the atoms and molecules of these elements. Atoms of many other elements (such as oxygen) do not exist free but combine with other atoms of the same element to form molecules (e.g., O_2, i.e., O + O). It happens because atoms of some elements strongly interact with other atoms of the same element to exist as molecules which are relatively weakly interacting with other molecules.

Molecule and Compound

All substances consist of exceedingly small particles called molecules. There are about 10^{19} molecules in 1 mL of air under normal conditions of temperature (T) and pressure (P). A molecule possesses the distinctive properties of the parent element or compound. A molecule is found to consist of two or more atoms of same kind or of different kinds.

The number of molecules comprising a macroscopic quantity of a gas is enormous typically around 10^{23} molecules. The number of molecules per unit volume and their velocity determine many properties of gases.

A compound is composed of two or more elements united chemically to form a substance different from the individual elements forming that compound. For example, carbon dioxide is a compound of carbon and oxygen. On subdivisions, the compound loses its properties and may resume those of the constituent elements. Both elements and compounds exist as molecules as smallest component.

Molecular Movement

All the molecules of matter are in a state of incessant motion. This is known as Brownian movement and forms the basis of kinetic theory of matter. This motion results from temperature—the higher the temperature, the larger the velocity of the molecules. At absolute zero temperature, the velocity of a classical molecule goes to zero. Molecules of a gas have great mobility and travel longer distances before colliding with other molecules. It is because of this mobility that a gas has no fixed shape and mixes readily with other gases.

Atomic and Molecular Weights

The mass of an atom is concentrated at its nucleus, which contains a definite number of neutrons and protons of almost identical masses. The neutrons or protons are also called nucleons. The mass of a nucleon is $\approx 1.6 \times 10^{-24}$ g (sometimes also called atomic mass unit, amu). Therefore, total number of nucleons of an atom determines the mass of an atom and is usually called atomic weight. This H atom has atomic weight equaling 1, whereas O atom has atomic weight equaling 16. Though their actual masses are around $1 \times 1.6 \times 10^{-24}$ g and $16 \times 1.6 \times 10^{-24}$ g, respectively. Similarly, molecular weight is determined by summing up atomic weights of the constituent atoms forming that molecule. As an example, H_2 molecule has a molecular weight = 2, and H_2O molecule has a molecular weight = 2 + 16 = 18. For obtaining their actual weights, we multiply those weights by amu (= 1.6×10^{-24} g) to get the mass in grams.

If M is the molecular weight of given substance, then 1 molecule of that substance weighs $M \times 1.6 \times 10^{-24}$ g. This gives us that M grams of the substance will have $1/1.6 \times 10^{-24}$ molecules, which is called Avogadro number No. $\approx 6.02 \times 10^{23}$. It is thus clear that M grams (also called 1 mole) of any substance will have N_0 molecules.

Gaseous substance (which behave like an ideal gas) follow an equation $PV = \eta RT$.

One can easily calculate the volume at NTP (normal temperature 0°C, and pressure ≡ 760 mmHg) from η = 1 mole. It comes out to be 22.4 liters for any gas. Therefore, a quantity of any substance equaling molecular weight as grams has 6.02×10^{23} molecules and as a gas, occupies 22.4 liters at NTP.

PHYSICAL PROPERTIES OF GASES

Volume

Volume is the space occupied by a gas. The volume of a cuboid shape vessel is determined by the multiplication of internal length, width and height of the vessel. It is expressed in cubic centimeters (cc), cubic feet or liters (L), etc. (1 L ≡ 1000 cc or mL).

Volume = Length × Width × Height

A 10 cm cube has the volume equaling 1 L. Volume of a container of uniform cross-sectional area A and height is given by V = A h.

The gas shall occupy the available volume irrespective of the amount (mass) of gas. For example, if a small vessel containing oxygen is emptied in a larger vessel, the entire volume of the larger vessel will be occupied by the same amount of gas **(Fig. 2.1)**.

Mass and Weight

Mass is the bulk or the total mass of number of molecules of the gas. In the above mentioned example, the mass of the gas in two cylinders shall remain the same, although the volume has changed. The number of molecules per unit of volume in the two vessels has changed, i.e., lesser number of molecules per unit volume in the larger vessel **(Fig. 2.1)**.

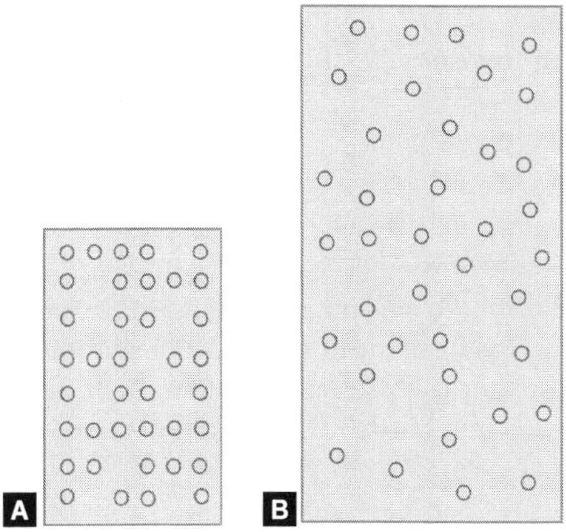

Fig. 2.1: Mass of a gas such as O_2 (i.e., number of molecules in vessels A and B is unchanged, but the volumes are different therefore, the density of the gas in vessel A is greater than that in vessel B.

Weight is often used synonymously with mass. Weight is determined by the pull of gravity on mass (i.e., m × g). Since the force of gravity on the earth is nearly constant, mass is equivalent to weight on the surface of the earth. In fact, weight is scaled to indicate mass and therefore both represent the same thing.

$$W \equiv \text{force} = mg$$

Density

Density is expressed as the weight in grams of one liter of a gas. Since the weight of 22.4 liters of a gas is that of a gram molecule of that gas, one liter of the gas shall weigh molecular weight/22.4 grams. When expressed this way, the density will be measured in g/L. It is also measured in g/cc which will equal 1/1000 in value to that in g/L.

Molecular weight of oxygen = 32

$$\begin{aligned} \text{Density} &= 32/22.4 \\ &= 1.43 \text{ g/L} \end{aligned}$$

The density of a gas is also expressed as relative to the density of air. Density of air shall vary depending upon its composition. For all practical purposes, it comprises of 1 volume of oxygen (about 20%) and 4 volumes of nitrogen (about 80%). At NTP, the density of air is $(32 \times 1/5 + 28 \times 4/5) / 22.4 = 1.3$ g/L. Therefore, the density of oxygen relative to that of air is 1.1. When expressed this way, it becomes unimportant if the density of individual gases was calculated in g/L or g/cc.

Pressure

The gas molecules are always in a state of motion and constantly bombard the walls of the container. The force applied to (or acting upon) a unit area of the wall is called the gas pressure. The closer the molecules, the greater the number which strike each unit area and therefore the greater the pressure applied. Also, larger the velocity (or temperature), larger is the impact on the walls, leading to greater pressure.

Gas pressure is generally considered as that of a stationary gas when the pressure exerted is the same at any point in a gas container. The pressure is usually expressed in millimeters of mercury (mm Hg) or centimeters of water (cmH_2O) or pounds per square inch (psi).

One mm Hg means force on a unit area (1 cm^2) on which 1 mm of height of Hg is placed. The volume of height h cm on unit area is A × h = h cm^3 and in mass is hd where d is the density of the liquid. The force on unit area due to this is hdg which is also the pressure p. Thus p due to a height h of a liquid of density d, p = hdg. The pressure due to 1 mm Hg can be calculated by putting h = 0.1 cm, d = 13.6 g/cc and g = 980 cm/s^2 CGS units or $dynes/cm^2$.

One mm Hg ≡ 1334 CGS units or $dynes/cm^2$. Practical unit of pressure is also $Newtons/M^2$ and is called Pa or Pascal. 1 Pa =10 CGS units or $dynes/cm^2$, that makes 1 mm Hg as 133.4 Pa. Expressing mm into inches and gram into pounds gives us the equivalence of 1 mm Hg as 0.0193368 psi (pounds per square inch).

Atmospheric Pressure

Atmospheric air is pulled to the earth by gravity and generates a force upon the surface of the earth, resulting in atmospheric pressure. Atmospheric pressure is the sum of pressures of all gases (e.g., N_2, O_2 and CO_2) present in air. It is measured with the help of a glass tube filled with either mercury or water (manometer). The height of the column of mercury (or water) multiplied by its density is a measure of the atmospheric pressure. Standard pressure is measured at sea level and expressed in mm Hg (torr) or cm H_2O. A torr is 1/760th of 1 atm.

One atmospheric pressure, also called 1atm is equal to 760 mm Hg or 1.013×10^6 CGS units or $dynes/cm^2$ or 1.013×10^5 Pa. Sometimes, pressure is also expressed in bars.

1 bar = 10^6 CGS units and is approximately 1 atm.

Equivalently, 1 atm equals 14.7 psi. It is also equivalent to 1030 cm H_2O pressure as hdg for water of height 1030 cm is equal to 76 cm of Hg.

It will be useful to express commonly used units of pressure for the readers of this book in **Table 2.1** in terms of other units.

One bar is approximately 1 atm or 760 mm Hg and 1030 cm H_2O or 10^5 Pa.

It is relevant here to mention that the lungs are subject to atmospheric pressure all the time. Since the alveoli are in direct

Table 2.1: Hg and H_2O unit heights in other pressure units.

1 mm Hg	1334 CGS	133.4 Pa	0.019 psi	1.33 mbar
1 cmH_2O	980 CGS	98 Pa	0.01 psi	0.98 mbar

communication with atmosphere through the tracheobronchial tree, the alveolar pressure is the same as the atmospheric pressure. The changes in alveolar pressure during inspiratory and expiratory phases of respiration are relative to the atmospheric pressure. During inspiration when the alveolar pressure is –10 cmH_2O, it implies the presence of atmospheric pressure minus 10 cmH_2O (i.e., 1030–10 cmH_2O). Similarly, when positive pressure is administered to a patient through a ventilator, the ventilator gauge pressure of 10 or 20 cmH_2O refers to a total pressure of 1040 or 1050 cmH_2O (i.e., atmospheric pressure + gauge pressure).

Partial Pressure

In a mixture of gases in a container, each gas exerts the same pressure which it would if it alone occupied the container. There is no interference from the presence of other gas/es. The pressure exerted by each individual gas is called the partial pressure. The total pressure exerted by the mixture of gases is equal to the sum of the partial pressures of all the gases contained in the mixture (Dalton's Law). The partial pressure is determined by the fraction of the concentration of the gas in the mixture.

The atmospheric air has a total pressure of 760 mm Hg when dry at sea level. The partial pressures of N_2 (79%) and O_2 (21%) therefore, are as follows:

PN_2 = 79% of Patm = 600.4 mm Hg

PO_2 = 21% of Patm = 159.6 mm Hg

Temperature

Temperature is the thermal state of a substance which determines whether the substance will give or receive heat from another substance in contact. It is an indication of the level of molecular activity. Heat is the thermal energy of a substance which can be given to or abstracted from it. Temperature is the measurement of heat.

Calorie (cal) is the unit of heat. It is defined as the quantity of heat required to raise the temperature of 1 g of water by 1°C.

To raise the temperature to a given range, similar weights of different substances require different quantities of heat. The number of calories required to raise the temperature of 1 g of that substance by 1°C is the specific heat of that substance.

The specific heat depends on the state of the matter—solid, liquid or gas. Specific heat of water is 1 (it follows from the definition of 1 calorie).

For gases such as O_2 and air, it is 0.0603 cals per cc, it is quite high when expressed per gram.

We can calculate the total quantity of heat required to raise the temperature of a given volume by multiplying the volume with specific heat and temperature rise, i.e., volume (cc) × specific heat (cals per cc) × temperature rise (°C).

THE GAS LAWS

There is a definite relationship between the gas properties described above. These relationships are described in different laws to understand the behavior of gases. These laws are valid for ideal gases only, where the assumption that the gas particles are very small and do not interact with each other is valid.

Boyle's Law

Pressure (P) of a gas is inversely proportional to its volume (V) provided the absolute temperature (T) of the mass of gas is kept constant. In other words the product of pressure and volume remains constant. It follows immediately from the ideal gas equation:

$$P \propto \frac{1}{V} \text{ if T is constant, or } PV = \textit{constant}$$

$$\text{Or } P_1V_1 = P_2V_2$$

The application of this law in respiratory physiology is best exemplified in the use of body plethysmography to measure total lung capacity. It is also employed in many mechanical ventilators whereby the gas is driven into patient's lungs or into the cylinder of the ventilator by the up-stroke and down-stroke movements of the piston.

Charles' Law

When pressure and mass of a gas are kept constant, the volume of the gas will vary directly with its absolute temperature. Again from gas equation:

$$\frac{V}{T} = K \quad \text{K is a constant (if P is constant)}$$

It is because of this reason that volumes measured with the help of lung function equipment (at room temperature) are a little lower than those at body temperature (37 °C) and need to be corrected for the same. If the temperature of a container of a gas is lowered, the volume shrinks. Therefore, more gas can be stored in the same cylinder at a lower temperature.

Gay-Lussac Law

Temperature and pressure of a gas are directly proportional when the volume and mass are kept constant.

$$P \propto T, \text{or} \frac{P}{T} = K, \text{at constant V}$$

It implies an increase in pressure if the temperature is increased. For this reason safety valves are provided with devices using high pressure gases to vent high pressures in case there is an accidental heating.

The General Gas Law

Assume N ideal non-interacting molecules of a gas each of mass m are contained in a cube of volume V. They are in motion if the temperature is above 0°K (0°K = - 273°C). If the temperature is T in Kelvin, the kinetic energy from each molecule is of the order of kT, where K is called Boltzmann constant ($K = 1.38 \times 10^{-16}$ CGS units). Because of this kinetic motion, the molecules of the gas keep bombarding the walls of the cube and exert pressure. The pressure increase results in extra energy (obtainable from force X distance or p × volume relation). In this way, it is quite evident that one can equate the energy because of pressure PV as resulting from kinetic energy of N molecules, PV = NkT.

If N is expressed in N_0 (Avogadro No.), PV = η N_0kT, where η = N/No.

This is the famous gas equation valid for all ideal gases. η is the number of moles of the gas, N_0k is also called gas constant R. $R \simeq 6 \times 10^{23} \times 1.38 \times 10^{-16}$ erg/deg K.

$$\simeq 2 \text{ cal/deg K}$$

The gas equation can be used to determine how the given initial state (P_1, V_1, T_1) relates to (P_2, V_2, T_2), some final state by using P_1V_1 ($T_1 = P_2V_2/T_2$).

$$\frac{P_1V_1}{T_1\eta_1} = \frac{P_2V_2}{T_2\eta_2}$$

It may be stated here that under conditions of lower temperature and high pressure the gas changes its state to a liquid. This is because the gas molecules get attracted to each other (Van der Waal's force) rather than being repelled. The higher pressure condenses the molecules and the lower temperature reduces their activity.

The temperature at which the gas turns into liquid is the "Critical temperature" of that gas. For oxygen, it is -116°C. A pressure of 50 atmospheres is required to liquefy oxygen at -116°C. To keep the oxygen in a liquid form at 1 atmosphere in a flask open to the atmosphere, the temperature is lowered to below -183°C. This principle forms the basis of availability of oxygen in the liquid form for storage and ambulatory use.

Henry's Law

The amount of gas that enters into physical solution in a liquid is directly proportional to the partial pressure of the gas above the liquid. For example, the greater the partial pressure of oxygen in the alveoli, the greater the solubility in plasma. Similarly, at high altitude, the pressure of oxygen reduces, leading to reduced dissolving of inhaled oxygen and opposite happens when deep diving under water takes place.

Graham's Law

The rate of diffusion (D) of a gas is inversely proportional to the square root of its density (d). This is evident from the ideal gas equation that the kinetic energy of a gas is only determined by the temperature. So at constant temperature, the kinetic energy of a gas with mass m_1 and velocity v_1 is equal to the other one with mass m_2 and velocity v_2.

$\frac{1}{2} m_1v_1^2 = \frac{1}{2} m_2v_2^2$, leading to lighter gases moving faster as squared velocities, or equivalently, diffusing as square root of masses. We express this as diffusion law:

$$\frac{D_1}{D_2} = \sqrt{\frac{d_2}{d_1}}$$

Therefore a light gas (such as helium) will diffuse at a faster rate than a heavier gas (such as oxygen).

Bernoulli's Principle

Flow of a gas through a partially obstructed tube can be described by Bernoulli's principle, i.e., the pressure required to produce flow is the difference in velocity at two points and the density of the gas **(Fig. 2.2)**. It derives from conservation of energy, if the velocity is higher, the quantity is appropriately lowered.

GAS SOLUTION AND TENSION

The amount of gas dissolved in a liquid is directly proportional to the pressure of the gas (Henry's Law). It also varies with the temperature—lesser amount is dissolved at the same pressure if temperature is increased. A state of equilibrium is reached when no further gas dissolves in the liquid. This is a state of full saturation with the gas at a given temperature and pressure. The gas in solution is said to exert the same "tension" as the partial pressure of the gas over the liquid in equilibrium with it. For example, when the partial pressure of oxygen in alveoli is 100 mm Hg, the tension of O_2 in alveolar capillaries is 100 mm Hg. At this pressure, 0.3 mL of oxygen at NTP dissolves in 100 cc of water. The weight of oxygen dissolved in 100 mL water is $0.3 \text{ x } \frac{1.3}{1000} = 0.0004$ g (1.3 g/L is the density of oxygen).

The amount of oxygen dissolved in plasma or water is the same (0.004 g/100 mL). This is quite sufficient to supply all the oxygen necessary for the metabolism of the body.

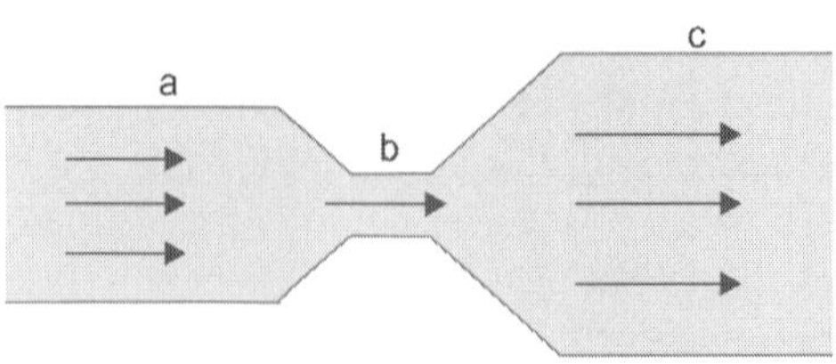

Fig. 2.2: Bernoulli principle.

VAPOURS

Vapour is defined as the gaseous state of a substance which at room temperature and pressure is a liquid. On the other hand a gas at room temperature exists only in the gaseous state. Like any other gas, the molecules of a vapour are continuously in violent motion and bombard the walls of the container. The force exerted on each unit area is called the pressure of the vapour (Vapour Pressure). A vapour in a mixture of gases obeys the same laws as the gases. The partial pressure of the vapour in a mixture bears the same proportion to the total pressure as the volume, i.e., it depends on the percent (or fractional) concentration in the mixture. For example, the concentration of about 16% of water vapours in air at NTP which is sufficient to saturate air with water vapours exerts a pressure of 16% of 760 mm Hg (47 mm Hg).

The presence of water vapours in air or oxygen is referred to as humidity. It is largely through the process of evaporation that the molecules of water (or any other liquid) evaporate into the overlying air (or any other gas in a container).

The molecules leave the liquid substance when their kinetic energy exceeds the surface tension of the liquid. If a liquid is kept in a closed container for long, a state of equilibrium is reached when the number of molecules returning to the liquid (condensation) is exactly equal to the number leaving it (evaporation). This is called the saturation-point. This is further dependent upon temperature; if the temperature increases, the number of molecules leaving the liquid also increase and the saturation-point is raised, i.e., there is a greater amount of vapours in the same amount of gas. Reverse happens with a fall in temperature.

The air we breathe is normally humid due to the presence of water vapour. The actual amount of water vapour present in air is expressed as "relative humidity" which is defined as the ratio of the amount of water vapour present in a given volume with the amount of water vapour which the air (or the gas) is capable of holding at the given temperature, in the same volume.

The humidity of air varies with the atmospheric conditions. Once inhaled in the lungs, air gets fully saturated. The amount of water vapour required to saturate the alveolar air at body temperature and pressure is the body humidity.

The presence of water vapour in the inhaled air exerts its own partial pressure, and lowers the pressures of constituent gases of air - oxygen and nitrogen. Therefore, PN_2 or PO_2 is calculated as a proportion of the atmospheric pressure minus water vapour pressure, i.e., Patm - PH_2O.

When fully saturated, PH_2O of atmospheric air is equal to 47 mm Hg. Therefore, PO_2 = (Patm - PH_2O) × 21% = (760 - 47) × 0.21 = 150 mm Hg. The rest, i.e., 760 – (150 + 47) would be approximately the PN_2.

EXPRESSION OF GAS VOLUMES AND PRESSURES

In view of the effects of temperature, pressure and humidity on all gases, these are expressed with reference to those conditions. Some of the common expressions are:

- Standard (or normal) temperature and pressure (STP) or NTP Temperature 0°C; Pressure 760 mm Hg
- STPD: D indicates 'dry' = complete absence of water vapour.
- Ambient temperature and pressure - dry or saturated (ATPD or ATPS). Ambient implies the room conditions.
- Body temperature and pressure saturated (BTPS): Body temperature (usually 37°C), ambient pressure and water vapour pressure (47 mm Hg).

Normally, gas volume measurements are made in the ambient conditions. Conversion is required to express the volume at BTPS or STPD. STPD is used for uniformity of expression. This is done by multiplying with conversion factors. Tables of conversion factors from ATPS to STPD, STPD to BTPS or BTPS to ATPS are available in most laboratories. Such corrections are also required to express volume of a gas (such as O_2) produced in the laboratory. The volume is expressed at STPD which is different than that produced at ATPS.

FLOW OF GASES

Flow is the movement of particles of a liquid or a gas from higher to lower pressure. It is expressed in terms of volume per unit time, e.g., liters per minute or per second (L/min or L/sec). The movement of air into the lungs during inspiration and out into the atmosphere during expiration is accomplished by the flow of air through tracheobronchial tree. Similarly, oxygen flows from a container cylinder to the lungs or a ventilator through connecting tubes as long as there is a pressure difference.

The flow is described as laminar if it is smooth and gas particles move along lines parallel to the walls of the tube **(Fig. 2.3A)**. But it is turbulent if the lines of flow are irregular, broken up and disorderly **(Fig. 2.3B)**. Whether the flow is laminar or turbulent, it has to meet a certain resistance while moving from one to the other end of the tube. The laminar flow is described by the Hagen-Poiseuille equation, i.e., $V = \prod \Upsilon^4 \Delta P)/(8\ \eta l)$. The resistance is dependent on the tube length (l) and diameter. It is also directly proportional to the velocity of flow (∇) or rate in case of laminar flow. The flow is also viscosity (η) dependent and density-independent. When the flow is turbulent, the resistance rises for steeply.

In this way the laminar flow through a straight tube of uniform size is inversely proportional to the length (l) of the tube and directly to the fourth power of radius (r).

When the flow exceeds a "Critical flow rate", the laminar flow is replaced by the turbulent flow throughout the length of the tube. Turbulent flow is less efficient since the ΔP varies directly with V^2. Turbulent flow is density dependent and viscosity-independent. The critical flow varies directly with the internal diameter of the tube—the larger the diameter, the greater the flow. At a flow below the critical rate, local turbulence may occur as a result of irregularities in the pathways of the gas. During oxygen administration this may occur due to constriction of kinking of the tubes.

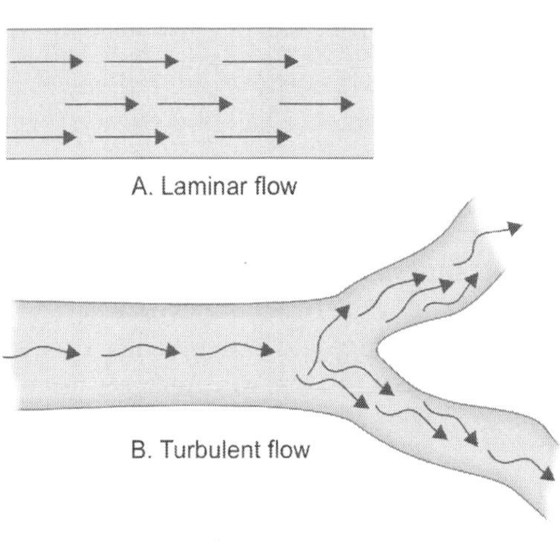

Figs. 2.3A and B: Patterns of flow.

Turbulence in a flowing system can also be predicted by Reynold's number. It is the ratio between inertial (density dependent, viscosity independent) and viscous (viscosity dependent, density independent) forces - a dimensionless number.

In case of Pipes,

$$\text{Reynold's number} = \frac{\text{Density} \times \text{Velocity} \times \text{Diameter}}{\text{Viscosity}}$$

Flow is laminar when the number is less than 2000 and turbulent when it is more than 3000. Turbulent flow is dominated by inertial forces producing random eddies and flow fluctuations. Between 2000–3000, the flow is transitional, i.e., neither fully laminar nor fully turbulent.

While administering oxygen, it is important that resistance is kept at a minimum so that the effort of breathing is reduced. Therefore, the breathing tube should be as wide and as short as possible and have smooth walls. There should be no kinks and constrictions and bends should be gradual.

Flow Through Orifices

An orifice is a narrow opening of a tube. Unlike a tube, the diameter of the fluid pathway of the orifice exceeds the length. The greater the diameter compared to the length, the more does the opening approach the 'ideal' orifice. The flow through an orifice depends on the diameter (or the cross section area) of the orifice and the difference in pressures on either side of the orifice.

The intrinsic property of a liquid which influences its flow which we earlier termed as resistance is called viscosity. It is attributed to the internal friction between different layers which move at different speeds. While the laminar flow largely depends on viscosity, it is the density which determines the flow when turbulent. The coefficient of viscosity is equal to the force per unit area necessary to maintain unit difference of velocity between two parallel planes.

The flow through an orifice is at least partially turbulent. The lower the density, i.e., the lighter the gas, the greater is its volume flow for any given pressure difference on either side of the orifice.

Wave Speed

Wave speed (c) is the speed at which a small disturbance (wave) travels in a compliant tube filled with a gas. In the airways, it depends upon the cross sectional area of the airway (A). The density of the gas (p) and the slope of the pressure area curve of the airway (dP/dA):

$$c^2 = \frac{A/p}{dP/dA}$$

Maximum flow (V_{max}) of a gas in an airway is the product of the gas velocity at wave speed and the airway area (cA). It increases as the density of the gas decreases.

Thermal Conductivity

It is a measure of a substance's capacity to conduct heat. The high thermal conductivity is likely to result in a higher skin heat loss. But respiratory heat loss depends on heat capacity not conductance.

Heliox

Heliox is a mixture of oxygen with helium (He) in varying concentrations, commonly as 20% oxygen and 80% helium. It has a lower density than that of air, i.e., oxygen (21%) with nitrogen (79%). Resistance offered to flow of heliox is lower than that of air and of oxygen and depends on the fractional concentrations. It diffuses 1.8 times faster than oxygen. This fact is exploited in clinical practice for treatment of acute respiratory distress of obstructive airway diseases such as asthma when the flow is highly turbulent. Heliox diffuses fastly than oxygen through partially obstructed airways. In view of the lower resistance offered to heliox, the breathing effort is considerably reduced and the crisis tide over.

SUGGESTED READING

1. Dawson SV, Elliott EA. Wave Speed Limitation on Expiratory Flow: A Unifying Concept. J Appl Physiol. 1977;43:498-515.
2. Egan DF. Fundamentals of Respiratory Therapy, St. Louis: CV Mosby Company, 1966.
3. Emsley J. Nature's Building Blocks: An A-Z Guide to the Elements. New York: Oxford University Press; 2001.
4. Hess DR, Fink JB, Venkataraman ST, Kim IK, Myers TR, Tano BD. The History and Physics of Heliox. Respir Care. 2006;51:608-12.
5. Macintosh RR, Mushin WW, Epstein HG. Physics for the Anaesthetist, Philadelphia: FA Davis Company, 1970.
6. Riggs JH. Respiratory Facts. FA Davis Company, 1989.

7. Thomas G, Stamatakis S. Physics of Gases. Anaesthesia and Intensive Care Medicine. 2009;10:48–51.
8. Varma YS. Applied Physics for the Anaesthetist, Rajan Publishers, Chandigarh, 1988.
9. West JB. Ventilation/Blood Flow and Gas Exchange, Philadelphia: FA Davis Company, 1970.
10. Young JA, Crocker D. Principles and Practice of Respiratory Therapy, 2nd ed., Chicago Year Book Medical Publishers Inc. 978.

Part B Physiological Considerations

Chapter Outline

Chapter 3

Respiratory Physiology of Gas Exchange

Uma Maheswari K

INTRODUCTION

The respiratory system is intricately designed to serve the purpose of gas transfer and transport. During breathing, oxygen is transferred from atmospheric air to blood for participating in the vital process of cellular respiration while carbon dioxide, the main byproduct of cellular respiration, egresses from the lung into the atmosphere.

Gas transfer can be conceptualized as a four part process consisting of:

1. Ventilation—physical movement of air in and out of the lungs.
2. Diffusion of gases across the alveolocapillary membrane.
3. Gas transport in blood in their dissolved and protein-bound forms
4. Diffusion across the cell membrane during cellular respiration.

In this chapter, design features of the lung and processes facilitating gas exchange will be discussed.

Section 1: Design of the Human Lung for Gas Exchange

The respiratory system consists of air passages, alveoli, interstitium and pulmonary vasculature housed within the thoracic cavity. During ventilation, atmospheric air is transported from the airway opening to alveoli across a pressure gradient created by expansion of the thorax. Thereafter, gas diffuses through the gas-liquid interface in the alveoli and alveolo-capillary membrane to blood in the pulmonary capillaries. The design features of the airways, parenchyma and vasculature that facilitate efficient gas transfer will be discussed.

ORGANIZATION OF THE AIRWAYS

The bronchial tree consists of about 23 generations of branching tubes ending in roughly 8 million alveolar sacs. Hypotheses about airway branching have evolved from the pure dichotomous branching theory (Weibel) to the widely accepted irregular dichotomous branching theory according to which airway branching shows considerable variability, with a dichotomous pattern predominating till the conducting airways and trifurcation or irregular branching patterns occurring thereafter.

Airway branches have a variable diameter and structure corresponding to the functions they subserve- gas conduction by convection or gas transfer by diffusion. Classification of airways and their anatomical features are depicted in **Tables 3.1 and 3.2**.

Two aspects are important in the understanding of gas transfer. Firstly, airway diameter decreases with each successive generation and the resultant increase in resistance to airflow is offset by increase in total cross-sectional area **(Fig. 3.1)**. Secondly, pattern of airflow changes from turbulent in the larger airways to laminar in the smaller airways to facilitate diffusion.

To put this into numerical perspective, cross-sectional area of the trachea is about 2.5 cm^2, that of the 10th generation airways is 13 cm^2 and acinar airways 300 cm^2. As the same volume of air flows through the bronchial tree, mean flow velocity falls 100-fold from 1 m/s in the trachea to <1 cm/s in the first-order respiratory bronchioles.

Airway structure is also adapted to facilitate gas transfer, from the nearly non-collapsible conducting airways with a cartilaginous-muscular envelope which transitions to a thin muscular layer in the smaller airways. While patency of cartilage containing airways is

Table 3.1: Classification of airways.

Generation 0	Trachea
Generations 1 to 4	Main, lobar and segmental bronchi
Generations 5 to 11	Small bronchi
Generations 12 to 14	Terminal bronchioles
Generations 15 to 18	Respiratory bronchioles
Generations 19 to 22	Alveolar ducts
Generation 23	Alveolar sacs

Table 3.2: Structural characteristics of air passages.

Airway	*Name and generation*	*Number*	*Cartilage*	*Muscle*
Trachea	Conducting airways (generation 1–14)	1	U shaped	Links open end of cartilage
Main bronchi		2		
Lobar bronchi		4 ↓ 8	Irregular shape	Helical bands
Segmental bronchi		16		
Small bronchi		32 ↓ 2000		
Terminal bronchioles		4000 ↓ 16,000	Absent	Strong helical muscle bands
Respiratory bronchioles	Acinar airways (generation 15–23)	32,000 ↓ 260,000		Muscle bands between alveoli
Alveolar ducts		520,000 ↓ 4,000,000		Thin bands in alveolar septa
Alveoli	Gas exchanging area	8,000,000		

Source: Nunn's Applied Respiratory Physiology, 8th edn. P8.

influenced by atmospheric and intra-thoracic pressures, terminal and respiratory bronchioles, which traverse the pulmonary parenchyma are influenced by lung volume and kept open by the fiber scaffold of the lung.

THE PULMONARY ACINUS (FIG. 3.2)

A pulmonary acinus the region of lung supplied by a first-order respiratory bronchiole and includes respiratory bronchioles, alveolar ducts, and alveolar sacs distal to a terminal bronchiole. An acinus represents generations 15 to 23 of the airway but can have between 6 and 12 divisions beyond the terminal bronchiole depending on its location. There are about 30,000 acini, each of which contains more than 10,000 alveoli.

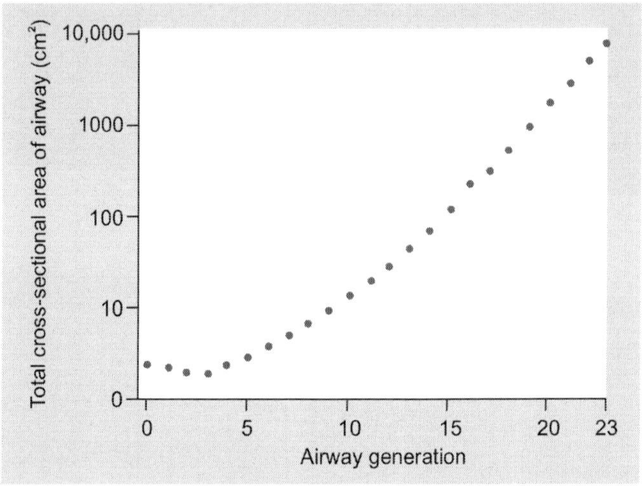

Fig. 3.1: Total cross-sectional area (CSA) of the air passages at different airway generations with minimum CSA at generation 3.

Source: Nunn's Applied Respiratory Physiology, 8th edn. P7.

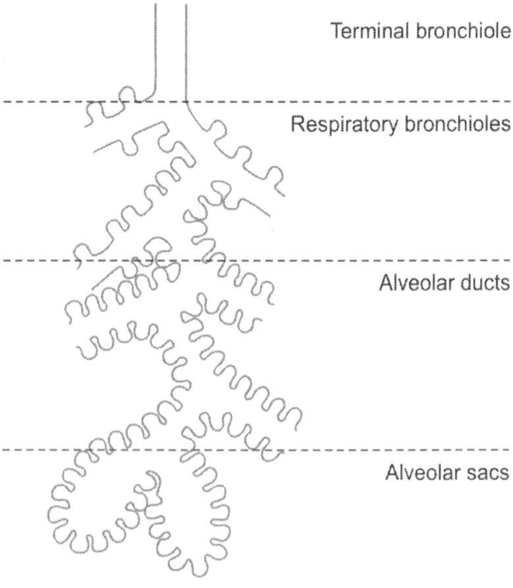

Fig. 3.2: Diagram of a pulmonary acinus.

Source: Nunn's Applied Respiratory Physiology, 8th edn. P7.

ALVEOLI AND ALVEOLAR SEPTA (FIG. 3.3)

Alveoli

Average number of alveoli in the human lung is about 400 million. Alveolar size depends on lung volume with the largest alveolar sizes in the upper lung. Differential ventilation and capability to recruit alveoli ensures optimal gas transfer during diverse physiological and pathological conditions.

Alveolar Septa

Alveolar septa are made of collagen and elastin fibers and are usually stretched out due to tension created by these fibers and surface tension at the air-fluid interface. They are perforated by the pores of Kohn which facilitate collateral ventilation between alveoli.

On the 'active' gas exchanging side of the alveolar wall, which is only 0.3 μm thick, the capillary endothelium and alveolar epithelium are closely apposed with almost no interstitial space and the capillary bulges into the alveolar wall. However, the opposite wall of the capillary, the 'service' side, is thicker (1–2 μm) and has considerable

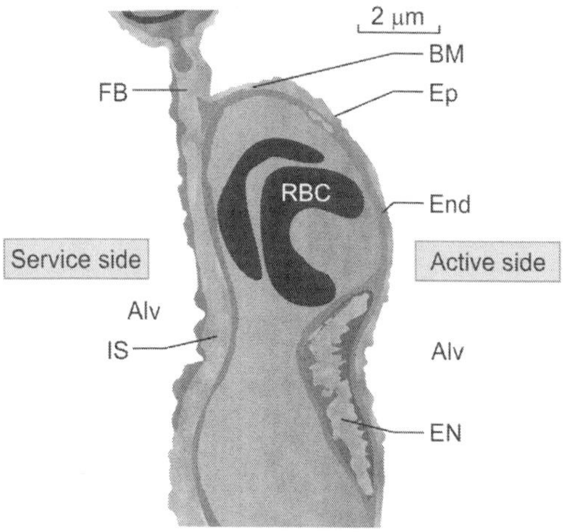

Fig. 3.3: The alveolo-capillary membrane.

(Alv: alveolus; BM: basement membrane; EN: endothelial nucleus; End: endothelium; Ep: epithelium; FB: fibroblast process; IS: interstitial space; RBC: red blood cell)

Source: Nunn's Applied Respiratory Physiology, 8th edn. P11.

interstitial space. Thus, the active side is protected from interstitial edema and can efficiently transfer gases even in pathological conditions.

INTERSTITIAL FIBER SYSTEM

There are three types of fibers criss-crossing the interstitium, these include:

1. **Axial spiral fibers:** Running from the hilum along airways.
2. **Peripheral fibers:** From visceral pleura extending inwards into the lung.
3. **Septal fibers:** Interweaving 'basket-like structures' in the alveolar septa, through which the pulmonary capillary network passes.

All these fibers are constantly in tension; this 'tensegrity structure' confers support to the interstitium and maintains alveolar and small airway patency. These fibers also aid in alveolar recruitment as lung volume increases from residual volume to total lung capacity.

PULMONARY VASCULATURE

The pulmonary vasculature is a low resistance, high compliance system and accommodates the same volume of blood as the systemic circulation. Pulmonary arterial pressure and vascular resistance are normally only 1/6th of the systemic circulation. This is achieved by the thinner arterial media (half as thick as systemic vessels). Besides, media of pulmonary arterioles is devoid of smooth muscle and has elastic tissue making them very distensible. Arterioles give rise to the extensive pulmonary capillary network which weaves through the fiber system and lies very close to the alveolar walls. One capillary network traverses multiple alveolar septa, increasing the efficiency of gas exchange.

Section 2: Physiology of Gas Transfer

VENTILATION

Ventilation is the physical process of air moving in and out of the lungs. Ventilation is facilitated by respiratory muscles and mechanical properties of the conducting airways and lung parenchyma. Mechanical properties may be 'static' (at zero airflow and constant volume) or 'dynamic' (when airflow is present).

Respiratory Muscles (Fig. 3.4)

From a functional standpoint, respiratory muscles can be classified as muscles of the upper airway and those of the trunk and abdomen. While upper airway muscles play an important role in maintaining upper airway patency, the latter are the 'muscles of respiration' and play an important role in the process of breathing.

The main inspiratory muscle is the diaphragm and is assisted by the external intercostals and scalenii during quiet breathing and by accessory muscles (sternomastoids, vertebral column extensors, pectoralis minor, trapezii and serratii) when ventilatory demand increases during exercise and disease. Inspiratory muscle contraction expands the ribcage antero-posteriorly, laterally, and upwards generating a negative intrathoracic pressure which creates a pressure gradient for air to flow into the respiratory tract.

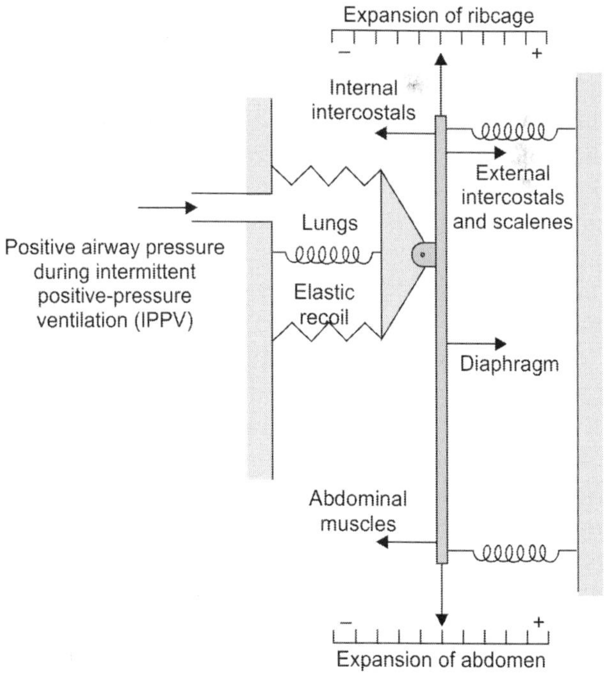

Fig. 3.4: Role of respiratory muscles in ventilation.

Source: Nunn's Applied Respiratory Physiology, 8th edn. P78.

Expiration is usually a passive process aided by elastic recoil of the lung; however, it becomes active during talking, singing, coughing/ sneezing and in flow limitation caused by airway disease. Main expiratory muscles are the rectus abdominis, external and internal obliques and transversalis abdominis.

Mechanical Properties of the Respiratory System

Ventilation is influenced by three mechanical properties of the lung-resistance, compliance and inertance. Resistance is mainly offered by the airways and influences airflow, compliance is determined by distensibility of the lung and inertance contributes to acceleration of airflow. The role of each of these factors in ventilation are discussed below.

RESISTANCE

The 80% of the airflow resistance is offered by conducting airways **(airway resistance)**; the remaining 20% is offered by tissue **(elastic resistance)**. While airway resistance is an important factor influencing ventilation and gas transfer, elastic resistance is only operational in conditions of zero airflow and is contributed by lung tissue, chest wall and surface tension at the gas-liquid interface. The role of airway resistance in regulating ventilation will be discussed.

As mentioned earlier, airflow decreases progressively down the bronchial tree, and it is almost zero in the terminal bronchioles. As flow velocity decreases, the driving pressure and resistance fall and airflow switches from turbulent to laminar. Thereafter, Brownian motion of air molecules in the respiratory bronchioles facilitates diffusion across the alveolocapillary membrane. Characteristics of turbulent and laminar flow and respiratory gas transport are depicted in **Figures 3.5 and 3.6**.

Turbulent flow occurs with high gas flow rates through unbranched/ irregular tubes, with formation of local eddies. Turbulent flow has a square advancing front and the volume of gas entering the tube is equal to the volume of the tube. Driving pressure is proportional to the square of the gas flow rate and density of gas, inversely proportional to the fifth power of the tubing's radius but independent of viscosity **(Fanning's equation)**.

Laminar and turbulent flow

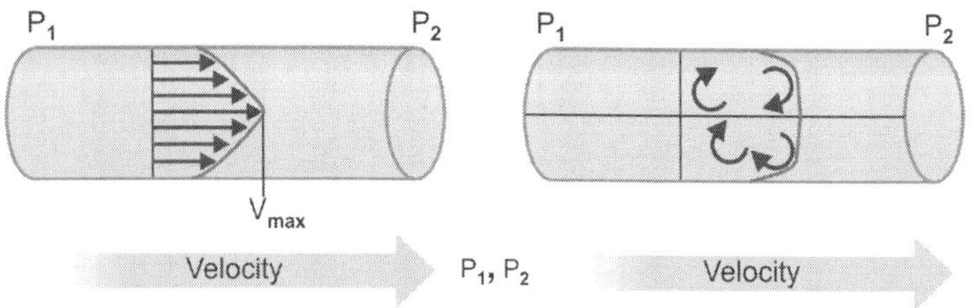

During laminar flow (smooth, steady flow) the flow profile is parabolic, with the fluid traveling most quickly at the centre of the tube and not moving at the edges of the tube. During turbulent flow (fluctuating and agitated flow) the flow profile is essentially flat, with all fluid traveling at the same velocity except at the tube edges where flow velocity is zero.

Fig. 3.5: Laminar and turbulent flow.

Source: Reference 3.

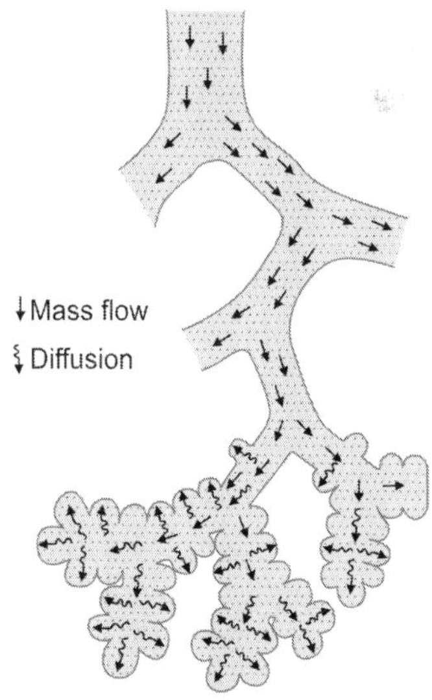

Fig. 3.6: Gas transport within the respiratory tract.

Source: Fishman's Pulmonary Diseases and Disorders, 5th edn. P158.

In laminar flow, gas flows along a straight unbranched tube as a series of concentric cylinders sliding over one another, with stationary peripheral cylinder and an advancing conical central cylinder. This implies that some gas will reach the end of the tube even if volume of gas entering the tube is less than the volume of the tube. In a straight unbranched tube, the **Hagen-Poiseuille equation** quantifies gas flow as follows:

$$\text{Flow rate} = \frac{\Delta P \times \pi \times (\text{radius})^4}{8 \times \text{length} \times \text{viscosity}}$$

$$(\text{where } \Delta P = \text{flow rate} \times \text{resistance})$$

$$\text{Resistance} = \frac{8 \times \text{length} \times \text{viscosity}}{\pi \times (\text{radius})^4}$$

Thus, resistance is inversely related to the fourth power of radius in laminar flow. If tube dimensions are constant, viscosity is the only property of gas that is relevant during laminar flow.

Transition from turbulent to laminar flow is determined by the Reynolds' number (N_R). Flow is laminar with $N_R < 2000$ and becomes turbulent at $N_R > 4000$. If NR is 2000–4000, both types of flow coexist; a critical length of tubing is necessary before laminar flow is established. Thus for gases with low N_R, resistance will be less during turbulent flow and laminar flow will occur faster after airway narrowing.

COMPLIANCE

Pulmonary compliance is defined as the change in volume of lung per unit change in transpulmonary pressure. Compliance is expressed in Litres/kiloPascal (l/kPa) or mL/cmH_2O with a normal value of 1.5 L/kPa.

Compliance may be static or dynamic depending on the conditions of measurement. Static compliance is measured after the lungs have been held at a fixed volume for as long as practicable, whereas dynamic compliance is measured during normal breathing. Elastance is the reciprocal of compliance and is expressed in kilopascals per liter. Elastic recoil of the lung tends to collapse the lung even at residual volume. Thus, the lungs would collapse to an almost airless state if removed from the thoracic cage.

The pressure-volume graph obtained during compliance measurement is curvilinear **(Fig. 3.7)** and exhibits 'hysteresis' due to which pressure-volume curve is slightly greater during deflation than inflation. Hysteresis is influenced by elasticity of the lung parenchyma and surface tension in alveolar spaces.

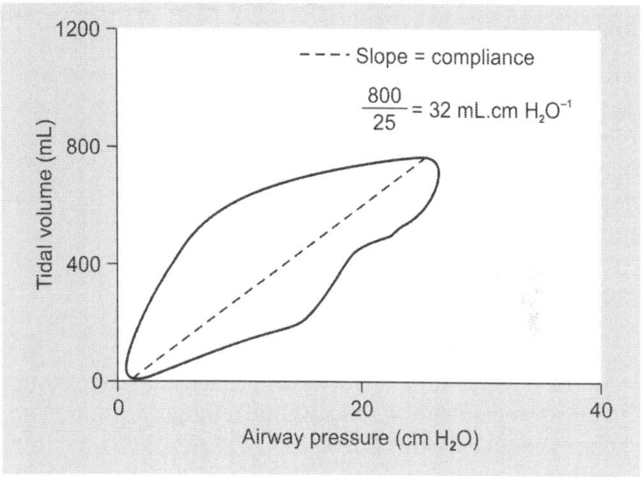

Fig. 3.7: Pressure volume graph during dynamic compliance measurement.
Source: Nunn's Applied Respiratory Physiology, 8th edn. P30.

FACTORS AFFECTING LUNG COMPLIANCE

- **Recruitment:** At low lung volumes, some small airways remain closed lowering compliance. However, they sequentially open-up as transpulmonary pressure rises, a phenomenon called recruitment. Recruitment in the initial phase of inspiration increases compliance and contributes to hysteresis.
- **Surface tension:** Surface tension present at the air-fluid interface is considerably reduced by surfactant produced by type II alveolar cells. At low lung volumes, as diameter of the alveoli decreases, pressure within them increases in accordance with Laplace's Law (Pressure = 2 × surface tension/radius), increasing propensity for alveolar collapse. This is prevented by surfactant which decreases surface tension despite decreasing alveolar radius and allows gas flow from larger to smaller alveoli and helps maintain stability of alveoli at lower lung volumes.
- **Physical characteristics of lung tissues:** Elastic properties of lung are due to elastic fibers in the interstitium. Lung expansion occurs due to unfolding and geometric re-arrangement of elastic fibers. Ageing alters elastin and collagen fibers in the lungs and increases lung compliance.

INERTANCE

As respired gases, lungs and chest wall have mass and therefore inertia, they offer impedance to change in direction of gas flow. This component called inertance, is difficult to measure but offers resistance to airflow that increases with respiratory frequency. For practical purposes, inertance is negligible and gas flow depends primarily on compliance and resistance.

Components and Distribution of Ventilation

Total and Alveolar Ventilation

Inhaled air gets distributed in the lungs depending on resistance and compliance of regional lung units. While a major portion of inhaled air reaches the alveoli and participates in gas exchange (alveolar ventilation, V_A), another portion called dead space volume (V_D) never reaches the alveoli. Total ventilation is the sum of dead space ventilation and alveolar ventilation **(Fig. 3.8)**.

Dead space comprises 2 components, the **anatomical dead space**, which is fixed and comprises the air in the conducting airways (~ 150 mL or 1/3rd of tidal volume) and **physiological dead space,**

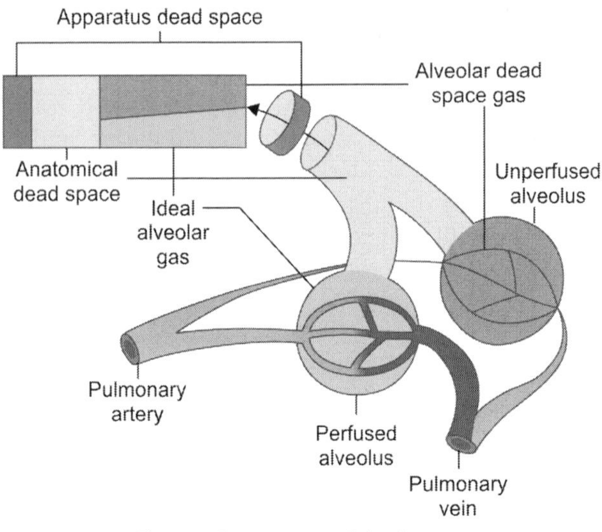

Fig. 3.8: Components of dead space.
Source: Nunn's Applied Respiratory Physiology, 8th edn. P120.

which is variable and includes alveoli that are adequately ventilated but not perfused. The sum of anatomical and physiological dead space is **'total dead space'** and is given by the formula:

$$V_D/V_E = 1 - P_ECO_2/P_ACO_2$$

where V_D = total dead space, V_E = minute ventilation, P_ECO_2 = partial pressure of CO_2 in expired air, P_ACO_2 = partial pressure of CO_2 in alveolar air (which is assumed to be equal to arterial PCO_2).

Distribution of Ventilation

Distribution of alveolar ventilation is essentially a function of the **"RC time constant"** of regional lung units. The latter is the product of regional compliance and resistance. The relative distribution of ventilation between two neighboring lung units can be easily understood with the two compartment lung model wherein RC time constant of adjacent lung units is equal resulting in normal distribution of ventilation.

In a diseased lung, time constants in different units may vary because of increased resistance, reduced compliance, or both. In a lung unit with abnormal RC time constant, ventilation will be maldistributed. A lung unit with a large time constant (slow alveolus) fills and empties slowly whereas one with a small time constant (fast alveolus) fills and empties rapidly **(Fig. 3.9)**. When a 'slow alveolus' is located adjacent to a 'fast alveolus,' the former may withdraw gas from the latter. Besides, a 'fast alveolus,' may receive a higher proportion of dead space gas, reducing its alveolar ventilation.

Uneven ventilation of small lung units can also occur due **stratified inhomogeneity**, which occurs due to varying alveolar distance from conducting airways and variable small airway caliber. A case in point is emphysema where altered airway caliber results in better ventilation of alveoli that are closer to conducting airways.

Some mechanisms that ensure uniform distribution of ventilation are **collateral ventilation** and **interdependence of peripheral lung units**. Collateral ventilation can occur between alveolo-alveolar pores of Kohn, bronchiolo-alveolar canals of Lambert, and bronchiolo-bronchiolar foramina of Martin. As contiguous lung units are attached to each other by connective tissue, behavior of one unit influences the behavior of its neighbors. This **interdependence** also helps in overcoming ventilation inhomogeneity.

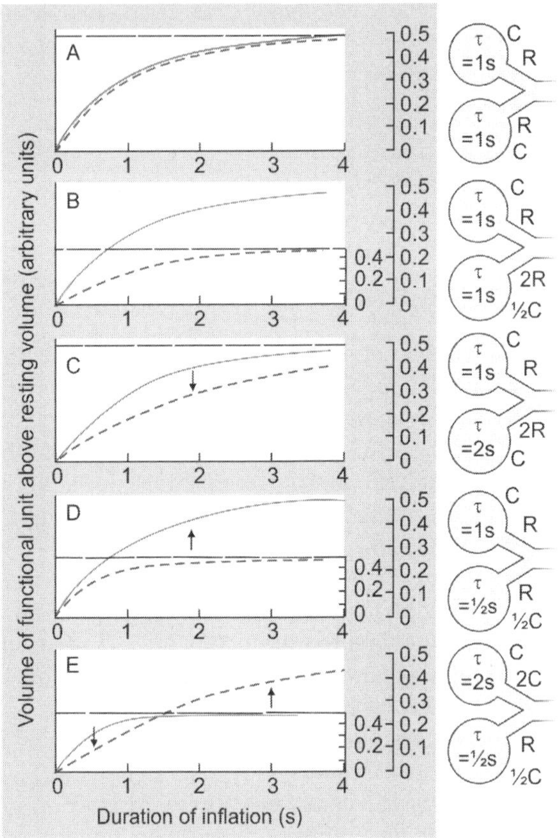

Fig. 3.9: Differential rates of filling of alveoli based on RC time constants.
Source: Nunn's Applied Respiratory Physiology, 8th edn. P112.

PERFUSION

Pulmonary vasculature structure and differences between pulmonary and systemic circulation have already been enumerated. In this section, ventilation-perfusion relationships will be discussed. The pulmonary bed is a low pressure circuit comprising a dense network of capillaries which can accommodate up to 5 times the resting cardiac output without appreciable increase in pulmonary arterial pressure. These is possible due to two mechanisms—**recruitment** of previously non-perfused capillaries in the upper zones, and **distension** of the pulmonary vasculature.

Distribution of Perfusion

There is an apico-basal gradient in perfusion due to gravity, with the lower zones being better perfused than upper zones. Based on these pressure differences, West subdivided the lung into four zones with differing patterns of blood flow **(Fig. 3.10)**.

- **Zone 1:** Located near the apex of the lung; alveolar pressure exceeds both pulmonary arterial and venous pressures **($P_A > P_a > P_v$)**, thus alveolar vessels are collapsed with no pulmonary blood flow.
- **Zone 2:** Pulmonary arterial pressure is more than alveolar pressure, but alveolar pressure exceeds venous pressure **($P_a > P_A > P_v$)**. Thus, resistance to blood flow is determined by the difference between pulmonary arterial and alveolar pressures. This behavior is called the **waterfall or sluice effect**. Additionally, in Zone 2, blood flow increases progressively down the lung because of increasing hydrostatic effect on pulmonary arterial pressure.

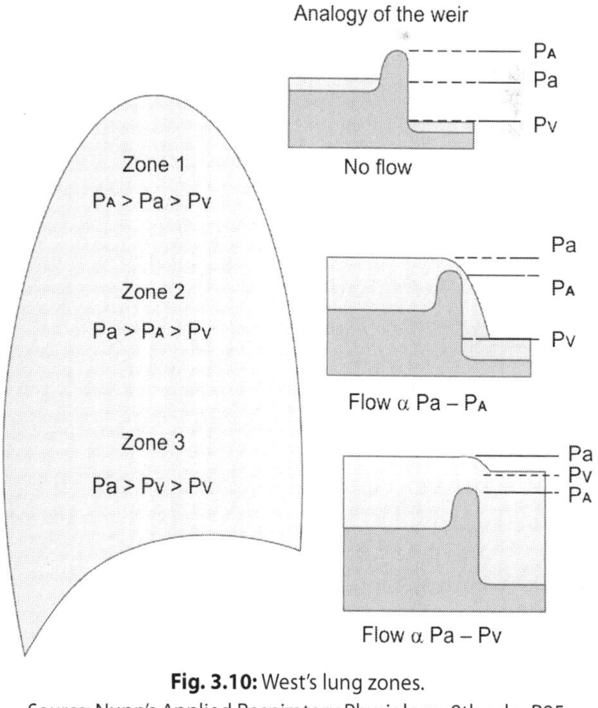

Fig. 3.10: West's lung zones.
Source: Nunn's Applied Respiratory Physiology, 8th edn. P95.

- **Zone 3:** Pulmonary venous pressure exceeds alveolar pressure ($P_a > P_v > P_A$), blood flow is maximal and dependent on the arterio-venous pressure difference. There is also a progressive increase in the perfusion because of the progressive 'distension' of vessels due to increase in P_a and P_v, while P_A remains constant.
- **Zone 4:** Relationship between intravascular and alveolar pressures are the same as zone 3, but blood flow **decreases** slightly. Zone 4 occurs in the lowermost region of the upright lung and diminishes as lung volume increases and increases as lung volume decreases. Thus, at residual volume, zone 4 extends nearly all the way up the lung, so that blood flow at the apex exceeds that at the base. Reduced blood flow in zone 4 is due to narrowing of extra-alveolar vessels at the lung base due to lower lung inflation caused by airway closure at 'closing volume'.

Ventilation Perfusion(V/Q) Relationships

The ratio of ventilation (4–6 L/min) to perfusion (5–6 L/min) at rest is 0.8 to 1 and is an important determinant of gas exchange. The spectrum of V/Q ratios in a healthy lung can vary between zero (perfused but not ventilated) to infinity (ventilated but not perfused). An area of lung that is well perfused but under-ventilated behaves like a right to left shunt (**physiological shunt**) whereas an area that is well ventilated but under-perfused behaves like dead space (**physiological dead space**). In an alveolar-capillary unit with a V/Q ratio of 0 (physiologic shunt), blood leaving the unit has a composition like mixed venous blood entering pulmonary capillaries, (PO_2-40 mm Hg, PCO_2-46 mm Hg) whereas in an alveolar-capillary unit with a high V/Q ratio (physiologic dead space) the small amount of blood leaving the unit has partial pressures of O_2 and CO_2 of 150 mm Hg and 0 mmHg similar to that of inspired gas.

Due to the sigmoid shape of the oxyhemoglobin dissociation curve, hemoglobin is almost fully (> 90%) saturated at a PO_2 of 60 mm Hg, and little additional O_2 binds to hemoglobin at PO_2 > 60 mm Hg (**Fig. 3.11**). However, significant desaturation of hemoglobin occurs when PO_2 falls below 60 mm Hg in the steep descending limb of the curve. Thus, blood coming from regions of the lung with a high V/Q ratio has a high PO_2 but causes only a small elevation in O_2 content and cannot compensate for blood coming from regions with a low

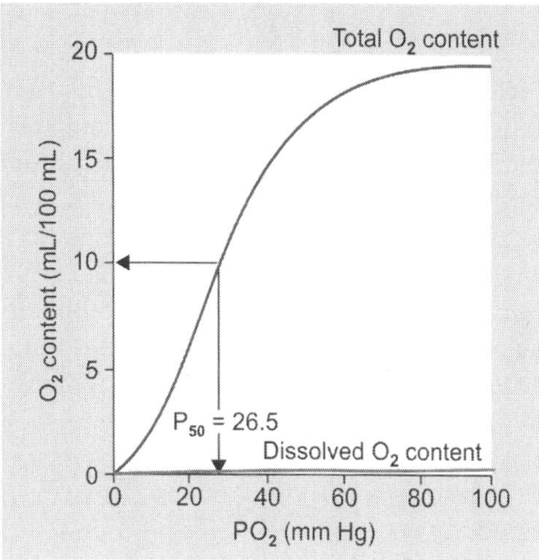

Fig. 3.11: Oxygen hemoglobin dissociation curve.

Source: Fishman's Pulmonary Diseases and Disorders, 5th edn. P489.

V/Q ratio and a low PO_2, which has a decreased O_2 content. Although V/Q mismatching can influence PCO_2, this effect is less marked as it is overcome by increasing minute ventilation.

Alveolar PO_2 appears to be the most important factor involved in the ventilation-perfusion distribution. The occurrence of hypoxic pulmonary vasoconstriction is an example of how V/Q is optimized. For example, in lung units with low V/Q ratio, fall in the local alveolar PO_2 results in local vasoconstriction thus reducing blood flow and restoring local V/Q ratio.

Section 3: Diffusion of Gases

GENERAL PRINCIPLES OF DIFFUSION

Diffusion of a gas is a process of transfer of gas molecules from a higher partial pressure to lower partial pressure zone. It occurs by random movement of molecules. Partial pressure of a gas in a gas mixture is the pressure it would exert if it occupied the space alone. Net gas transfer is proportional to the difference in partial pressure between the two zones.

OXYGEN TRANSFER (FIG. 3.12)

Oxygen is carried in the blood in two forms, dissolved form and that bound to hemoglobin. In general, transfer of gases from alveoli to capillary blood can be **perfusion-limited** or **diffusion-limited**. Gases that do not chemically combine with hemoglobin for transport (example N_2O) rapidly cross the alveolocapillary membrane based on partial pressure gradient; their transport is thus perfusion-limited. Transport of gases that avidly combine with hemoglobin requiring time for transfer across the membrane is diffusion-limited (example-carbon monoxide—CO). Oxygen is intermediate between N_2O and CO; it is taken up by hemoglobin although with lesser rapidity than CO and reaches equilibrium with capillary blood in about 0.25s that is roughly 1/3rd the total transit time of 0.8s. Thus, oxygen uptake is perfusion-limited.

The diffusing capacity of the lung for a gas is directly proportional to surface area of the alveolocapillary membrane and inversely proportional to its thickness. Factors that influence movement of gas from an area of higher partial pressure to lower partial pressure are governed by Fick's law:

$$V = Ad/T\,(P1-P2)$$

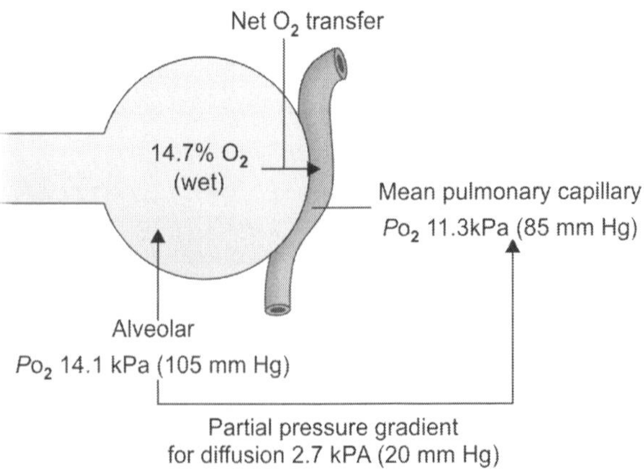

Fig. 3.12: Oxygen transfer across the alveolo-capillary membrane.

Source: Nunn's Applied Respiratory Physiology, 8th edn. P138.

where, V = volume of gas diffusing per unit time, A = area available for diffusion, d = diffusion coefficient of the barrier, (P1–P2) = pressure difference of gas on the two sides; T = membrane thickness.

Diffusion coefficient (d) is related to the solubility of the gas and the square root of its molecular weight. Assuming that other factors are constant, partial pressure difference is the most important factor determining oxygen transfer across the alveolo-capillary membrane. When this pressure falls, oxygen delivery to the tissues becomes diffusion limited. Normal capillary transit time across the alveolar walls is usually 0.8s but in healthy individuals only 0.25s is required for gas exchange to be completed, giving an adequate buffer for gas exchange to occur even with a diffusion defect.

Carbon Dioxide Transfer

Carbon dioxide has a much higher water solubility than oxygen and thus crosses the alveolocapillary membrane 20 times as rapidly as oxygen. Reactions involved in the release of chemically combined CO_2 into the alveolar space include— (a) release of CO_2 from carbamino carriage and (b) conversion of bicarbonate ions to carbonic acid followed by its dehydration to release molecular CO_2 (catalysed by carbonic anhydrase). Equilibrium of CO_2 is nearly complete within the normal pulmonary capillary transit time and CO_2 excretion is finely regulated by varying minute ventilation.

SUGGESTED READING

1. Hillman DR, Finucane KE. A Model of the Respiratory Pump. J Appl Physiol. 1987;63:951–961.
2. Hughes JMB, Glazier JB, Maloney JE, et al. Effect of Lung Volume on the Distribution of Pulmonary Blood Flow in Man. Respir Physiol. 1968;4: 58–72.
3. Laminar and Turbulent Flow: Mitchell V, and Cheesman K. (2014). Gas, Tubes and Flow. Anaesthesia and Intensive Care Medicine, 15(5), 225–228. doi:10.1016/j.mpaic.2014.02.006.
4. Lumb AB. In: Nunn's Applied Respiratory Physiology, 8th edn, Elsevier 2017.
5. Ochs M, Weibel RE. Functional Design of the Human Lung for Gas Exchange. In: Grippi MA, Elias JA, Fishman JA (Eds). Fishman's Pulmonary Diseases and Disorders 5th edition. McGraw-Hill, 2015.

6. Wagner PD. The Physiological Basis of Pulmonary Gas Exchange: Implications for Clinical Interpretation of Arterial Blood Gases. Eur Respir J. 2015;45(1):227–43.
7. West JB, Dollery CT. Distribution of Blood Flow and the Pressure-Flow Relations of the Whole Lung. J Appl Physiol. 1965;20:175–83.

Chapter 4

Oxygen and Carbon Dioxide Transport

Uma Devaraj

Oxygen contributes to 21% of the atmospheric air and to two-thirds the mass of the human body. Cellular metabolism produces energy in the form of adenosine triphosphate (ATP). In the presence of oxygen, each glucose molecule yields 38 molecules of ATP, whereas anaerobic condition yields only two ATP molecules. Therefore, all animals and humans are dependent on oxygen for normal function and survival. As there is no storage system for oxygen in the body, a continuous supply of oxygen is essential.

The key steps in oxygen cascade are the following:

- Uptake in the lungs
  - Atmospheric air to alveoli
  - Alveoli to arterial blood
- Oxygen carriage in blood
- Delivery from capillary blood to interstitium
- Delivery from interstitium to individual cells
- Cellular/mitochondrial use of oxygen.

Significant challenges to oxygen transfer are between:

- Inspired and alveolar gas
- Alveolar to arterial transfer and
- Diffusion from the capillaries to the cellular mitochondria. The transport of oxygen takes place down the partial pressure gradients from the inspired air (159 mm Hg), through the respiratory tract-humidified with water vapor (149 mm Hg), the alveolar gas (104 mm Hg), the arterial blood (100 mm Hg), the systemic capillaries(40–50 mm Hg), the tissues and the cell (3.8–22.5 mm Hg) **(Fig. 4.1)**.

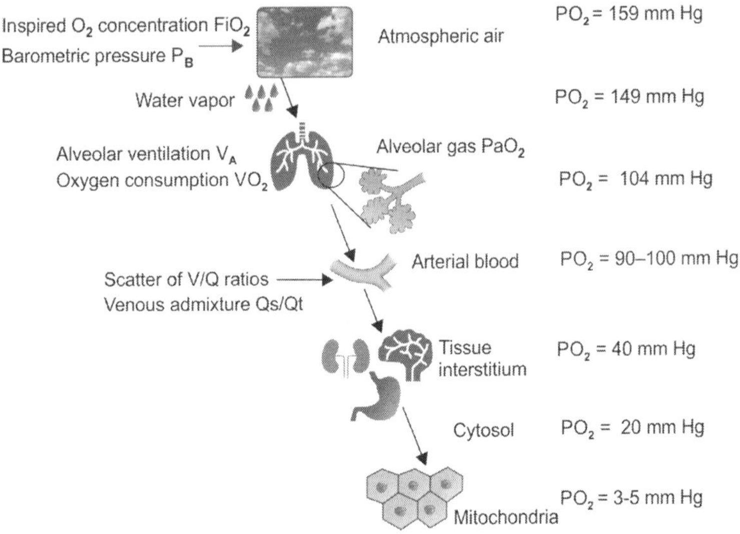

Fig. 4.1: Oxygen cascade.

UPTAKE IN THE LUNGS

Atmospheric Air to Alveoli

The first step in oxygen transport is from atmosphere to alveoli. The alveolar oxygen tension is determined by atmospheric pressure, the concentration of inspired oxygen, oxygen consumption and alveolar ventilation.

Atmospheric Pressure

In a mixture of gases, the concentration of a gas is determined by the partial pressure of the respective gas. Dalton's Law of Partial Pressures states that "the total pressure of all gases is equal to the sum of the partial pressures of each gas." The total atmospheric pressure of air is 760 mm Hg. When computed as an equation:

$$P(N_2) + P(O_2) + P(CO_2) + P(HOH) = P(\text{total atmospheric air})$$

$$594.7 + 160 + 0.3 + 5.0 = 760 \text{ mm Hg}$$

From the above equation, the concentration of oxygen in dry atmospheric gas is 20.94%, at a partial pressure of 159 mm of Hg. During inspiration, gas becomes humidified with water vapor at body temperature and dilutes the oxygen to 149 mm Hg. A progressive fall in alveolar PO_2 can be noted with increasing altitude as alveolar PO_2 is directly proportional to barometric pressure.

Concentration of Inspired Oxygen

The alveolar PO_2 either rises or reduces corresponding to the change in the inspired gas PO_2.

Oxygen Consumption

Although oxygen consumption at rest is calculated to be approximately 250 mL per minute, it may vary depending on many factors. Conditions such as restlessness, pain, increased work of breathing, shivering or fever, sepsis, thyrotoxicosis or convulsions lead to increased O_2 consumption whereas general anesthesia, hypothyroidism or hypothermia lead to reduced O_2 consumption.

Alveolar Ventilation

As ventilation increases, the alveolar PO_2 rises towards the PO_2 of the inspired gas. The equation relating to the hyperbolic relationship between alveolar PO_2 and alveolar ventilation is given by:

$$\text{Alveolar } PO_2\ (PAO_2) = (PB-PH_2O)\ FiO_2-(PaCO_2 \div R)$$

$$= (760-47) \times 0.21-(40/0.8) = 100 \text{ mm Hg}$$

Where PB = atmospheric pressure; PH_2O = water vapor pressure; FIO_2= fractional concentration of inspired oxygen; $PaCO_2$= partial pressure of alveolar CO_2; R= respiratory quotient.

Due to the shape of the curve, alveolar PO_2 is minimally affected when change in ventilation is above the normal level, whereas a marked effect is noted when changes in ventilation occur in the steep part of the curve (below the normal level).

Alveoli to Arterial Blood

The passage of oxygen from the alveoli onto the arterial blood is an important step in the oxygen cascade. The most common cause of arterial hypoxemia in clinical practice is due to increased alveolar/arterial PO_2 difference or the A-a gradient. While breathing room air, the A-a gradient is usually within 15 mm Hg in young healthy adult, but can be greater than 37 mm Hg in healthy aged subjects.

The main cause for alveolar/arterial PO_2 difference is venous admixture secondary to shunt and scatter of *V/Q* ratios. Oxygen uptake is perfusion dependent in the pulmonary capillaries as the hemoglobin is fully saturated within the first third of transit time. Inadequate oxygenation rarely results from inadequate pulmonary capillary transit time because of the presence of a 200% reserve. Impaired diffusion of oxygen from alveoli into blood in pulmonary capillaries is a less common cause for arterial hypoxemia.

Effect of Shunt

The (A-a) gradient increases in a non-linear manner with increasing alveolar PO_2, due to the shape of the oxygen dissociation curve. When oxygenation is diminished due to a true shunt, for each 1% of shunt, the arterial PO_2 rises with increasing inspired oxygen to reach a plateau value of 15–22 mm Hg concentration. For small shunts at a constant alveolar PO_2, the A-a gradient is proportional to the scale of shunt. The A-a gradient reaches a plateau at high alveolar PO_2. However, when the shunt is large, a higher alveolar PO_2 is required to reach the plateau.

Effect of V/Q Scatter

With varying V/Q ratios, when the inspired oxygen concentration is increased, the arterial PO_2 approaches the normal value for the inspired oxygen concentration. The PO_2 of mixed arterial blood tends towards the direction of the poorly oxygenated blood from areas of low V/Q ratio, as more blood flows through the under-ventilated and over-perfused alveoli. The ventilation from areas of high V/Q regions cannot compensate for this, as the amount of blood flowing through these areas is much smaller. Similarly, due to the sigmoid shape of the O_2 dissociation curve, the drop in saturation occurring in the areas of low V/Q is greater than the rise in oxygen saturation from the areas with high V/Q ratio.

The shunt fraction increases and decreases corresponding to increased or decreased cardiac output. This change counteracts the effect of mixed venous desaturation, hence change in cardiac output has little effect on arterial PO_2. Hemoglobin concentration, temperature, pH and base excess of the patient's blood influence the oxyhemoglobin dissociation curve and thus the A-a gradient.

Increase in alveolar ventilation results in raised PAO_2 and thus an increased A-a gradient.

OXYGEN CARRIAGE IN BLOOD

The next important step in the oxygen cascade is carriage of oxygen in the blood. Majority of the oxygen is transported in a reversible chemical combination with hemoglobin (Hb), while a small proportion is carried dissolved in plasma.

O_2 carriage bound to hemoglobin: The human red blood cells are mainly filled with hemoglobin with about 280 million molecules of Hb in a single RBC. Adult hemoglobin (HbA) consists of 2 alpha (α) and 2 beta (β)chains with heme group (a porphyrin ring containing iron) attached at the histidine residue in each chain, while HbA_2 (the minor adult Hb) contains 2 alpha and 2 delta (δ) chains. The heme group lies in the crevices formed by the alpha/ beta chain loops, which are held by electrostatic forces. The electrostatic forces hold the hemoglobin in its quaternary structure, which plays an important role in its reaction with oxygen. The electrostatic bonds are strong in deoxyhemoglobin, and hemoglobin is present in the tense (T) form, whereas in oxyhemoglobin the bonds weaken, resulting in the relaxed (R) state of the hemoglobin. The T or R conformational form has the effect of reduced or increased affinity of hemoglobin to bind oxygen respectively. The chemical reaction binding oxygen to hemoglobin has complex kinetics. The velocity of binding of oxygen to heme group increases from first to fourth heme moiety, resulting in rapid filling up of the heme groups with oxygen.

When pH drops or CO_2 increases, there is a change in the electrostatic bonds resulting in stabilizing the hemoglobin molecule in the T quaternary structure, thereby reducing oxygen affinity. This is called the **Bohr effect**, where oxygen release is facilitated when there is acidosis or hypercarbia. On the other hand the reduction in the capacity of oxyhemoglobin to carry carbon dioxide, due to the conformational change in the oxyhemoglobin to the R state, is called **Haldane effect**.

O_2 carriage dissolved in plasma: About 0.00314 mL/dL/mm Hg of oxygen is carried in blood in solution at 37°C. Thus, slightly more than 1% of the total oxygen is carried in physical solution which is about 0.25 to 0.3 mL/dL at normal arterial PO_2. The amount of dissolved oxygen can be increased when breathing either 100% oxygen (to 2 mL/dL) or at increased barometric pressure (6 mL/dL at 3 atmospheric pressure) or with decreasing temperature with same PO_2.

Oxygen Content

The oxygen binding capacity of hemoglobin or the Hüfner constant is 1.39/g in total, which is marginally reduced to 1.34 when accounting for carboxy hemoglobin and methemoglobin.

The oxygen content per 100 mL of blood is the total amount of oxygen bound to hemoglobin and dissolved in plasma. The main determinants are Hb level, PaO_2 and oxygen saturation (SaO_2). It is calculated as follows:

$$\text{Oxygen content } (CaO_2) = \{SaO_2 \times \text{Hb (g\%)} \times 1.34\} + (PaO_2 \times 0.003)$$
$$= \{0.97 \times 15 \times 1.34\} + (100 \times 0.003) = 19.8 \text{ mL.}$$

The oxygen hemoglobin dissociation curve: The relationship between PO_2 and percentage saturation of hemoglobin (SaO_2) is given by a sigmoid shaped curve **(Fig. 4.2)**. On the other hand, the O_2 content dissolved in plasma bears a linear relationship with PaO_2 **(Fig. 4.3)**. The average values of PO_2 and SaO_2 in arterial blood are 95 mm Hg and 97% and values in venous blood are 40 mm Hg and 75%.

Determination of PO_2 required for 50% of hemoglobin to be saturated (P50) helps to identify the shift of the dissociation curve. Normally, the P50 is 26.3 mm Hg. Displacement of the oxygen-hemoglobin dissociation curve along the x-axis to the right or left

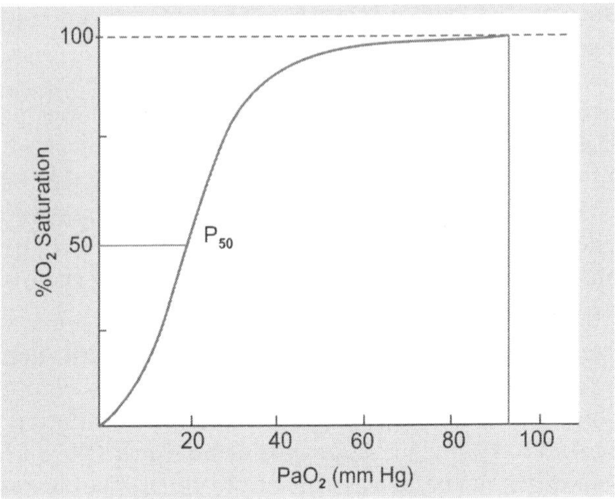

Fig. 4.2: The oxygen dissociation curve. It shows relationship between PaO_2 and percent saturation of oxygen.

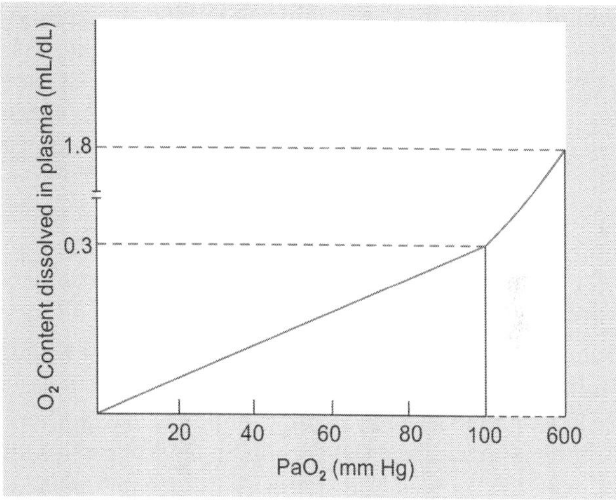

Fig. 4.3: Relationship between PaO_2 and O_2 dissolved in plasma.

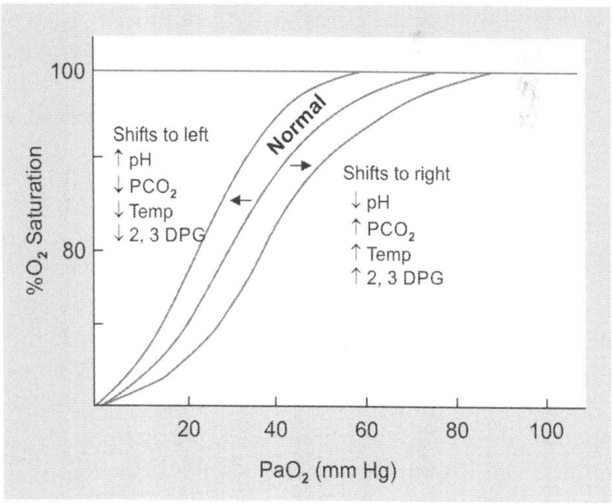

Fig. 4.4: Factors influencing the shift of hemoglobin dissociation curve for oxygen.

influences release of oxygen to the tissues. Any shift to the right benefits tissue oxygenation. The shift of the oxygen dissociation curve is influenced by pH, PCO_2, temperature, 2,3 – DPG, percentage of fetal hemoglobin and the altitude **(Fig. 4.4)**.

PCO_2 and pH: Almost 25% of the oxygen uptake or release is due to the Bohr effect. In venous circulation setting, the increase in PCO_2 leads to reduced O_2 binding and release of O_2 to the tissues. The opposite happens in the lungs, where CO_2 diffuses out of the blood and simultaneously H^+ concentration also decreases, leading to a left shift of the curve and enhanced O_2 binding.

Transfer of carbon dioxide leads to alteration in the pH of the blood and also shifts the dissociation curve. Fall in pH from 7.4 to 7.2 causes shift of the dissociation curve by 15% to right. A similar shift to the left occurs with an increase in pH of the same magnitude.

Temperature: The dissociation curve shifts to the right with fever or hyperthermia. This results in better delivery of oxygen to the tissues with rise in temperature and vice versa happens in hypothermia.

2,3-diphosphoglycerate (DPG) influences P50 profoundly. 2,3-DPG binds to the β-chain and stabilises the Hb in T state, thereby reducing its oxygen affinity and results in right shift of the curve.

Fetal hemoglobin is tailored to function at a lower PO_2 than adult blood, with a left shift of the curve, so as to improve oxygen delivery to the fetus. On the contrary, presence of high fetal hemoglobin in adults can result in tissue hypoxia.

Progressive respiratory alkalosis at high altitude causes a leftward shift of the hemoglobin dissociation curve.

OXYGEN DELIVERY FROM CAPILLARY BLOOD TO INTERSTITIUM

Oxygen transfers into the tissues by simple diffusion rapidly down the large pressure gradient, from 95 mm Hg in blood to 40 mm Hg in the interstitium. Several factors affect the interstitial PO_2: hemoglobin concentration, rate of blood flow and rate of tissue metabolism. Increase in blood flow to four times normal increases PO_2 from 40 to 66 mm Hg, and with further increase in flow, the PO_2 approaches that seen in the arterial blood of around 95 mm Hg. The rate of tissue metabolism has an inverse relationship with interstitial fluid PO_2, while hemoglobin concentration has an effect similar to that of blood flow.

DELIVERY FROM INTERSTITIUM TO INDIVIDUAL CELLS

The largest fall in PO_2 is in the last step of the oxygen cascade, between capillary and mitochondrial PO_2. The final tissue PO_2 is determined by the capillary PO_2, tension gradient between the capillary and the tissue, and the distance between the capillary and the cell.

The constant metabolism in the cells consume oxygen, keeping the intracellular PO_2 always lower than the surrounding interstitium. Depending on the capillary density, the distance between the capillaries and the cells also vary, sometimes as great as 200 μm. Oxygen diffusion is faster when capillary to cell distance is shorter and/or oxygen gradient between capillary and cell is greater. The average intracellular PO_2 is 23 mm Hg (ranges between 5 and 40 mm Hg), which is more than adequate for normal intracellular requirement of 3 mm Hg for maintenance of metabolic pathways.

The delivery of oxygen to tissues can be compromised in the following situations—most commonly in "hypoxic" hypoxia (a fall in PaO_2), and rarely in "stagnant" (a fall in flow) or "anemic" (reduced hemoglobin) hypoxia.

CELLULAR/MITOCHONDRIAL USE OF OXYGEN

The end user of oxygen is the individual cell, whereby energy is produced by oxidative metabolism of substrates. Most of the oxygen consumption occurs in the mitochondria, in the process of oxidative phosphorylation in the cytochromes. The intracellular metabolic rate determines the rate of oxygen consumption. The aerobic pathway, utilizing oxygen results in production of far greater energy output (38 ATPs) from glucose metabolism in comparison to the anaerobic pathway (2 ATPs).

Oxygen Delivery and Consumption

The circulatory and respiratory systems work in tandem to supply oxygen to all the cells of the body. Oxygen delivery (DO_2) is defined as the amount of oxygen supplied to the body in 1 minute, which is equal to the product of cardiac output and arterial oxygen content. The oxygen supply should be at a satisfactory partial pressure and at an adequate quantity to meet the metabolic demand of the tissues, failing which circulatory shock results.

On an average, the oxygen delivery is given as follows:

DO_2 (mL/min) = Qt × CaO_2

1000 mL O_2/min= 5000 mL blood/min × 20 mL O_2 per 100 mL of arterial blood

Where Qt = cardiac output and CaO_2 = oxygen content of arterial blood.

Of this 1000 mL/min, a resting subject uses approximately 250 mL/min for normal metabolism, which is termed as oxygen consumption (VO_2). Hence almost 70% of oxygen is still unextracted by the tissues when the blood reaches venous circulation. This unextracted oxygen is an important reserve under conditions of increased demand, such as exercise or fever, where the body adapts to stress by additional extraction of oxygen. Hypoxia sets in when there is imbalance between supply and demand, despite raised oxygen extraction.

Under normal circumstances, each 100 mL of blood transports 5 mL of O_2 to tissues, as evidenced by fall in O_2 content from 19.8 mL to 14.8 mL/100 mL of blood from arterial to venous side. This reflects a change in PO_2 from 95 mm Hg to 40 mm Hg (oxygen saturation of 97% and 75% respectively).

Physiological changes during exercise in O_2 transport:
Demand for oxygen increases up to 20 times the normal during strenuous exercise. The blood also remains in the capillary (transit time) for less than half the normal time because of increased cardiac output.

However the following physiologic parameters aid in maintaining the oxygen saturation in the blood:

- Blood gets fully saturated within the first third of the transit time in pulmonary circulation.
- Diffusion capacity increases up to 3 fold since:
  - Recruitment of hitherto non-functioning capillaries and dilation of capillaries.
  - Improvement in V/Q mismatch as perfusion improves to the upper lobes during exercise
  - Dilation of alveoli and the capillaries flattens the alveolar capillary membrane, thereby improving diffusion of oxygen.
- Oxygen extraction by tissues increases from normal 5 mL to 15 mL during exercise.
- The oxygen hemoglobin shifts to the right due to increased temperature of exercising muscles, increased release of CO_2 resulting fall in pH and increased levels of 2,3- DPG.

Carbon Dioxide Transport

Carbon dioxide (CO_2) is the main output of aerobic cellular metabolism. This CO_2 needs to be eliminated from the body by transport to the lungs and expired into the surrounding atmosphere.

In addition to renal regulation of pH, the complex process of CO_2 production, transport, and elimination is an important method by which the body regulates the blood's pH.

Carbon dioxide takes the reverse pathway of the oxygen cascade to be expired from the lungs. On an average, tissue metabolism results in production of about 200 to 250 mL of carbon dioxide each minute. At a cardiac output of 5 L/min, 4 to 5 mL of carbon dioxide is unloaded per 100 mL of blood passing through the lungs. Carbon dioxide is transported in the blood in three forms **(Fig. 4.5)**: as physical solution (5–10%), as carbamino compound (5–10%), and as bicarbonate ions (80–95%).

CO_2 in Physical Solution

CO_2 is carried dissolved in plasma according to Henry's law of solubility: $PCO_2 \times$ solubility coefficient (α) = CO_2 concentration in solution. The solubility coefficient varies according to temperature of the solution. In comparison to oxygen, CO_2 is approximately 20 times more soluble in the blood (in plasma and erythrocytes). CO_2 carried in physical solution constitutes about 5% to 10% of the total carbon dioxide transport. About 2.4 to 2.7 mL CO_2 is carried in physical

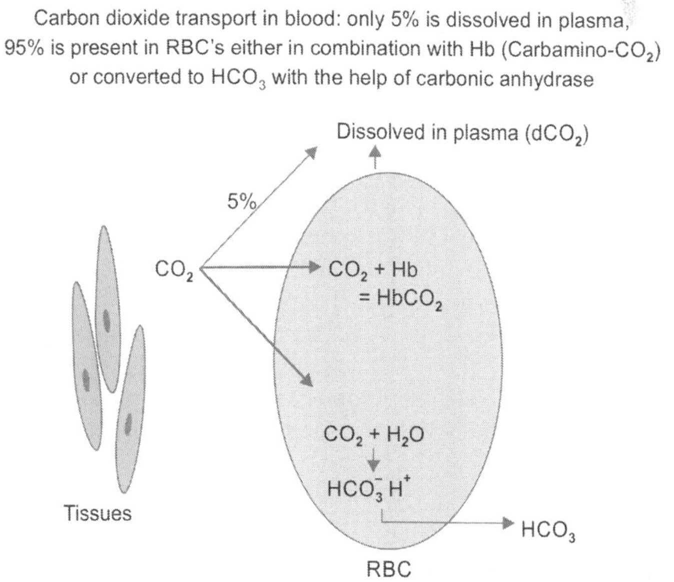

Fig. 4.5: CO_2 transport in blood.

solution per 100 mL of plasma or whole blood at a PCO_2 of 40 mm Hg. However, during heavy exercise, the contribution of dissolved CO_2 can increase up to sevenfold and then it is responsible for almost one-third of the total CO_2 exchange.

Carbamino Compounds

5–10% of total CO_2 is transported in combination with the terminal amine group of blood proteins, most importantly hemoglobin **(Fig. 4.6)**. Reaction of CO_2 with other plasma proteins is insignificant due to the smaller quantity of these proteins when compared to hemoglobin. CO_2 combines in a loose bond with the histidine group of hemoglobin to form carbamino-hemoglobin. This reversible bond benefits uptake of CO_2 at tissue level as well as unloading of CO_2 from the alveolar capillaries to the atmosphere. Haldane effect is when reduced hemoglobin binds more CO_2 than oxygenated hemoglobin. This facilitates the loading of carbon dioxide onto hemoglobin in the peripheral capillaries and tissues, where unloading of oxygen takes place. Similarly, the loose bond also facilitates the ready release of CO_2 into the alveoli where the PCO_2 is lower than in the tissue capillaries.

Bicarbonate Ions

Carbonic anhydrase (CA) acts as a catalyst, accelerating by many thousand folds, the combination of carbon dioxide with water to form carbonic acid. The reaction of CO_2 with water is very slow in the absence of carbonic anhydrase. The erythrocytes have abundant carbonic anhydrase (nil in plasma). The carbonic anhydrase is so efficient and is present in such a quantity that there is no apparent change in carbon dioxide transport even when 98% of its activity is blocked. Carbonic anhydrase is inhibited by some drugs such as thiazide diuretics and acetazolamide. Tissue PCO_2 can increase from 45 mm Hg to as high as 80 mm Hg when CA is blocked by acetazolamide.

Carbonic acid subsequently ionizes into hydrogen and bicarbonate ions. About 96% of the carbonic acid is dissociated under physiological conditions.

$$CO_2 + H_2O \xrightleftharpoons{\text{Carbonic anhydrase}} H_2CO_3 \rightleftharpoons H^+ + HCO_3$$

The hydrogen ions thus produced are quickly buffered by hemoglobin. Large amounts of bicarbonates are formed within the erythrocytes due to the above reaction **(Fig. 4.7)**. To maintain electrical neutrality across the erythrocyte membrane, the excess bicarbonate ions are exchanged for chloride ions present in the plasma by active transport. The membrane bound protein, band 3 exchanges the bicarbonate and the chloride ions in a ping-pong fashion where first an ion is shifted out, followed by the other ion entering the cell, rather than a simultaneous exchange seen in most other ion pumps. This ionic exchange described in 1918 by Hamburger as chloride shift explains the higher chloride content of venous RBCs than that of arterial cells.

Carbon Dioxide Dissociation Curves

The relationship between PCO_2 and total carbon dioxide concentration more linear unlike the sigmoid shaped the oxygen dissociation curve **(Fig. 4.6)**. For a given PCO_2, the CO_2 concentration increases corresponding to the drop in SpO_2.

The Bohr and Haldane effects can be explained on the following basis: Deoxygenated hemoglobin is a weaker acid compared to oxyhemoglobin. Deoxyhemoglobin combines more readily with

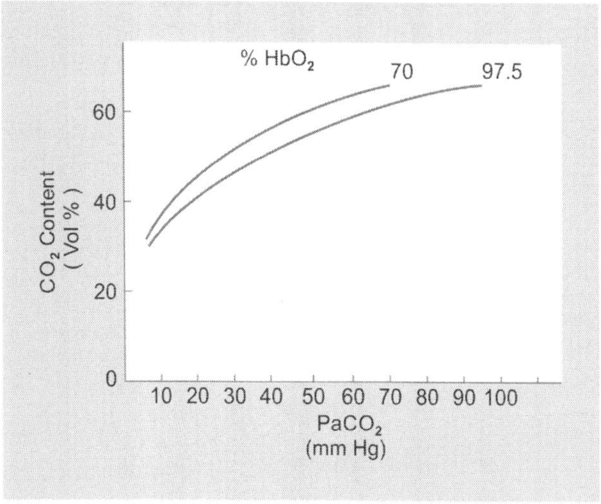

Fig. 4.6: Carbon dioxide dissociation curve: The upper and lower curves represent deoxygenated and oxygenated blood respectively.

hydrogen ion released by the dissociation of carbonic acid, than oxyhemoglobin. This facilitates more CO_2 transport in the form of bicarbonate ion. On the contrary, the association of hydrogen ions with hemoglobin lowers the affinity of hemoglobin for oxygen, resulting in right shift of the oxyhemoglobin dissociation curve, at low pH or high PCO_2, thereby more readily releasing oxygen to the tissues.

The Haldane effect leads to increased uptake of CO_2 in the tissues (when O_2 is released) and increased release of CO_2 in the lungs (when O_2 gets bound to hemoglobin). The Haldane effect approximately doubles the amount of CO_2 released from the blood in the lungs and that picked up in the tissues.

The effect of CO_2 on pH: Most cell membranes including blood brain barrier are impervious to H^+ and bicarbonate ions but allow rapid diffusion of CO_2. CO_2 diffuses across these membranes and within the cells combine with water to form carbonic acid that dissociates into H^+ and bicarbonate ions. Hence intracellular H^+ ion concentrations are relatively unaffected by changes in extracellular pH but changes in PCO_2 can cause significant alterations in their values. Therefore CO_2 strongly influences intracellular pH.

The pressure gradients during diffusion of CO_2, during ascent from tissues to the lungs and atmosphere (Fig. 4.7).

Carbon dioxide takes the reverse pathway of the oxygen cascade to be expired from the lungs. At each point, CO_2 diffuses twenty times

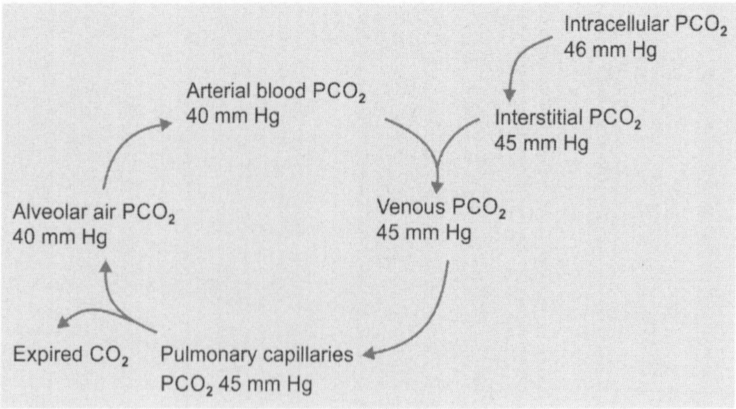

Fig. 4.7: The pressure gradients during diffusion of CO_2, during ascent from tissues to the lungs and atmosphere.

faster in the opposite direction to O_2. Consequently, the CO_2 diffusion requires smaller pressure differences as compared to O_2 diffusion:

- A pressure gradient of only 1 mm Hg is enough to transfer CO_2 from intracellular (PCO_2 about 46 mm Hg) to interstitial (PCO_2 about 45 mm Hg) compartment.
- PCO_2 of arterial blood entering the tissues is about 40 mm Hg and that of the venous blood leaving the tissues is about 45 mm Hg and hence the tissue capillary blood PCO_2 comes almost exactly to equilibrium with the interstitial PCO_2.
- PCO_2 of venous blood entering the pulmonary capillaries is around 45 mm Hg and PCO_2 of alveolar air is around 40 mm Hg thus causing only a 5 mm Hg pressure gradient which is responsible for the diffusion of entire amount of CO_2 out of the pulmonary capillaries into the alveoli. The fall in its level in capillary blood takes place before it has passed one-third of the distance through the capillaries (similar to O_2).

SUGGESTED READING

1. Geers C, Gros G. Carbon dioxide transport and carbonic anhydrase in blood and muscle. Physiological Reviews. 2000; 80: 681–715.
2. J-OC Dunn, MG Mythen, MP Grocott. Physiology of oxygen transport. BJA Education. 16(10): 341–8 (2016).
3. John B West. Pulmonary Pathophysiology. The Essentials, 8th edition. Lippincott Williams & Wilkins; Wolters Kluwer, 2012.
4. John B West. Respiratory Physiology: The Essentials, 9th edition. Lippincott Williams & Wilkins; Wolters Kluwer, 2012; ISBN 978-1-60913-640-6.
5. Joseph Feher. Quantitative Human Physiology: An Introduction., Elsevier; ISBN: 9780128011546.
6. Lumb AB. In: Nunn's Applied Respiratory Physiology, 8th edition. Edinburgh, Elsevier, 2017.
7. Michael G Levitzky. Pulmonary Physiology, 7th edition. MacGraw Hill.
8. Murray & Nadel's. Textbook of Respiratory Medicine, 6th edition. Elsevier Saunders.

Chapter 5

Tissue Oxygenation

Ruchi Singh, Poonam Chaudhary, Abhishek Goyal

INTRODUCTION

Continuous supply of oxygen is essential to meet the constant cellular energy demand. Cardiorespiratory systems function in a coordinated manner to meet these cellular oxygen demands. Cellular consumption of oxygen is dependent on the metabolic needs of the organism which depends on the metabolic substrates. Rarely ever, the metabolic substrates like oxygen, fat, sugars and their metabolites act as limiting factors. However, adenosine triphosphate (ATP) is the common limiting factor and depends on the metabolic needs of the individual.

Cytochrome oxidase is the single enzyme which utilizes 90% of the body's oxygen consumption during oxidative phosphorylation. It is the most efficient means of generating ATP, by a series of oxidation-reduction reactions. Oxygen acts as the terminal electron acceptor during aerobic respiration in electron transport chain resulting in generation of 38 molecules of ATP per molecule of glucose. Under aerobic conditions, ATP is continuously hydrolyzed to adenosine diphosphate (ADP), inorganic phosphate (Pi), and H^+, and these metabolites, together with O_2 are in turn reutilized by the mitochondria to regenerate ATP. However, hypoxia and accumulation of AMP stimulates glycolysis, leading to production of lactate. During anaerobic metabolism, i.e., in absence of oxygen only 2 molecules of ATP are formed per glucose molecule, in addition to H^+ ions which can lead to systemic metabolic acidosis. In sustained hypoxia, increase in cytosolic ADP stimulates adenylate kinase reaction:

$$[ADP] + [ADP] = [ATP] + [AMP]$$

Further, breakdown of AMP by 5-nucleotidase produces adenosine which is a strong vasodilator. It escapes from the cell in the microvasculature and provides a metabolic feedback to increase the blood flow in hypoxic areas.

Thus, tissue oxygenation regulation is critical for maintaining the cellular activities and hence essential for survival of an organism. An imbalance between normal parameters of oxygen demand and supply **(Table 5.1)** occurs in critically ill patients with poor cardiopulmonary reserves. Optimization of oxygen delivery meeting the oxygen demands or reducing the oxygen demands (i.e., metabolic rate) has the potential to improve the outcomes of these patients. Several physiological processes are involved in the delivery of oxygen from the environment to the cells including oxygenation, oxygen delivery and oxygen consumption. This involves diffusion of oxygen through the alveolar-capillary membrane in blood, transportation as it binds to hemoglobin in RBCs along with some amount being dissolved in plasma and unloading in the peripheral tissues to be utilized as to fuel for aerobic cellular metabolism. Thus, cellular metabolic rate determines the oxygen demand. A balance between the oxygen demand (oxygen consumption - VO_2) and supply (oxygen delivery - DO_2) is regulated by control of ventilation as well as blood flow or cardiac output.

Table 5.1: Normal values and equations of tissue oxygenation parameters.

Parameter	*Equation*	*Normal range*
Arterial O_2 content (CaO_2)	$CaO_2 = (1.34 \times Hb \times SaO_2) + (0.0031 \times PaO_2)$	20 mL/dL
Cardiac output (Q)	$Q = HR \times SV$	4–8 L/min
Cardiac index (CI)	$CI = Q/BSA$	2.4–4.0 L/min/m^2
Oxygen delivery (DO_2)	$Q \times 1.34 \times Hb \times SaO_2$	900–1000 mL/min
Oxygen delivery index (DO_2 index)	DO_2/BSA	520–570 mL/min/m^2
Oxygen uptake (VO_2)	$Q \times 1.34 \times Hb \times (SaO_2–SvO_2)$	180–280 mL/min/m^2
Oxygen uptake index (VO_2 index)	VO_2/BSA	110–160 mL/min/m^2
Oxygen extraction ratio (O_2ER)	$(SaO_2–SvO_2/SaO_2) \times 100$	20–30%

(BSA = body surface area; Hb = Hemoglobin; HR = heart rate; PaO_2 = partial pressure of O_2 in arterial blood; SaO_2 = arterial O_2 saturation; SvO_2 = mixed venous O_2 saturation; SV = stroke volume)

Source: Dunn J, Mythen MG, Grocott MP. Physiology of oxygen transport. BJA Education, (2016);16, 341–348.

OXYGEN DELIVERY (DO_2)

Oxygen delivery is the rate of oxygen carried by the blood to the tissues. It is controlled by the oxygen demand (metabolic rate) of the tissues. It is the product of cardiac output (Q) and arterial oxygen content (CaO_2).

Thus, oxygen delivery = cardiac output × arterial oxygen content

$$DO_2\,(mL/min) = Q \times CaO_2$$

Oxygen delivery is also designated as systemic oxygen transport (SOT), total oxygen transport (TOT), transport of oxygen (TO_2) and delivery of oxygen (QO_2) but the concept remains the same. Interestingly, the term oxygen delivery is bit incorrect as it depicts the amount of oxygen delivered to tissues and utilized for metabolism. Though, at rest the oxygen extraction ratio is only 25% which rarely increases to 75% during exceptional metabolic stress. Increases in oxygen demand are met by increases in blood flow and oxygen extraction. Thus, sometimes the term "oxygen dispatch" has also been utilized instead. However, to maintain consistency we will be using the term "oxygen delivery". Normal DO_2 is approximately 1000 mL/min. However, if cardiac index (cardiac output per square meter of body surface area) is substituted for cardiac output than the value is approximately 500 mL/min/m^2. It should be noted that this is an overall measurement of oxygen delivery and does not describe regional differences. The microcirculation responds to altering tissue metabolic demands by varying the regional and local blood flow.

Factors Affecting DO_2

Arterial O_2 Content (CaO_2)

It is the sum of oxygen bound to hemoglobin and the amount of oxygen dissolved in plasma. The amount of oxygen dissolved in plasma is proportional to the partial pressure exerted by oxygen on the plasma at a given temperature, according to Henry's law.

$$CaO_2 = \text{Hb bound oxygen} + \text{dissolved oxygen}$$

$$CaO_2 = (Hb \times SaO_2 \times 1.34) + (0.003 \times PaO_2)$$

where CaO_2 = arterial oxygen content; Hb = hemoglobin level; SaO_2 = arterial oxygen saturation; PaO_2 = partial pressure of oxygen in arterial blood in kilopascals (kPa)

This gives the amount of oxygen in each 100 mL of blood. If blood is equilibrated with 100% O_2, hemoglobin becomes 100% saturated. Each gram of hemoglobin contains 1.39 mL of O_2 when fully saturated. But due to the presence of inactive hemoglobin derivatives (e.g., carboxyhemoglobin and methemoglobin), the value is slightly lower. However, the directly measured maximum oxygen-carrying capacity per gram of hemoglobin is 1.34 mL. SaO_2 is the arterial hemoglobin oxygen saturation expressed as a fraction (i.e., 1.0 instead of 100%).

Thus, at a Hb level of 15 g/dL and SaO_2 of 98% (Hb at the end of pulmonary capillaries is only 98% saturated with O_2 due to admixture of venous blood that bypasses the pulmonary capillaries), the oxygen carried by Hb will be:

$$1.34 \times 15 \times 0.98 = 19.7 \text{ mL}/100 \text{ mL}$$

The amount of dissolved O_2 is a linear function of PaO_2. The second part of the equation shows that, at PaO_2 of 100 mm Hg the expected concentration of dissolved O_2 in blood is:

$$0.0031 \times 100 = 0.3 \text{ mL}/100 \text{ mL}$$

The arterial blood therefore contains a total concentration of 20 mL/100 mL of O_2 (19.7 + 0.3 = 20 mL/100 mL). Thus, it is clear that CaO_2 primarily depends on Hb and SaO_2 and to a lesser extent on PaO_2.

Cardiac Output (CO)

The output of the heart per unit of time is known as cardiac output. It is the product of **stroke volume** (amount of blood ejected out of heart per beat) and **heart rate per minute** of the individual.

Cardiac output = stroke volume × heart rate

Normal value of stroke volume is about 70 mL. Thus, if heart rate is 72 beats/minute, the CO is 70 mL × 72 = 5,040 mL, i.e., approximately 5 L/min.

CO can be measured by direct and indirect methods.

- **Direct methods:**
  - CO can be measured directly by placing electromagnetic flow meter in the ascending aorta. This is an accurate method but is applicable in experimental animals.
  - In humans, CO is usually determined by using echocardiography.
- **Indirect methods:** This includes Fick method, indicator dilution and thermodilution method.

Any alterations in the stroke volume or heart rate affect the cardiac output. The factors effecting stroke volume are as follows:

Preload

It is the load applied on the muscle just before contraction. The end-diastolic volume (EDV) is considered the preload of the ventricles. Increases in the EDV increases the stroke volume in accordance with the Frank-Starling's Law which states that *"the force of contraction is directly proportional to the initial length of the muscle fiber, within the physiological limit".* Thus, increase in preload increases the initial muscle length causing a more forceful cardiac contraction. This emphasizes the value of prompt correction of hypovolemia leading to reduction of cardiac output. The relationship between preload and cardiac output is however not linear and is also influenced by changes in ventricular compliance and geometry. Since ventricular EDV is not easily measured at the bedside, end-diastolic pressure (EDP) and central venous pressure (CVP) are more commonly used as reflections of preload in clinical practice.

After Load

The force against which ventricular fibers shortens is known as after load. It is the resistance offered against ejection of blood from ventricles. Thus, it depends on the aortic and pulmonary arterial pressures, systemic and pulmonary vascular resistance as well as compliance of ventricular muscle. CO is inversely proportional to the after load. Determination of these forces is complex thus systolic left ventricular pressure is usually used as a reasonable measure of afterload. Being a transmural force, afterload is influenced by the pleural pressures at the surface of the heart. Positive pleural pressures can promote ventricular emptying by facilitating the inward displacement of the ventricular wall during systole and this is one of the mechanisms by which noninvasive positive pressure ventilation is beneficial in cardiogenic pulmonary edema.

Myocardial Contractility

Myocardial contractility is the intrinsic property of cardiac myocytes and exerts a major influence on the CO. It depends mainly on the ventricular muscle mass, state of autonomic activity, concentration of various hormones and chemicals in blood, drugs and heart rate. It is measured indirectly by impedance cardiography and doppler echocardiography.

Steps Involved in DO_2

Tissue oxygenation and systemic blood flow play an important role in prevention of tissue hypoxia. Abnormalities of oxygen delivery may involve a reduction in total oxygen transport or changes in regional distribution. This may account for disturbances in organ system function. The mechanisms by which oxygen is involved in the local regulation of blood flow remains unclear to an extent. However, oxygen transport should be viewed with two perspectives:

1. Molecular or biochemical perspective in which oxygen and other molecules like hemoglobin, cytochrome c oxidase, etc., interact and
2. Cellular interaction in which oxygen interacts with cells and organelles like mitochondria where energy is generated to support cellular activities.

Microcirculation has a strategic location as it is the interface between the parenchymal cells in a tissue (consumers) and the circulatory system (supplier) which is responsible for maintaining nutrient supply and removal of metabolic wastes. Microcirculatory level of integration constitutes the smallest number of system components that retain the complete integrated function of both the circulatory and cellular systems. The main role of microcirculation is to maintain the physiological matching of oxygen supply to the metabolic demands of cells and tissues. O_2 delivery thus involves cellular O_2 supply as well as cellular O_2 utilization.

- **Cellular oxygen supply:** As oxygen is exchanged between the intravascular and extravascular compartments without any significant restriction due to its high solubility and diffusibility, all arteries in body are considered to carry identical concentrations of O_2 but the distribution of O_2 is not equal to all cells. This is due to the fact that tissue oxygenation strongly depends on mechanisms which regulate the blood flow through the microvessels and microcirculation. The cylinder of Krogh must be considered to understand the function of microcirculation in maintenance of tissue oxygenation. In Krogh's cylinder single straight capillary is assumed from where oxygen diffuses to the volume of tissue in reach. Each cylinder has a small diameter when all the capillaries are open and oxygen pressure is high and uniform in the dependent cells. As the number of functioning capillaries reduces, the remaining capillaries assume compensatory function.

The diameter of the cylinders largely increases along with the increase in the gradient of oxygen pressure within the center and the periphery. The oxygen concentration in cells becomes low and O_2 consumption becomes "flow dependent". The prognostic value of increasing O_2 delivery and consumption is thus obvious and it means that the microcirculatory network is able to increase its exchange area and to supply adequate oxygen to the cells. The regulation of microcirculation is quite complex and in healthy conditions involves nerves, catecholamines, acetylcholine, serotonin, histamine, and kinins all together modulating constriction, dilatation and permeability. The oxygen status of the cell is impacted due to microcirculatory, tissue diffusion, and cellular factors. Thus, global measurements may fail to identify local tissue hypoxemia.

- **Cellular O_2 utilization:** Eukaryotic cells are dependent on aerobic metabolism as mitochondrial respiration offers greater efficiency for extraction of energy from glucose compared to anaerobic glycolysis. Metabolic utilization of O_2 in cells occurs by oxidation of pyruvic acid in Krebs cycle taking place in mitochondria and resulting in production of 38 ATP molecules. Maintenance of oxidative metabolism is dependent on complex mechanisms of microvascular oxygen distribution and cellular oxygen uptake. Reduced blood flow in a tissue is evolved as an energy conserving mechanism when substrate, specifically molecular oxygen, are scarce. Thus, in absence of O_2 only 2 molecules of ATP are generated by anaerobic glycolysis along with production of lactic acid, which may lead to systemic metabolic acidosis.

OXYGEN CONSUMPTION (VO_2)

Oxygen consumption (VO_2) is the amount of oxygen consumed by the tissues per minute. Thus, it is the product of cardiac output and arteriovenous difference of oxygen content in blood.

Calculation of VO_2 can be performed in following ways:

- Indirectly, by using Fick's equation, by measuring the oxygen content of mixed venous blood (which requires placement of a pulmonary artery catheter), CvO_2.

  $CvO_2 = (1.31 \times Hb \times SvO_2 \times 0.01) + (0.0225 \times PvO_2)$

  $VO_2\ (mL\ O_2/min) = Q \times (CaO_2 - CvO_2)$

- By measurement of inspired and expired minute ventilation (Vi and Ve) and of fractional concentrations of O_2 (FiO_2 and FeO_2) in the two samples. This is a non-invasive method but is relatively unreliable in mechanically ventilated patients on high FiO_2.

  $VO_2 = (Vi \times FiO_2) - (Ve \times FeO_2)$

- Direct measurement of VO_2 can be done by re-spirometry. During re-spirometry, the patient breathes through a chamber filled with oxygen. Measurement of the oxygen depleted from the chamber, as well as the carbon dioxide and water vapor produced in the chamber, is used to determine VO_2. Respirometry can be used in mechanically ventilated patients, but the accuracy of direct measurement of VO_2 diminishes at high oxygen concentrations (i.e., ≥80 percent).

  Regardless of the method used, measurement should be performed when the patient is clinically stable and resting quietly because many routine procedures (e.g., physiotherapy and suctioning) and physiologic parameters (e.g., fever, pain, and anxiety) can result in sharp variations in VO_2. Normal VO_2 in a conscious, resting person is approximately 250 mL O_2/min.

Calculated VO_2

VO_2 is often not measured directly and is usually derived from Fick's equation. These derived methods have certain limitations as significant errors can occur in measurement of both CO as well as the difference between CaO_2 and CvO_2. In thermodilution CO measurement technique there is an error of about 5% to 10%. The precision of hemoglobin measurements is also about 5%, and hemoglobin saturation is about 2%. There can be an overestimation of true VO_2 by 17%, underestimation by 13% when these factors are considered. Thus, changes of VO_2 less than 20% cannot be detected reliably. Another limitation of derived method is that lung VO_2, is not considered. Directly measured VO_2 is slightly greater than the derived value which does not include alveolar oxygen consumption. In normal conditions lung VO_2 is less than 5% of the total VO_2 but during inflammatory processes it may be as high as 20% as suggested by experimental studies. Also, mathematical coupling may occur because CO will be a common variable if both DO_2, and VO_2, are calculated with the Fick's equation, and this situation may incorrectly suggest a relationship between DO_2 and VO_2. Thus, while studying the relationship between

VO_2 and DO_2 it is important to use the directly measured rather than the derived value to avoid problems of mathematical linkage.

O_2 Extraction Ratio (O_2ER)

This is the fraction of oxygen delivered via the cardiovascular system that is utilized by the tissues, and is therefore the ratio of oxygen consumption to oxygen delivery:

$$O_2ER = VO_2/DO_2$$

It is also expressed as the proportion of arterial oxygen that is removed from the blood as it passes through the microcirculation:

$$O_2\,ER = (CaO_2 - CvO_2)/CaO_2$$

In health, only 20–30% of the oxygen delivered to tissues is utilized (an O_2ER 0.2–0.3) and if we substitute the values presented earlier (namely VO_2 250 mL/min and DO_2 1000 mL/min), an adult male has an O_2ER 0.25 at rest. Thus, oxygen consumption under conditions of rest is said to be 'supply independent' and VO_2 is maintained even in the face of a decreasing DO_2. However, at a critical DO_2 (DO_2crit) of ~4 mL/kg/min, the O_2ER becomes maximal (O_2ER 0.6–0.8) and VO_2 becomes 'supply dependent'. If DO_2 decreases further below the DO_2crit, or if VO_2 increases for a given DO_2crit, tissue hypoxia ensues with resultant anaerobic respiration and lactate production secondary to an imbalance between ATP supply and demand (producing a type A hyperlactatemia).

The DO_2-VO_2 Curve

Figure 5.1 describes the biphasic relation between DO_2 and VO_2. The solid line 'ABC' depicts the normal relationship in health while the dashed line 'DEF' depicts the condition during critical illness. As metabolic demand (VO_2) increases or DO_2 diminishes (C–B), O_2ER rises to maintain aerobic metabolism and consumption remains independent of delivery. Points B and E depict DO_2crit in health and critical illness, respectively. At these points maximum O_2ER is reached. This is believed to be 60–70% and beyond this point, any further increase in VO_2 or decline in DO_2 leads to tissue hypoxia. In health, VO_2 is 'supply independent' between B and C and 'supply dependent' between A and B.

In critical illness, the slope of maximum O_2ER falls (DE v AB), reflecting the reduced ability of tissues to extract oxygen. The

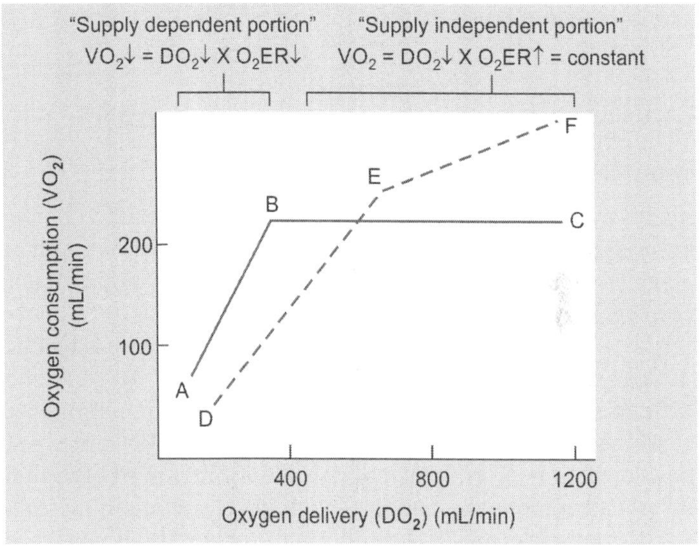

Fig. 5.1: The biphasic relation between DO_2 and VO_2.

relationship does not plateau as in the normal relationship. Hence consumption continues to increase (E–F) to "supranormal" levels of DO_2, demonstrating so called "supply dependency" and the presence of a covert oxygen debt that would be relieved by further increasing DO_2. This is termed a 'pathological DO_2 dependency' and O_2ER may not increase proportionately with VO_2. O_2ER increases during exercise, with a peak maximal exercise at 0.8. This is because although DO_2 increases, it does not match the increase in VO_2 required by exercise.

Factors Influencing VO_2

Causes of Decreased VO_2

- Sedation/analgesia/neuromuscular blocking agents/antipyretics
- Hypovolemia/shock states
- Mechanical ventilation
- Hypothermia

Factors that Increase VO_2

- Exercise
- Trauma (including surgery and burns)

- Inflammation/sepsis/pyrexia
- Shivering
- Pain
- Agitation

Oxygen Debt (O_2 Deficit or O_2D)

Oxygen serves as a critical carbon acceptor in generation of energy from metabolic fuels and thus oxygen consumption is regulated during health. In a cardiogenic, vasodilatory, or hemorrhagic shock, oxygen delivery may be sufficiently reduced to decrease VO_2 below a critical level. When this critical level of oxygen restriction is reached, an oxygen debt (O_2D) occurs. Thus, oxygen debt or 'oxygen deficit' is defined as the integral difference between the prehemorrhage/pretrauma resting normal VO_2 and the actual VO_2 during the hypovolemic or hemorrhage period. It is the difference between the metabolic demand for O_2 and the actual VO_2. As demand increases, VO_2 must increase to preserve aerobic metabolism. This is met with by increasing DO_2 either by physiological compensation, e.g., an increase in cardiac output or O_2ER or by therapeutic interventions such as intravenous fluids or inotropes. Extent of an O_2D is further highlighted by an increase in the unmetabolized metabolic acids generated by the anaerobic processes. The congruence of O_2D and related metabolic acidemia permits precise quantification of the severity of the ischemic shock process. If this increase in DO_2 is delayed, O_2 debt continues to grow and a stage is reached from where recovery is not possible.

Assessment of Tissue Oxygenation

Tissue hypoxia is defined as abnormal O_2 utilization by cells; unlike hypoxemia (defined by low PaO_2) has standard normal and abnormal values, there are no normal values for tissue PO_2 and it cannot be routinely measured at the bedside.

There are three ways to detect tissue hypoxia.

Clinical Assessment

Although clinical examination should be the first step in assessing tissue oxygenation, it is a crude and insensitive method as they occur late during the course of tissue hypoxia. Signs like mental obtundation, oliguria, abnormal vital signs, delayed capillary refill often indicate specific organ dysfunction due to tissue hypoxia. Direct or indirect measurements of local tissue oxygenation of an organ suspected to suffer from hypoxia will facilitate the assessment.

Local tissue oxygen probes have been used in critical care areas in some instances (e.g., brain and intestine). External probes placed on forehead to measure oxidative status using near infrared technology are theoretically attractive but subjects to artifacts from muscle metabolism on the scalp.

Similarly, some monitors now commercially available utilize intestinal luminal pH (PCO_2) sensors to determine oxygenation status.

Physiological Parameters

Mixed Venous O_2 Saturation (SvO_2)

Mixed venous blood represents blood returning from all the venous beds of the body "mixed" together in the right ventricle. It is obtained from the distal end of the pulmonary artery with pulmonary artery catheter, the tip of which emits infrared light and records light reflected back from hemoglobin in circulating erythrocytes. This technique is called *reflectance spectrophotometry* (whereas pulse oximeters use *transmission spectrophotometry*). SvO_2 can also be measured intermittently by withdrawing blood from the catheter. In the proximal part of the pulmonary artery, blood from the two venae cavae is not fully blended and so it is not true representative of total body venous gas values.

SvO_2 is a marker of the balance between whole body oxygen delivery and O_2 demand and is normally between 65% and 75%, i.e., O_2 demand is usually about 25–35% that of O_2 delivery.

Mixed venous PO_2 >40 mm Hg or SvO_2 >70% (so called goal directed therapy) might suggest presence of adequate oxygenation.

It has been recently been shown that measurement of central venous oxygen saturation ($ScvO_2$), and its manipulation in patients with severe sepsis has improved survival. Patients with $ScvO_2$ levels higher than 70% usually have lower serum lactate levels, higher pH and base deficit and improved survival. Also $ScvO_2$ has been shown to correlate well with SvO_2 measurements and both serum lactate and $ScvO_2$ appear to be independent predictors of poor outcome. The advantage of $ScvO_2$ lies in the fact that it can be easily measured by insertion of a catheter in the internal jugular or subclavian vein whereas the measurement of SvO_2 requires the placement of a pulmonary arterial catheter.

Causes of decreased SvO_2

- Decrease in DO_2: Which may occur due to hypovolemia, decreased cardiac output, low Hb, low PaO_2 and SaO_2.
- Increase in O_2 demand: Critical illness, sepsis, thyrotoxicosis, etc.

Causes of increased SvO_2

- Increased DO_2: Increased cardiac output (e.g. exercise, use of inotropes), increased Hb (polycythemia)
- Decrease in O_2 demand: Deep sedation and paralysis in ventilated patients
- Decreased tissue O_2 utilization: Cyanide and CO poisoning, sepsis
- Left to right shunts: These can usually be diagnosed by an abnormal "step-up" of SvO_2 at the level of the defect as the pulmonary artery catheter is passed into the right atrium or ventricle.

Limitation of SvO_2

Normal or increased values do not always mean that tissue oxygenation is adequate. For example, in sepsis and CO poisoning, impaired tissue O_2 utilization results in a normal or high SvO_2. In addition, pathologic vasodilatation and increased cardiac output in sepsis also tend to increase SvO_2 even though tissue hypoxia is ongoing.

Dual Oximetry

By simultaneously measuring SaO_2 by pulse oximetry one can get a continuous measurement of whole body O_2 extraction, i.e., SaO_2 – SvO_2. This method is known as dual oximetry and normal value of O_2 extraction is 20 to 30% (as explained above in **oxygen delivery**).

Biochemical Markers of Hypoxia

Blood Lactate Level

Lactate is end product of anaerobic metabolism and it is normally metabolized by liver. It is intermediate of carbohydrate metabolism which is derived mainly from muscle cells and erythrocytes. Therefore lactate production depends upon rates of production and metabolism, both of which are dependent on tissue perfusion.

Type A lactic acidosis

Blood lactate levels increase due to tissue hypoperfusion (most commonly seen in shock, anemia).

Type B lactic acidosis

Occurs due to non-hypoxemic causes like delayed clearance of lactate due to liver disease, thiamine deficiency (blocks pyruvate metabolism) and metabolic alkalosis (stimulates glycolysis).

Lactate levels ≥4 mmol/L defines lactic acidosis. It is easy to measure and can be followed sequentially to assess prognosis as well as response to therapy. Blood lactate concentrations are a better prognostic indicator than oxygen-derived physiological variables.

Gastric Tonometry

Physiological variables of oxygen transport and lactate are indices of global tissue oxygenation and cannot identify oxygen deficits in individual organs. This led to development of gastric tonometry to measure regional perfusion in the gut that employs a balloon in the stomach to measure intramucosal pH. Gastric PCO_2, like derived gastric intramucosal pH (pHi) and the gradient or gap between gastric PCO_2 and arterial PCO_2 has been shown to be a reliable index of hypoperfusion with prognostic value in critically ill patients. Despite its complexity, gastric tonometry is a reasonably good prognostic indicator in critically ill patients.

Sublingual Capnography

Sublingual capnometry is a non-invasive technique to measure sublingual mucosal PCO_2 ($PslCO_2$) using carbon dioxide-sensing optodes or microelectrodes. $PslCO_2$ correlates with organ blood flows and systemic markers of hypoperfusion such as MAP, cardiac index, and arterial lactate value. Normal range for $PslCO_2$ is 43 to 47 mm Hg.

Nuclear Magnetic Resonance Spectrometry

Metabolomics is upcoming discipline that aims to identify changes in concentrations of the metabolites in a biological sample, such as blood, urine, or saliva. Metabolites are chemical fingerprints that cellular processes leave behind. Nuclear magnetic resonance (NMR) spectroscopy is a quantitative high throughput method that needs only minimal sample preparation. Alterations in concentrations correlates with metabolic derangements in sepsis and severity of illness and mortality. 3-hydroxybutyrate, citrate, glycine, histidine, and AGP are candidates for further studies to enable identification of phenotype association in the early stages of sepsis.

Potential Biochemical Markers of Hypoxia

Various proteins like hypoxia induced factor (HIF1-alpha), CA-9, PI3K, MAPK, BNIP3, GLUT1 and PDK1 are induced by hypoxia and are potential markers of tissue hypoxia.

Carbonic anhydrase-9 (CA-9) has crucial role in pH regulation and it is most widely expressed gene in response to hypoxia. HIF1-alpha stabilizes in hypoxemic condition, it moves into cell nucleus and increase rate of transcription of genes that control oxygen delivery. This leads to induction of BNIP3, which further induces PDK1 protein (which has important role in maintain ATP production). In the last step, GLUT1 [(Glucose Tranporter1) transmembrane protein for facilitated glucose transport across membrane] is induced under hypoxemic conditions.

These potential markers of hypoxia can be measured by various imaging techniques like immunostaining, PET and SPECT; but these are currently limited to research due to cost and availability.

SUGGESTED READING

1. Dunn J, Mythen M, Grocott M. Physiology of oxygen transport. BJA Education. 2016;16:341–8.
2. Krogh A. The number and distribution of capillaries in muscles with calculations of the oxygen pressure head necessary for supplying the tissue. J Physiol. 1919;52:409–15.
3. Leach RM, Treacher DF. The pulmonary physician and critical care. 6. Oxygen Transport: The relation between oxygen delivery and consumption. Thorax. 1992;47(11):971–8.
4. Leach RM, Treacher DF. The pulmonary physician in critical care* 2: Oxygen delivery and consumption in the critically ill. Thorax. 2002; 57(2):170–7.
5. Rixen D, Siegel JH. Bench-to-bedside review: Oxygen debt and its metabolic correlates as quantifiers of the severity of hemorrhagic and post-traumatic shock. Crit Care. 2005;9(5):441–53.
6. Samsel RW, Schumacker PT. Oxygen delivery to tissues. Eur Respir J. 1991;4(10):1258–67.

Part C Clinical Considerations

Chapter Outline

Chapter 6

Blood Gases and Acid-Base Balance

Sourabh Pahuja, Saurabh Mittal, Karan Madan

Blood gas analysis is a commonly used diagnostic tool to evaluate patients in the emergency rooms and intensive care units. Typically parameters measured in arterial blood gas (ABG) are partial pressure of oxygen (pO_2), partial pressure of carbon dioxide (pCO_2) and pH. Other derived values such as HCO_3^-, base excess, anion gap and the alveolar-arterial gradient are obtained from the ABG. It is a vital laboratory tool that can assist clinicians in the timely detection and management of metabolic and respiratory disorders.

ARTERIAL VS VENOUS BLOOD GAS ANALYSIS

Arterial blood is commonly used for assessment, and values obtained are considered the gold standard. Venous blood taken through peripheral veins or central venous catheters can serve as an alternative to ABG when evaluating patients with metabolic and respiratory disturbances. Advantages of venous blood over arterial blood are less incidence of vascular injury, nerve damage and lesser pain. VEINART trial by Chauvin et al. demonstrated that venous blood gas is less painful than ABG. Venous blood gas may be used in place of ABG in non-hypoxemic patients.

The question remains whether values (pH, pCO_2 and HCO_3) measured via venous blood are reliable. Zeserson et al. conducted a prospective cohort study of 156 critically ill patients in the ED and ICU setting to evaluate the correlation between pH and pCO_2 when derived from ABG compared to VBG with added pulse oximetry for estimating PaO_2. They and concluded pH and pCO_2 on VBG analysis correlated with pH and pCO_2 on ABG analysis. The SpO_2 correlated well with pO_2 on ABG analysis. A meta-analysis by Byrne et al., including 1768 subjects from 18 individual studies, found that peripheral VBG correlates well with ABG for pH but found an unacceptably wide 95% prediction interval when looking at the pCO_2. **Table 6.1** summarizes the correlation of VBG and ABG values as seen in various studies.

Therefore, VBG is an acceptable alternative to ABG in many cases when supplemented with pulse oximetry.

Parameters Measured during ABG

Partial Pressure of Oxygen (PaO_2)

Partial pressure of oxygen gives us an estimate about the tissue oxygenation and helps us decide on further oxygen therapy. PaO_2 indicates the partial pressure of dissolved oxygen present in the blood. In a healthy adult breathing air at sea level (760 mm Hg), PaO_2 is about 97 mm Hg. It decreases with age and approaches 80 mm Hg in a 60-year-old man. There is a fall of about ten mm Hg for every 10 years of age after that. A PaO_2 of 80 mm Hg in an adult is relatively acceptable at sea level as it does not affect blood oxygen saturation. Factors on which it depends are—a fraction of inspired oxygen (FiO_2) and barometric pressure (PB).

Fraction of Inspired Oxygen (FiO_2)

Any change in inspired oxygen changes the Alveolar oxygen partial pressure (P_AO_2), which itself affects the partial pressure of oxygen (PaO_2) in blood. This equation can determine the relationship of FiO_2 and P_AO_2:

$$P_AO_2 = [FiO_2(P_B - PH_{20}) - PaCO_2]/R$$

(P_B = barometric pressure; R = respiratory gas exchange ratio, i.e., CO_2 output/O_2 uptake).

On room air (at sea level), P_AO_2 = [0.21 (760–47)–40]/0.8 = 100 mm Hg.

Table 6.1: Correlation between ABG and VBG values.

Variable	*Bias (ABG-VBG)*	*95% CI*
pH	0.035	–0.11 to 0.02
pCO_2	5.7 mm Hg	–17.4 to 23.9
HCO_3	–1.41 mmol/L	–5.8 to 4.3
pO_2	36.9 mm Hg	27.2 to 46.4
Base excess	0.089	–0.97 to 0.55

As the FiO_2 is increased, the P_AO_2 (hence PaO_2) increases. Therefore, in a person breathing 40% oxygen, PAO_2 = [0.4 (760–47)–40]/0.8 = 235 mm Hg.

Barometric Pressure

Atmospheric pressure is constant (760 mm Hg) at sea level. It decreases at high altitudes. As altitude increases, the decrease in P_B leads to a reduction in the amount of inspired oxygen, leading to a fall in partial pressure of alveolar oxygen (P_AO_2).

For example: On the summit of Mt. Everest (8848 m), the barometric pressure is 253 mm Hg. $PaCO_2$ decreases due to hypoxic drive, and it is ten mm Hg at around 8000 m.

P_AO_2 = [0.21 (253–47)–10]/0.8 = 30 mm Hg

Consequently, P_AO_2 is only about 30 mm Hg (hence PaO_2 also decreases). Alveolar PO_2 at sea level is 100 mm Hg.

The Partial Pressure of CO_2 in the Blood ($PaCO_2$)

$PaCO_2$ produced depends on minute ventilation and dead space. Minute ventilation (MV) consists of two components:

1. Amount of ventilation taking part in gas exchange in alveolar ventilation (VA).
2. Volume not taking part in ventilation, i.e. dead space ventilation (VD).

$MV = V_A + V_D$

The equation can best describe the relationship between dead space ventilation and $PaCO_2$.

$$V_D / V_T = \frac{PaCO_2 - P_ECO_2}{PaCO_2}$$

V_D = dead space volume, V_T = tidal volume, $PaCO_2$ = partial pressure of CO_2 in blood, P_ECO_2 = partial pressure of CO_2 in exhaled gases.

Therefore, $PaCO_2$ shall depend on MV, provided the V_D is relatively constant. In an average healthy person, the physiological dead space is generally unchanged. In the presence of an adequate cardiopulmonary reserve, an increase in minute ventilation due to any cause can decrease $PaCO_2$, provided the VD is unaltered. If there is an increase in $PaCO_2$ in the presence of hyperventilation, a dead space producing disease (e.g. COPD) should be suspected.

Hydrogen Ion Concentration and pH

Hydrogen ion concentration [H+] in aqueous solutions is traditionally expressed by the pH, which means the power of hydrogen, and is a logarithmic function of the [H+]. Systemic arterial pH is maintained between 7.35 and 7.45 by extracellular and intracellular chemical buffering together with respiratory and renal regulatory mechanisms. The control of arterial CO_2 tension ($PaCO_2$) by the central nervous system (CNS) and respiratory system and the control of plasma bicarbonate by the kidneys stabilize the arterial pH by excretion or retention of acid or alkali. The Henderson-Hasselbalch equation describes the metabolic and respiratory components that regulate systemic pH:

$$pH = 6.1 + \log_{10}\left(\frac{[HCO_3^-]}{0.0307 \times PCO_2}\right)$$

FACTORS AFFECTING ABG INTERPRETATION

Delayed Analysis

Oxygen decreases, and carbon dioxide increases even after blood is withdrawn. Therefore sample should be iced quickly and should be processed within 1–2 hours. **Table 6.2** shows the change in parameters with time.

Excess Heparin

Heparin is a weak acid, and excess of it will cause dilutional effects leading to a fall in bicarbonate and $PaCO_2$ values. Hence syringe should be appropriately flushed before taking the sample.

Presence of Air Bubble

Partial pressure of O_2 and CO_2 in the air is 150 mm Hg and 0 mm Hg, respectively. The addition of an air bubble will lead to a fall in $PaCO_2$

Table 6.2: Change in ABG parameters with time at different temperatures.

Parameter	*Change every 10 min at 37°C*	*Change every 10 min at 4°C*
pH	Decreases by 0.01	Decreases by 0.001
$PaCO_2$	Increases by 1 mm Hg	Increases by 0.1 mm Hg
PaO_2	0.1 vol %	0.01 vol %

and a rise in PaO_2. So precaution should be taken while withdrawing samples, and samples with excessive air should be discarded.

WBC Count

Hyperleukocytosis leads to increased oxygen consumption more than usual (0.1 mL per decilitre blood per 10 min with normal leukocyte count). Hence immediate processing of the sample is recommended to avoid errors.

Type of Syringe

Glass syringes are preferred to plastic syringes as the PO_2 values drop more rapidly in plastic syringes while the pH and PCO_2 values are unaffected.

INTERPRETATION OF ABG

Blood Gases in Respiratory Disturbances

Assessment of PaO_2 and $PaCO_2$ in blood samples helps in categorizing a patient with respiratory disturbance. The three most common patterns of the respiratory disorder are: Type 1 respiratory failure, Type 2 respiratory failure (respiratory acidosis) and hyperventilation (respiratory alkalosis).

Type 1 Respiratory Failure

It is defined as low PaO_2 with normal or low $PaCO_2$. It signifies defective oxygenation despite adequate ventilation. The majority of the cases have V/Q mismatch as the predominant mechanism responsible for it, whereas in some instances, shunt, diffusion limitation, low inspired FiO_2 and hypoventilation may also contribute. $PaCO_2$ is often low due to compensatory hyperventilation.

If arterial blood gas (ABG) is drawn from a patient on supplemental O_2, the PaO_2 may not be below the normal range but will be inappropriately low for the FiO_2. As a rough guide, if PaO_2 is less than five times the FiO_2, the patient is probably hypoxemic on room air. Hypoxemia can be classified based on the level of PaO_2 **(Table 6.3)**.

Type 2 Respiratory Failure

It is defined by a high $PaCO_2$ (hypercapnia) with usually a low PaO_2. PaO_2 may be normal if the patient is on supplemental oxygen. The

Table 6.3: Severity of type 1 respiratory failure.			
Assessing severity of type 1 respiratory impairment			
Variables	*Mild*	*Moderate*	*Severe*
PaO_2 (kPa)	8–10.6	5.3–7.9	<5.3
PaO_2 (mm Hg)	60–79	40–59	<40
SaO_2 (%)	90–94	75–89	<75

Table 6.4: ABG in different patterns of type 2 respiratory failure.			
	$PaCO_2$	*HCO_3*	*pH*
Acute	↑	→	↓
Chronic	↑	↑	→
Acute on chronic	↑	↑	↓

Table 6.5: Causes of respiratory acidosis.	
Conditions causing respiratory acidosis	
Central	Drugs (anesthetics, sedatives)
	Stroke, infection
Airway	Asthma, COPD
Parenchyma	Emphysema, advanced ILD, ARDS
Neuromuscular disorders	Poliomyelitis, kyphoscoliosis, myasthenia
Miscellaneous	Obesity, hypoventilation

predominant mechanism for this entity is inadequate ventilation, and as the oxygenation also depends on ventilation, the PaO_2 is low. The rise in CO_2 can be acute or chronic depending upon the underlying aetiology. ABG parameters help in distinguishing between these entities. An acute increase in CO_2 leads to a falling in pH with no significant change in bicarbonate, whereas a chronic rise in CO_2 leads to a rising in bicarbonate with maintained pH. In the case of chronic respiratory failure, the acute rise can lead to a fall in pH.

Table 6.4 shows the changes in ABG parameters during these conditions. Common causes for type 2 respiratory failure are documented in **Table 6.5**.

Hyperventilation

It is characterized by low $PaCO_2$ (hypocapnia) and a corresponding rise in blood pH. In acute cases, it is usually not associated with significant change in HCO_3, whereas in chronic cases, it is associated with decreased serum bicarbonate levels. Usually, PaO_2 is normal in the disorders associated with hyperventilation. It can be primary or secondary (compensatory response associated with metabolic acidosis). Common causes for the same are given in **Table 6.6**.

Assessment of Acid-Base Disturbances

Acid-Base Status

Acid is a substance capable of providing a hydrogen ion (proton donor). At the same time, a base can accept or remove a hydrogen ion from a solution (proton acceptor). Based on $[H^+]$, acidosis and alkalosis are defined as the conditions in which $[H^+]$ are above or below the normal range. To prevent this extreme change in $[H^+]$ concentration, we need a buffer system. A buffer consists of a combination of a weak acid (or a base) and the salt of that acid (or base). Various buffer systems are hemoglobin, bicarbonate, phosphate ions and serum proteins. Among these, the carbonic acid anhydrase-bicarbonate buffer system is most important.

Acidemia is a reduction in arterial pH < 7.36, while alkalemia is an increase in arterial pH >7.45. Changes in $PaCO_2$ or HCO_3 can cause these disorders. An increase in $PaCO_2$ causes acidosis, whereas a decrease in its value causes alkalemia. In HCO_3, a reduction in its value causes acidemia, whereas an increase in its value causes alkalemia. Any change in $PaCO_2$ causes a secondary adaptive response by a change in HCO_3 values and vice versa.

Table 6.6: Conditions causing hyperventilation.

Common causes of hyperventilation	
Primary	***Secondary***
Anxiety (psychogenic), pain, fever, cerebrovascular accident	Metabolic acidosis (of any etiology)
Hypoxaemia	
Salicylate toxicity	
Hepatic cirrhosis	

Acid-base homeostasis has to be maintained for normal physiological functioning. It can sometimes be challenging to establish its correct diagnosis. But if we follow a stepwise approach to assess these disorders, we are likely to achieve an accurate diagnosis. Three different approaches are there to identify these disorders. These are:

1. Physiological approach
2. Base excess approach
3. Physiochemical approach (Stewart method).

The physiological approach is a commonly used method to assess these disorders. Studies done previously in metabolic acidosis patients have shown that all three methods perform equally good. It is not clear that further delineation of complex metabolic acid-base disorders using the Stewart physiochemical or the modified base excess methods is clinically beneficial. The physiological approach uses the carbonic acid-bicarbonate buffer system.

Steps of Identifying Acid-Base Disorder

History and Physical Examination

Careful history taking and clinical evaluation are of paramount importance in identifying the acid-base disorder. Presentation of the patient and the condition leading to the current presentation gives a clue to the acid-base disturbance. For example, a patient with a known history of type 1 diabetes mellitus presenting in an emergency with acidosis usually suffers from ketoacidosis (metabolic origin). So the history of underlying medical conditions should be elicited with caution. A history of drugs or intoxication should also be noted, as certain disorders are common with specific medications. For example, salicylate toxicity patients usually present with respiratory alkalosis. Similarly, physical evaluation such as vital signs (for shock, fever, tachypnea, hypoxia) should be measured to guide an underlying disturbance.

Identifying the Primary Acid-Base Disorder and Secondary Compensatory Response

Primary Acid-Base Disorder

Determining the primary acid-base disturbance is the first step in interpreting ABG. Whether the primary disorder is respiratory or metabolic is determined by the change in $PaCO_2$ and HCO_3 values, respectively. The disorder is characterized as respiratory acidosis if a decrease in pH (<7.38) is associated with an increase in $PaCO_2$ (> 45 mm Hg), and respiratory alkalosis if a rise in pH (>7.42) is associated with a decrease in $PaCO_2$ (<35 mm Hg) **(Table 6.7)**. Similarly, the primary metabolic disorder is characterized by a change in HCO_3 in the same direction as pH. A decrease in pH with an associated decrease in HCO_3 (<22 mmol/L) is described as primary metabolic acidosis. In contrast, an increase in pH (>7.42) with an associated increase in HCO_3 (>26 mmol/L) is characterized as primary metabolic alkalosis.

Secondary Compensation Response

Compensation is the normal response of the respiratory system or kidneys to a change in pH induced by a primary acid-base disorder. In acidosis or alkalosis, regulatory mechanisms occur that attempt to maintain the arterial pH in the physiologic range. These processes result in the return of pH towards, but generally just outside, the normal range. Disturbances in HCO_3^- (metabolic acidosis or alkalosis) result in respiratory compensation (by a change in $PaCO_2$) while changes in $PaCO_2$ (respiratory acidosis/alkalosis) are counteracted by renal compensation (change in HCO_3).

Respiratory compensation usually occurs immediately by alteration of ventilation. On the other hand, renal compensation takes time. Full renal compensation usually takes 2–5 days. The amount of change in values of HCO_3 and $PaCO_2$ in response to primary disorder is given in **Table 6.8**.

Mixed Acid-Base Disorder

Simple disorders are characterized by a single primary disorder with a compensatory response as per the values given in **Table 6.8**. Mixed acid-base disorders are defined as independently coexisting disorders, not merely compensatory responses. They are often seen in patients

Table 6.7: The characteristics of primary acid-base disorders.

Disorder	*Primary changes*			*Compensatory response*
Metabolic acidosis	↑ $[H^+]$	↓ pH	↓ HCO_3^-	↓ pCO_2
Metabolic alkalosis	↓ $[H^+]$	↑ pH	↑ HCO_3^-	↑ pCO_2
Respiratory acidosis	↑ $[H^+]$	↓ pH	↑ pCO_2	↑ HCO_3^-
Respiratory alkalosis	↓ $[H^+]$	↑ pH	↓ pCO_2	↓ HCO_3^-

Table 6.8: Renal and respiratory compensations to primary acid-base disturbances.

Disorder	*Compensatory response*
Metabolic acidosis	$PaCO_2 = 1.5 \times [HCO_3] + 8 \pm 2$ mm Hg or $[HCO_3]$ + 15 mm Hg
Metabolic alkalosis	$PaCO_2 = 0.7 \times ([HCO_3]–24) + 40 \pm 2$ mm Hg or $[HCO_3]$ + 15 mm Hg
Respiratory acidosis (acute)	HCO_3^- ↑ by 1.0 mEq/L per 10 mm Hg ↑ in PCO_2
Respiratory acidosis (chronic)	HCO_3^- ↑ by 4.0 mEq/L per 10 mm Hg ↑ in PCO_2
Respiratory alkalosis (acute)	HCO_3^- ↓ by 2.0 mEq/L per 10 mm Hg ↓ in PCO_2
Respiratory alkalosis (chronic)	HCO_3^- ↓ by 4.0 mEq/L per 10 mm Hg ↓ in PCO_2

in critical care units and can lead to dangerous extremes of pH. Mixed acid-base disorders are usually diagnosed by the difference in the secondary response compared to what is expected. For example, if $PaCO_2$ is less or more than the expected compensatory response in metabolic acidosis, it signifies the presence of additional respiratory alkalosis or acidosis, respectively. Mixed disorders can be concomitant metabolic (alkalosis and acidosis) and respiratory (alkalosis and acidosis) disorders or two metabolic disorders coexisting.

Examples of Mixed Acid-base Disorders

Metabolic acidosis and respiratory alkalosis

Expected values of ABG in a patient presenting with metabolic acidosis as the primary disorder are:- pH <7.38 and HCO_3<22 mmol/L. The secondary response expected is a fall in $PaCO_2$ as per formula $[HCO_3]$ +15 mm Hg. If the value of $PaCO_2$ measured is less than expected, it signifies the presence of concomitant respiratory alkalosis.

For example: A patient with lactic acidosis or sepsis in ICU with hyperventilation has pH-7.37, HCO_3^-14, and $PaCO_2$-24. The expected $PaCO_2$ here was 29 ($[HCO_3]$ + 15 mm Hg), but the measured value here is 24. Measured $PaCO_2$ < expected $PaCO_2$ signifies concomitant respiratory alkalosis.

Metabolic acidosis and respiratory acidosis

Expected values of ABG in a patient presenting with metabolic acidosis as the primary disorder are: pH <7.38 and HCO_3<22 mmol/L. The secondary response expected is a fall in $PaCO_2$ as per formula $[HCO_3]$

+ 15 mm Hg. If the value of $PaCO_2$ measured is more than expected, it signifies the presence of concomitant respiratory acidosis.

For example: A patient with severe pneumonia presenting with ABG values pH:- 7.30, HCO_3-18 and $PaCO_2$-38; here, the primary disorder is metabolic acidosis, and the expected $PaCO_2$ is 33. Measured $PaCO_2$ > Expected $PaCO_2$ signifies the concomitant presence of respiratory acidosis.

Metabolic alkalosis and respiratory alkalosis

Expected values of ABG in a patient presenting with metabolic alkalosis as the primary disorder are: pH >7.42 and HCO_3>26 mmol/L. The secondary response expected is a rise in $PaCO_2$ as per formula $[HCO_3]$ + 15 mm Hg. If the value of $PaCO_2$ measured is less than expected, it signifies the presence of concomitant respiratory alkalosis.

For example: Patient with liver disease being administered diuretics concomitantly, presented with ABG values pH- 7.55, HCO_3-33 and $PaCO_2$-38. Here the primary disorder is metabolic alkalosis. Expected $PaCO_2$ was 48, whereas measured $PaCO_2$ is 38 (measured<expected). So this signifies the presence of concomitant respiratory alkalosis.

Metabolic alkalosis and respiratory acidosis

Expected values of ABG in a patient presenting with respiratory acidosis as the primary disorder are:- pH < 7.38 and $PaCO_2$ > 45 mm Hg. The secondary response expected is a rise in HCO_3 by 1 mEq/L per 10 mm Hg↑ in $PaCO_2$. If the value of HCO_3 measured is more than expected, it signifies concomitant metabolic alkalosis.

For example: Patient with COPD in type 2 respiratory failure, being treated with diuretics, presented with ABG values pH-7.37, $PaCO_2$-60 and HCO_3- 36. Here the primary disorder is respiratory acidosis with expected HCO_3, in this case, being 28. But measured HCO_3 here is 36 (measured > expected), signifying concomitant metabolic alkalosis.

Use of Gaps in Evaluating Metabolic Acidosis

Mixed metabolic disorders are common in critically ill patients. Calculation of anion gap and gap-gap ratio helps in the evaluation of these disorders.

Anion Gap

It is a rough estimate of the relative abundance of unmeasured anions. Normally the sum of the positive and negative ion charges in plasma are equal: $[Na^+] + [K^+] + [Ca^{2+}] + [Mg^{2+}] + [H^+]$ + unmeasured cations = $[Cl^-] + [HCO_3] + [CO^{2-}] + [OH^-]$ + albumin + phosphate+ sulfate + lactate + unmeasured anions (e.g., in-organic anions).

It is not recommended routinely to measure these ions in the plasma. Most of these ions are present in minimal quantities, and their change during pathological conditions is usually small. However, to measure this gap three most common ions are:

$[Na^+]–[Cl^-]–[HCO_3^-]$

The normal value of the anion gap varies significantly due to methods used to assess and inter-individual variations. The normal value of the anion gap ranges from 8–15 mmol/L. Low values most commonly indicate laboratory error or hypoalbuminemia but can denote the presence of paraproteinemia or intoxication with lithium, bromide, or iodide. Elevated values most commonly indicate metabolic acidosis but can reflect laboratory error, metabolic alkalosis, hyperphosphatemia, or paraproteinemia.

The effect of hypoalbuminemia is to be taken into consideration when calculating the anion gap. Corrections should be done for abnormal albumin concentration. The correction factor is 2.3–2.5 times the change in albumin concentration. For every decrement of 1 g per deciliter in the serum albumin concentration, the calculated anion gap should be increased by approximately 2.3 to 2.5 mmol per litre. The anion gap is used to determine if metabolic acidosis is due to an accumulation of non-volatile acids (e.g., lactic acid) or a primary loss of bicarbonate (e.g., diarrhea).

Metabolic acidosis based on anion gap is divided into two types (Table 6.9):

1. Normal anion gap metabolic acidosis
2. High anion gap metabolic acidosis

Gap-Gap Ratio

A gap-gap ratio is used to detect the presence of additional metabolic disorder (normal anion gap acidosis and metabolic alkalosis) in patients with high anion gap acidosis. The gap-gap ratio is calculated by the difference in anion gap excess (measured anion gap—normal anion gap) and HCO_3 deficit (measured bicarbonate—normal bicarbonate). In the setting of high anion gap acidosis, the ratio is used as follows:

Table 6.9: The causes of high and normal anion gap metabolic acidosis.

High anion gap acidosis	*Normal anion gap acidosis*
Ketoacidosis (diabetic ketoacidosis, alcoholic ketoacidosis, starvation)	Diarrhea
Lactic acidosis	Type 1 and 2 renal tubular acidosis
Advanced renal failure (acute and chronic)	Drugs (calcium chloride, magnesium sulfate, acetazolamide)
Impaired lactate clearance in liver failure	Ureteroenterostomy
Massive rhabdomyolysis	Early renal insufficiency
Toxins (ethylene glycol, methanol, salicylates, propylene glycol, pyroglutamic acid (5-oxoproline)	Isotonic saline infusion

Δ AG/Δ HCO_3^- = 1 → Pure high AG metabolic acidosis
Δ AG/Δ HCO_3^- > 1 → Associated metabolic alkalosis
Δ AG/Δ HCO_3^- < 1 → Associated normal AG metabolic acidosis.

Steps in ABG Interpretation

- History and physical examination
- Determining the primary disorder
- Assessing the adequacy of secondary response to identify mixed disorder if any
- Calculate anion gap and correct in regards to albumin concentration
- In the case of high anion gap acidosis, calculate the change in anion gap and change in bicarbonate (gap-gap ratio).

SUGGESTED READING

1. Berend K, de Vries APJ, Gans ROB. Physiological approach to assessment of acid-base disturbances. In: Ingelfinger JR (Ed). N Engl J Med. 2014 9;371(15):1434–45.
2. Byrne AL, Bennett M, Chatterji R, Symons R, Pace NL, Thomas PS. Peripheral venous and arterial blood gas analysis in adults: Are they comparable? A aystematic review and meta-analysis: Systematic review of PVBG and ABG analysis. Respirology. 2014;19(2):168–75.
3. Chauvin A, Javaud N, Ghazali A, Curac S, Altar A, Ali T, et al. Reducing pain by using venous blood gas instead of arterial blood gas (VEINART): A multicentrerandomised controlled trial. Emerg Med J. 2020;37(12): 756–61.

4. Feldman M, Soni N, Dickson B. Influence of hypoalbuminemia or Hyperalbuminemia on the serum anion gap. J Lab Clin Med. 2005;146(6):317–20.
5. Fidkowski C, Helstrom J. Diagnosing metabolic acidosis in the critically ill: Bridging the anion gap, Stewart, and base excess methods. Can J Anaesth. 2009;56(3):247–56.
6. Kraut JA, Madias NE. Serum anion gap: Its uses and limitations in clinical medicine. Clin J Am Soc Nephrol. 2007;2(1):162–74.
7. Morris CG, Low J. Metabolic acidosis in the critically ill: Part 1. Classification and pathophysiology. Anaesthesia. 2008;63(3):294–301.
8. Zeserson E, Goodgame B, Hess JD, Schultz K, Hoon C, Lamb K, et al. Correlation of venous blood gas and pulse oximetry with arterial blood gas in the undifferentiated critically ill patient. J Intensive Care Med. 2018;33(3):176–81.

Chapter 7

Blood Gas Monitoring

Ravindran Chetambath, Paramez Ayyappath, Jesin Kumar C

ABSTRACT

Monitoring of blood gases is fundamental to respiratory critical care and oxygen therapy. Since hypoxia and acid base imbalance lead to sudden and life-threatening changes in all the systems, a thorough understanding of blood gas derangement is mandatory for any treating physician. However, the understanding of blood gas measurements and their interpretation can sometimes be difficult and confusing. The proper application of the concepts of acid–base balance will help the healthcare provider to follow the progress of a patient, and to evaluate the effectiveness of care being provided. This chapter presents a logical and systematic approach to enable the reader to make an easier interpretation of blood gas measurement in the context of a clinical problem.

INTRODUCTION

Blood gas analysis (BGA) is an essential part of diagnosing and managing the oxygenation status and acid-base balance of the high-risk and critically ill patients treated in the intensive care units. Disorders of acid–base balance can create complications in many disease states, occasionally the abnormality may be severe and life-threatening. In such situations, therapeutic interventions are carried out after careful monitoring of blood gases. Accurate results for a blood gas measurement depend on the proper collection, handling, and analysis of the specimen. BGA is particularly vulnerable to procedural errors. Arterial blood gas (ABG) sampling by direct puncture is the procedure often practiced in the hospital setting. The relatively low incidence of major complications, ability to perform at the patient's bedside, and rapid analysis make it an important investigation to direct the treatment of patients, especially when they are critically ill. BGA is also useful to determine gas exchange levels in the blood related to respiratory, metabolic, and renal function.

ARTERIAL PUNCTURE FOR BLOOD GAS MEASUREMENTS

Indication

- Measurement of the partial pressures of oxygen and carbon dioxide during diagnostic evaluation of patients suffering from acute and chronic respiratory diseases.
- Assessment of the acid-base status of critically ill patients.
- Assessment of the response to therapeutic interventions such as oxygen therapy and mechanical ventilation in a patient with respiratory failure.
- Preoperative evaluation of high risk patients requiring general anesthesia.
- Evaluation of treatment responses in patients with respiratory, metabolic and renal disorders.

Contraindications

Absolute Contraindications

- Local infection or distorted anatomy at the potential puncture site (e.g. from previous surgical interventions, congenital or acquired malformations, burns).
- Presence of arteriovenous fistulas or vascular grafts, in which case arterial vascular puncture should not be attempted.
- Known or suspected severe peripheral vascular disease of the limb involved.

Relative Contraindications

- Severe coagulopathy.
- Anticoagulation therapy with warfarin, heparin and derivatives, direct thrombin inhibitors, or factor X inhibitors. Use of aspirin is not a contraindication for arterial vascular sampling in majority of the cases.
- Use of thrombolytic agents, such as streptokinase or tissue plasminogen activator.

Procedure

Blood for gas analysis is obtained by puncturing an easily accessible artery. Radial artery being superficial and easily accessible, is the most common site; femoral or brachial artery are considered as alternative sites. Rarely venous samples are used for blood gas analysis.

Sampling Methods

Whenever possible, the healthcare provider should obtain an informed consent after explaining the BGA sampling procedure, associated risks and benefits to the patient. The actual procedure focuses on the choice of a puncture site and accurate delineation of the vascular anatomy. If radial artery sampling is to be performed, the adequacy of the ulnar collateral circulation must be confirmed. Alternative sites such as femoral or brachial arteries can be used in cases where distal perfusion is compromised and distal pulses are diminished.

CONFIRMATION OF VASCULAR ANATOMY

ABG sampling can be difficult in patients with feeble pulses, distorted anatomic landmarks or in situations where sampling of a deep vascular structure such as femoral or brachial artery is required. In these scenarios, ultra-sonographically guided ABG sampling should be considered, especially when sampling by the standard approach has been unsuccessful or is not feasible.

Repeated arterial puncturing at the same site increases the risk of hematoma, laceration and scarring. It also increases the chances of inadvertent venous blood sampling. Alternate puncture sites should be preferred for recurrent sampling. If more frequent sampling is necessary, it is better to consider placing an indwelling arterial catheter through arterial cannulation.

ASSESSMENT OF COLLATERAL CIRCULATION (MODIFIED ALLEN TEST)

If puncture of the radial artery is planned, a modified Allen test should be performed beforehand to assess the collateral circulation. Although the anatomy of the radial artery in the forearm and the hand is variable, most patients have adequate collateral flow to maintain blood supply even if a radial artery thrombosis develops following the procedure. The modified Allen test is performed as follows:

Firm occlusive pressure is applied on both the radial artery and the ulnar artery **(Fig. 7.1A)**. The patient is asked to clench and unclench the fist several times until the palmar skin is blanched. Overextension of the hand or wide spreading of the fingers should be avoided, because it may cause false-normal results. The pressure on the ulnar artery is released while occlusion of the radial artery is maintained **(Fig. 7.1B)**. The time required for palmar capillary refill is noted. The test is then repeated, but this time the radial artery is released while the ulnar artery remains compressed **(Fig. 7.1C)**.

In an uncooperative or unconscious patient who cannot clench the first, the test is done in a similar fashion by obstructing both the arteries and raising the patient's hand above the level of the heart until blanching occurs. The hand is then lowered below the level of the heart and pressure removed from the ulnar artery when blanching disappears.

Other methods to assess patency of circulation are finger pulse plethysmography, Doppler flow measurements, and measurement of the arterial systolic pressure of the thumb.

Equipment

The following materials are needed for collection of arterial blood for analysis.

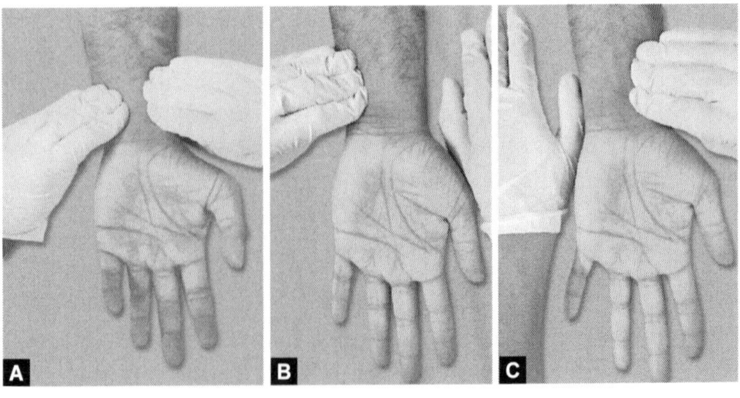

Figs. 7.1A to C: Modified Allen's test.

- Nonsterile gloves may be used and the operator should not touch the puncture site once it is cleaned for the procedure.
- Syringe and needle: 3 mL glass syringe with a 23 or 25-gauge needle is used for puncture. A 21-gauge needle may also be used. Glass syringes are generally preferred to plastic syringes unless analysis is done immediately. The plunger of the syringe should be left depressed to allow the arterial blood flow to fill up the syringe. Some ABG kits contain a prefilled heparinized syringe along with a protective needle sleeve and a syringe cap.
- Heparin: 0.2 mL heparin (1000 U/mL) should be aspirated into the syringe through the needle and then pushed out.
- Antiseptic skin solution: Commonly used chemicals for skin sterilization are chlorhexidine and povidone-iodine.
- Syringe cap: Usually included in the ABG syringe kit.
- Sterile gauze, adhesive bandage, bag with ice and lidocaine hydrochloride (1%) without epinephrine (optional) are the other ancillary materials to be kept at the procedure site.

Patient Preparation

Chances of a successful arterial sampling depend on proper positioning of the patient and a thorough knowledge of the vascular anatomy.

Positioning

For radial artery blood sampling, the patient should be in the supine position with the arm lying on a hard surface. The forearm should be supinated and the wrist dorsiflexed at 400. A gauze roll may be placed under the wrist to make the patient more comfortable and to bring the radial artery to a more superficial plane. For femoral artery blood sampling, the patient is supine on a stretcher, and the patient's leg is placed in neutral anatomic position. For brachial artery blood sampling, the arm is placed on a firm surface with the shoulder slightly abducted. The elbow is extended, with the forearm in full supination.

Anesthesia

The standard practice is direct puncture of the identified vessel. Some centers prefer local anesthesia with subcutaneous injection of 1% lidocaine hydrochloride to minimize the pain. The use of mepivacaine and cryo-analgesia has also been reported to significantly reduce pain.

Radial Artery Sampling

The arterial pulse is felt with the middle and index finger pads of the non-dominant hand. Both fingers should be proximal to the desired puncture site. Visualize the direction of the artery, and clean the desired puncture site in an outward circular motion with an antiseptic solution. If the ABG syringe is to be used, the protective needle sleeve and needle should be placed onto the syringe, the prefilled heparin expelled, and the vented plunger repositioned to the 2 mL mark. Arterial blood samples should be obtained in strict anaerobic conditions and should be placed on ice and held at 0° C until analysis. Uncap the ABG syringe, and hold it with two fingers of the dominant hand. The needle bevel should be facing upward. Insert the needle just under the skin at a 45° angle, aiming in the direction of the artery. Inserting the needle in this fashion help to reduce trauma to the vessel and allows smooth-muscle fibers to occlude the puncture site after the procedure. As the needle advances slowly and enters the lumen of the radial artery, blood starts to fill the syringe **(Fig. 7.2)**. Allow the blood to fill the syringe automatically and never apply suction pressure. At this point, remove the nondominant hand from the field.

After 2–3 mL of arterial blood has been obtained, remove the needle. At the same time, use a small piece of gauze, held in the nondominant hand, to apply firm occlusive local pressure at the puncture site for 5 minutes. Check for hemostasis, and apply an adhesive bandage over the puncture site. Patients should be asked not to manipulate the area involved in the procedure and should be instructed to alert healthcare personnel if new symptoms develop, such as skin color changes, persistent or worsening pain, active bleeding, impaired movement or sensation of the limb.

Remove the excess air in the syringe by holding it upright and gently tapping it, allowing any air bubbles present to reach the top of

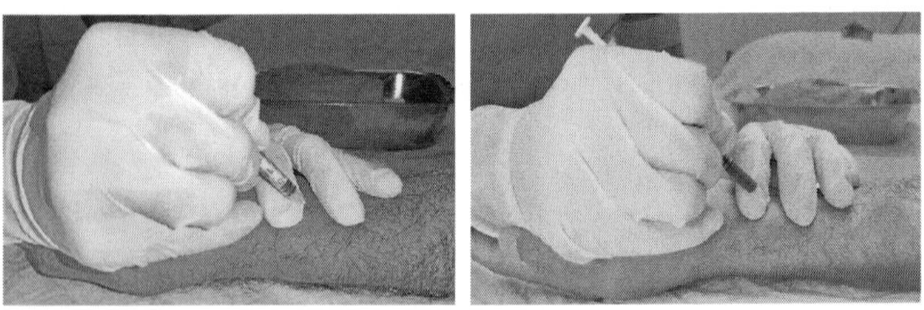

Fig. 7.2: Radial artery sampling.

the syringe, from where they can then be expelled. Any air bubbles introduced during the sampling procedure will lead to erroneous values. Cap the syringe, place it in the ice bag, and send it for analysis. Sample is kept at lower temperatures until analysis to minimize cellular metabolism and ongoing consumption of oxygen. This is especially important in patients with leukocytosis.

Femoral Artery Sampling

The femoral artery is best identified in the midline between the symphysis pubis and the anterior superior iliac crest, 2–4 cm distal to the inguinal ligament. The femoral artery is medial to the femoral nerve and lateral to the femoral vein. Possibility of peripheral arterial disease (PAD) should be ruled out before a femoral artery puncture.

Brachial Artery Sampling

The brachial artery is best identified between the medial epicondyle of the humerus and the tendon of the biceps brachii in the antecubital fossa. It can be felt higher in the arm in the groove between the biceps and triceps tendons. The basilic vein and the brachial nerve are located in close proximity.

Arterial Cannulation

Most patients requiring critical care need repeated arterial punctures, therefore many intensivists prefer indwelling arterial catheter/cannula to avoid repeated punctures. With the availability of an arterial cannula, samples can be repeatedly drawn as and when required. It is also useful in patients whose cardiopulmonary status is unstable. The pre-analytical errors related to improper sampling, handling and storage are minimal with samples obtained from arterial cannula. In addition, the arterial cannula can be used for systemic blood pressure monitoring and to obtain blood samples for other numerous clinical estimations such as electrolytes, urea, creatinine, etc.

However, arterial cannulation is not without risks. There is an increased chance of diminished or absent blood flow through a cannulated artery. This is often reversible, although necrosis and loss of tissue have been reported in some cases. Local infection and systemic sepsis can also occur. Another method to obtain arterial blood especially in infants and young children is the arterialized earlobe capillary blood sample (ELCS) which shows strong agreement with arterial blood pH and $PaCO_2$. Simultaneous measurements of oxygen saturation through pulse oximetry may also improve the accuracy of ELCS for PaO_2 assessment.

Post Procedure Monitoring

After the blood sampling procedure, operator should monitor the patient for early and late signs and symptoms of potential complications. These include:

- Local pain due to nerve lesions
- Local hematoma—often large enough to compromise regional circulation and cause compartment syndrome
- Vasovagal response
- Arterial vasospasm
- Arterial occlusion—which manifest in the form of limb skin color changes, absent pulses and distal coldness
- Air or thrombus embolism
- Local anesthetic anaphylactic reaction
- Infection at the puncture site causing regional erythema and fever
- Needle-stick injury to healthcare personnel
- Vessel laceration causing profuse bleeding
- Hemorrhage.

Venous Sampling for Blood Gas Analysis

The "gold standard" sample for BGA is arterial blood collected anaerobically by needle puncture of an artery or via an indwelling arterial catheter. Arterial puncture is technically more demanding and significantly more painful and hazardous for the patient. In intensive care settings most patients who require frequent blood gas monitoring have a central venous catheter inserted that allows easy and safe sampling of venous blood for laboratory testing, obviating the need for repeated venipuncture. It would be logistically convenient for clinical staff, and more comfortable and safer for the patient if this kind of venous blood sample could also be used for BGA. In this circumstance it is worthwhile to consider if venous blood might be a valid substitute for arterial blood in some circumstances. At the same time venous sample is affected by the metabolism, blood flow and many other factors of different tissues. However central venous samples have been shown to correlate well with arterial samples with respect to pH, $PaCO_2$ and base excess in mechanically ventilated trauma patients to reach clinically reliable conclusions **(Table 7.1)**. But central venous sample cannot substitute arterial samples for resuscitation and management. Many clinical studies investigating the validity of using venous blood for BGA have been conducted using venous blood obtained by conventional venipuncture of a peripheral vein. Venous blood gas values can potentially differ to some extent with site of sampling.

ANALYSIS AND INTERPRETATION OF BLOOD GAS

The arterial blood sample collected is analyzed by automated blood gas analyzers, which automatically transport the specimen to electrochemical sensors to measure pH, $PaCO_2$ and PaO_2. The $PaCO_2$ is measured using a chemical reaction that consumes CO_2 and produces a hydrogen ion. It is sensed as a change in pH. The PaO_2 is measured using oxidation-reduction reactions that generate measurable electric currents. The pH is measured indirectly with a pH calibrated electrode tip which determines the voltage using a reference potential. The voltage is directly proportional to the concentration of hydrogen ions **(Table 7.2)**. Bicarbonate is not measured directly, but is derived from measured pH and $PaCO_2$ using Henderson-Hasselbalch equation.

Arterial blood gas analyzers are affected by temperature; pH increases but PaO_2 and $PaCO_2$ decreases as temperature declines. Most automated analyzers report the pH, PaO_2 and $PaCO_2$ at either 37°C or at patient's body temperature.

Interpretation

Normal Values

- pH: 7.35 to 7.45
- $PaCO_2$: 35 to 45 mm Hg (4.7 to 6 kPa)

Table 7.1: Arterial and venous reference range for comparison during analysis.

Parameter	*Arterial*	*Venous*	*Arteriovenous difference*
pH	7.35–7.45	7.31–7.41	0.04
pCO_2 (mm Hg)	35–45	41–51	0.6
pO_2 (mm Hg)	80–100	30–40	55
Bicarbonate (mmol/L)	22–28	23–29	1
SaO_2 (%)	>95	75	>20

Table 7.2: H^+ Concentration and corresponding pH.

pH	*H^+ (mEq/L)*
7.00	100
7.10	79
7.20	63
7.30	50
7.40	40
7.50	32
7.60	25

- HCO_3: 21 to 27 mEq/L
- PaO_2: A resting PaO_2 > 80 mm Hg and SaO_2 > 95 % is considered normal (normal values are not defined because a threshold below which tissue hypoxia occurs has not been clearly identified).

Primary Acid-base Disorders

If the $PaCO_2$ and/or pH are outside the normal range, there is an acid-base disorder. It can be respiratory or metabolic. Respiratory acid-base disorders occur when the change in $PaCO_2$ causes a change in pH. If $PaCO_2$ increases, it is called respiratory acidosis and if $PaCO_2$ decreases, it is called respiratory alkalosis.

Metabolic acid-base disorders occur when a change in HCO_3 causes change in pH. If the HCO_3 decreases, it is called metabolic acidosis and if HCO_3 increases, it is called metabolic alkalosis.

A mixed disorder occurs when both metabolic and respiratory abnormalities occur concomitantly. For example—if respiratory acidosis and metabolic acidosis occurs simultaneously (e.g. COPD exacerbation with acute kidney injury), the fall in pH will be drastic resulting in rapid deterioration of clinical condition.

Secondary Responses/Compensatory Responses

When the acid-base homeostasis is disturbed compensatory mechanisms take place which tries to keep the pH to near normal limits. In metabolic acidosis, the respiratory compensation is immediate though it may take up to 12–24 hours for full compensation (a decrease in $PaCO_2$ of 1.2 mm Hg for each 1 mEq/L decrease in the serum bicarbonate) to occur (e.g. Kussmaul respiration in diabetic ketoacidosis). In metabolic alkalosis, hypoventilation may occur (not necessarily in critically ill cardio-pulmonary patients). The appropriate respiratory response is a 0.7 mm Hg increase in the $PaCO_2$ for each 1 mEq/L increase in the serum bicarbonate. In respiratory acidosis, the HCO_3 level increases and in respiratory alkalosis HCO_3 levels decreases as a compensatory response. Respiratory acid-base disorders can be acute or chronic and the compensatory mechanism varies accordingly.

How to Interpret an ABG Report

- **Step 1:** Assess the internal consistency of the values using the Henderson-Hasselbalch equation:

  $$[H^+] = 24(PaCO_2)/[HCO_3^-]$$

- **Step 2:** Is there alkalemia (pH > 7.45) or acidemia (pH < 7.35) present? This is usually the primary disorder. An acidosis or alkalosis may be present even if the pH is in the normal range (7.35–7.45).
- **Step 3:** The relationship between the direction of change in the pH and the direction of change in the $PaCO_2$ gives the clue whether the disorder is metabolic or respiratory. In primary respiratory disorders, the pH and $PaCO_2$ change in opposite directions; in metabolic disorders the pH and $PaCO_2$ change in the same direction **(Table 7.3)**.
- **Step 4:** Check for appropriate compensation. If the observed compensation is not the expected compensation, it is likely that more than one acid-base disorder is present **(Table 7.4 and 7.5)**.
- **Step 5:** Calculate the anion gap (if a metabolic acidosis exists): The difference between unmeasured anions and unmeasured cations is called anion gap (AG).

  $$AG = [Na^+]-([Cl^-] + [HCO_3^-])$$

Table 7.3: Relationship of pH and $PaCO_2$ with various acid-base disorders.

Acidosis	Respiratory	pH ↓	$PaCO_2$ ↑
Acidosis	Metabolic	pH ↓	$PaCO_2$ ↓
Alkalosis	Respiratory	pH ↑	$PaCO_2$ ↓
Alkalosis	Metabolic	pH ↑	$PaCO_2$ ↑

Table 7.4: Expected $[HCO_3^-]$ change in acute and chronic respiratory acid–base disorders (assume a baseline $[HCO_3^-]$ of 24 mEq/L).

Acute respiratory acidosis	Increase in $[HCO_3^-]$ = $\Delta PaCO_2/10$+/– 3	Decrease in pH = 0.08*[$\Delta PaCO_2/10$]
Chronic respiratory acidosis (3–5 days)	Increase in $[HCO_3^-]$ = 3*[$\Delta PaCO_2/10$]	Decrease in pH = 0.03*[$\Delta PaCO_2/10$] to 0.08*[$\Delta PaCO_2/10$]
Acute respiratory alkalosis	Decrease in $[HCO_3^-]$ = 2*[$\Delta PaCO_2/10$]	Increase in pH = 0.08*[$\Delta PaCO_2/10$]
Chronic respiratory alkalosis	Decrease in $[HCO_3^-]$ = 5*[$\Delta PaCO_2/10$] to 7*[$\Delta PaCO_2/10$]	Increase in pH = 0.03*[$\Delta PaCO_2/10$] to 0.08*[$\Delta PaCO_2/10$]

Table 7.5: Expected $PaCO_2$ and respiratory compensation for metabolic acidosis and alkalosis.

Metabolic acidosis	$PaCO_2 = (1.5 \times [HCO_3^-]) + 8$	pCO_2 = –1.2 mm Hg for every 1 mEq/L fall in $[HCO_3^-]$ (below 24 mEq/L)
Metabolic alkalosis	$PaCO_2 = 40 + 0.6\ (\Delta HCO_3^-)$	pCO_2 = + 0.6 + 0.7 mm Hg for every 1 mEq/L rise in $[HCO_3^-]$ (above 24 mEq/L)

A normal anion gap is approximately 12+/- 4 mEq/L. In patients with hypoalbuminemia, the normal anion gap is lower than 12 mEq/L; the "normal" anion gap in patients with hypoalbuminemia is about 2.5 mEq/L lower for each 1 g/dL decrease in the plasma albumin concentration (for example, a patient with a plasma albumin of 3.0 g/dL would be approximately 9.5 mEq/L). If the anion gap is elevated, calculate the osmolal gap (OSM gap) in clinical situations if elevation in AG is not explained by an obvious case like diabetic ketoacidosis, lactic acidosis, renal failure or if toxic ingestion is suspected.

OSM gap = measured OSM – (2[Na^+] – glucose/18–BUN/2.8)

The OSM gap should be < 10

- **Step 6:** If an increased anion gap is present, assess the relationship between the increase in the anion gap and the decrease in $[HCO_3^-]$. Assess the ratio of the change in the anion gap (ΔAG) to the change in $[HCO_3^-]$.

  $(\Delta[HCO_3\text{-}]) = \Delta AG/\Delta[HCO_3\text{-}]$

This ratio should be between 1.0 and 2.0 if an uncomplicated anion gap metabolic acidosis is present. If this ratio falls outside of this range, then another metabolic disorder is present. If $\Delta AG/\Delta[HCO_3^-] < 1.0$, then a concurrent non-anion gap metabolic acidosis is likely to be present. If $\Delta AG/\Delta\ [HCO_3^-] > 2.0$, then a concurrent metabolic alkalosis is likely to be present **(Table 7.6)**. Next step is assessment of arterial oxygenation. This includes evaluation of hypoxaemia as well as the arterial oxyhaemoglobin saturation along with the A-a gradient.

NON-INVASIVE METHODS OF BLOOD GAS MONITORING

Even though the direct measurement of blood gases would remain the gold standard in patient monitoring, it only provides a single measurement of a dynamic and rapidly changing clinical picture. Besides this, it also involves subjecting patients to a lot of discomfort. Hence, there is a necessity for continuous, non-invasive monitoring of blood gases.

Table 7.6: Selected mixed and complex acid-base disturbances.

Disorder	*Characteristics*	*Selected situations*
Respiratory acidosis with metabolic acidosis	↓ in pH ↓ in HCO_3 ↑ in $PaCO_2$	• Cardiac arrest • Intoxications • Multi-organ failure
Respiratory alkalosis with metabolic alkalosis	↑ in pH ↑ in HCO_3^- ↓ in $PaCO_2$	• Cirrhosis with diuretics • Pregnancy with vomiting • Over ventilation of COPD
Respiratory acidosis with metabolic alkalosis	pH in normal range ↑ in $PaCO_2$ ↑ in HCO_3	• COPD with diuretics, vomiting, NG suction • Severe hypokalemia
Respiratory alkalosis with metabolic acidosis	pH in normal range ↓ in $PaCO_2$ ↓ in HCO_3^-	• Sepsis • Salicylate toxicity • Renal failure with CHF or pneumonia • Advanced liver disease
Metabolic acidosis with metabolic alkalosis	pH in normal range HCO_3^- normal	• Uremia or ketoacidosis with vomiting, NG suction, diuretics, etc.

Non-invasive Oxygen Monitoring

Pulse Oximetry

Pulse oximetry, often referred to as the fifth vital sign, provides us a convenient means of monitoring the oxygen saturation of hemoglobin in arterial blood. This is done by the use of sensors which can be placed on the finger tips, ear lobes, toes, soles or palms. The readings thus obtained (SpO_2) provides an indirect estimation of the saturation of oxygen in arterial blood (SaO_2). Besides measuring the percentage of oxyhemoglobin and deoxyhemoglobin, it also displays the amplitude of pulse and heart rate.

Principles of Pulse Oximetry

Spectrophotometry and plethysmography form the basis for pulse oximetry.

- **Spectrophotometry:** Johann Heinrich Lambert and Pierre Bouguer first described the relationship between absorption of light and the amount of absorbent. This was further investigated by August Beer and the Beer- Bouguer-Lambert (BBL) law was formulated. This law states that when a ray of monochromatic light passes through an absorbing medium, its intensity decreases exponentially as the concentration of the absorbing species increases. In pulse oximetry, there are two photodiodes which emit light at 660 nm (red) and 940 nm (infra-red) wavelengths **(Fig. 7.3)**. This occurs phasically at several hundred times per second and is absorbed by different species of hemoglobin. Oxyhemoglobin absorbs greater amounts of infra-red light and lower amounts of red light than deoxyhemoglobin. This lower absorption and increased scattering of red light explains why oxygenated blood appears bright red in color. The light which is eventually transmitted through the finger is then detected by a photodiode on the opposite arm of the probe and the proportion of oxyhemoglobin is calculated.
- **Plethysmography:** The change in volume of arterial blood with each pulse beat can be detected and measured. This is done by measuring the variation in the transmission of light through the site during systole and diastole. Thus, the amplitude of the pulse and heart rate can be measured and displayed.

Advantages

- Provides a real time assessment of arterial oxygenation in patients with pulmonary and cardiac disorders.

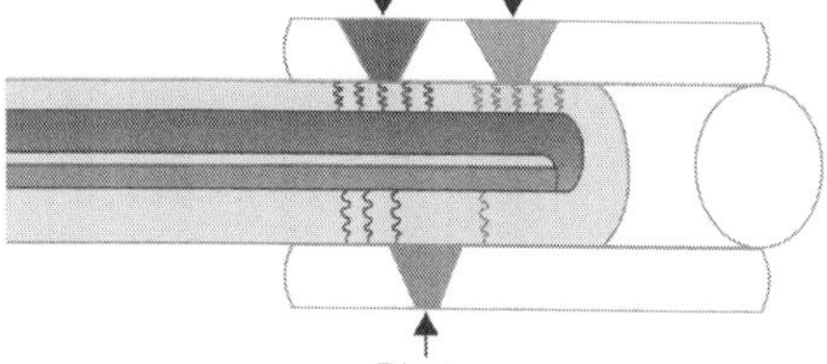

Fig. 7.3: Diagrammatic illustration of the principle of spectrophotometry utilized by a pulse oximeter.

- Can be used to assess oxygenation status during physiological states like sleep and exercise.

Disadvantages

- Does not provide any valuable information regarding ventilation.
- Cannot distinguish between oxyhemoglobin and dysfunctional hemoglobin's like carboxyhemoglobin, methemoglobin and Hb-S in sickle cell anemia. A blood gas analyzer like co-oximeter is needed for this purpose.
- Correlates poorly with the partial pressure of oxygen when the pressure is high.
- It is often unreliable in severe hypoxemia.
- SpO_2 is unreliable in critically ill patients due to hypoperfusion secondary to hypotension, hypothermia and vasoconstriction.
- The readings are unreliable in severely anemic patients (Hb < 5 g/dL).
- Conditions that hamper the transmission of light like skin pigmentation, peripheral edema, nail polish and hyperbilirubinemia can also affect the SpO_2 reading.

Pulse oximetry is one of the most important advances in the field of respiratory monitoring. Since it measures the arterial oxygenation with reliable precision, it is an important tool in the management of patients in acute medicine and intensive care settings.

Co-oximetry

Co-oximeter is a device that can also measure the abnormal forms of hemoglobin such as deoxygenated hemoglobin, carboxyhemoglobin, methemoglobin and sulfhemoglobin in addition to oxygenated hemoglobin. The absorption spectrum of each of these hemoglobins varies and this property is utilized by the co oximeter. Its use is warranted in cases where history consistent with toxin exposure is present.

Transcutaneous Oxygen Monitoring

The oxygen delivered to the skin via the underlying tissue is detected and measured in transcutaneous oxygen monitoring. It is done using heated electrodes which comprise of a platinum cathode and silver reference anode that is encased in an electrolyte solution and separated from the skin by an oxygen permeable membrane. These electrodes heat the underlying skin to 44°C causing dilation of the underlying vessels and increasing blood supply to the tissues thus enabling the measurement of the transcutaneous partial pressure of oxygen ($P_{tc}O_2$).

Applications

It has a wide range of applications among patients ranging from premature infants to adults. A drop in tissue perfusion can occur during hypotension, hypovolemia, hemorrhage, shock, ischemia or embolism. A low reading of $P_{tc}O_2$ warrants a thorough evaluation for these conditions. Its property to assess blood supply is used by surgeons to ensure that adequate blood supply exists to heal lower extremity wounds and ulcers. This property is also used by vascular surgeons to assess the need and determine the site of amputation. It also serves as a valuable tool for monitoring of patients during the perioperative phase.

Factors Influencing $P_{tc}O_2$

- Site of probe placement
- Skin thickness
- Sensor temperature
- Amount of contact gel used
- The state of peripheral perfusion.

Limitations

Despite its wide array of clinical applications, this method also has its limitations. There is a high propensity for calibration errors to occur. Hence, the sensors have to be calibrated every 4–8 hours and the

PO_2 measured during this period is unreliable. Since the electrode consumes oxygen during measurement, this method is rendered incapable of measuring low levels of oxygen particularly when it is done at room temperature. Due to its slow reaction time, sudden changes in oxygenation are often not picked up by this method. Hence, it needs to be used in tandem with pulse oximetry in conditions where a reliable detection of hyperoxemia is needed such as in low-birth-weight infants on supplemental oxygen.

Non-invasive Carbon Dioxide Monitoring

Capnography

The monitoring of the partial pressure of carbon dioxide in respiratory gases is known as capnography. This is plotted on a graph, known as capnogram, which can either be time-based or volume based. This serves as a snapshot and gives the physician an idea of the patient's condition and underlying disease. It is also frequently used by intensivists for ventilator-trouble shooting.

Capnogram

Capnogram is a waveform which depicts the amount of CO_2 present at each phase of the respiratory cycle. It normally has a rectangular shape **(Fig. 7.4)**.

The capnogram consists of various phases:

- **Phase I:** Inspiratory baseline.
  - Represents the first expired gas that normally occupies the conductive zone, i.e., the dead space of the lung. Hence, this is normally devoid of carbon dioxide.
- **Phase II:** Expiratory up stroke.
  - Represents the beginning of alveolar exhalation. It is denoted by a steep upslope.
- **Phase III:** Alveolar plateau phase.

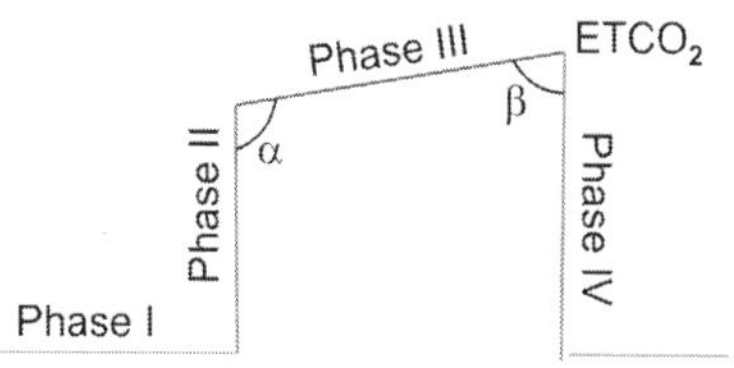

Fig. 7.4: Normal capnogram and its various phases.

  - Represents the phase of alveolar exhalation.
  - The peak seen at the end of the phase denotes the end-tidal carbon dioxide ($EtCO_2$).
- **Phase IV:** Inspiratory down stroke.
  - Denotes the washout of carbon dioxide seen during inspiration.

α angle: Denotes the transition from phase II to III. It can be used to assess ventilation/perfusion of the lung.

β angle: Denotes transition from phase III to IV. It can be used to assess rebreathing.

Waveform Interpretation and Abnormalities

The following parameters have to be analyzed when interpreting the capnogram **(Table 7.7)**:

- Height of the waveform ($EtCO_2$)
- Frequency (respiratory rate)
- Shape of the waveform
- Height of baseline.

Height of waveform ($EtCO_2$)

Denotes the point where the CO_2 level is at its maximum. In normal individuals it is 35–40 torr.

Application of Capnography

- Confirmation of tracheal (rather than esophageal) intubation.
- Ensuring patency of endotracheal or tracheostomy tube.
- Monitoring adequacy of ventilatory support.
- Assessing the severity of respiratory distress and ventilatory fatigue.
- Monitoring response to the treatment of bronchospasm.
- Monitoring patients with raised intra cranial pressure.
- Estimation of cardiac output and assessing degree of circulatory failure.
- Assessing the effectiveness of cardiopulmonary resuscitation (CPR).
- Identifying return of spontaneous circulation following cardiac arrest.

Typical Capnograms (Table 7.8)

Capnography is an investigation that is gaining popularity and is a useful tool utilized by intensivist, surgeon and anesthetists. Hence, a thorough knowledge of its various applications and interpretation of the waveforms is of paramount importance.

Table 7.7: Conditions causing an increase or decrease in $EtCO_2$.

Increased $EtCO_2$	*Decreased $EtCO_2$*
CO_2 production	
• Fever • Sodium bicarbonate • Tourniquet release • Venous CO_2 embolism • Overfeeding	• Hypothermia
Pulmonary perfusion	
• Increased cardiac output • Increased blood pressure	• Reduced cardiac output • Hypotension • Hypovolemia • Pulmonary embolism • Cardiac arrest
Alveolar ventilation	
• Hypoventilation • Bronchial intubation • Partial airway obstruction • Rebreathing	• Hyperventilation • Apnea • Total airway obstruction • Extubation
Apparatus malfunctioning	
• Exhausted CO_2 absorber • Inadequate fresh gas flow • Leaks in ventilator tubing • Ventilator malfunctioning	• Circuit disconnection • Leaks in sampling tube • Ventilator malfunctioning

Transcutaneous Carbon Dioxide Monitoring

Similar to transcutaneous oxygen monitoring, transcutaneous carbon dioxide ($TcCO_2$) monitoring also uses electrodes to warm the skin and measure the transcutaneous partial pressure of carbon dioxide ($P_{tc}CO_2$). Warming the skin induces vasodilation of the capillary bed and lead to close approximation of the capillary and arterial PCO_2.

However, the CO_2 levels measured transcutaneously is often an overestimation of the arterial CO_2 levels. The externally applied heat alters the solubility of carbon dioxide in blood and increases the metabolic rate of the tissues by approximately 5% for every 1°C rise in temperature. The local production of carbon dioxide by the epidermal cells also makes an, albeit slight, contribution in this aspect. The tc-artPCO_2 gradient can be minimized, to a certain extent, by temperature correction of the values obtained.

Table 7.8: Typical capnograms and associated conditions.

Hyperventilation	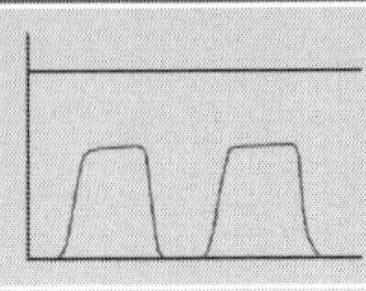	• Low $EtCO_2$ • High frequency • Good alveolar plateau
Hypoventilation	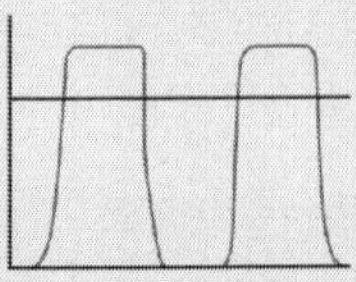	• Elevated $EtCO_2$ • Low frequency • Good alveolar plateau
Inadequate muscle relaxant reversal	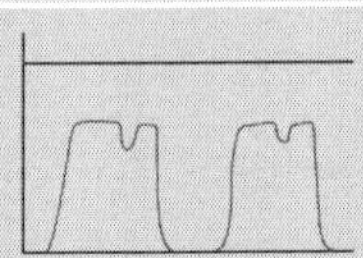	Notch seen in the last third of the plateau (Curare notch/cleft)
Cardiogenic oscillations (heart beating against lungs)	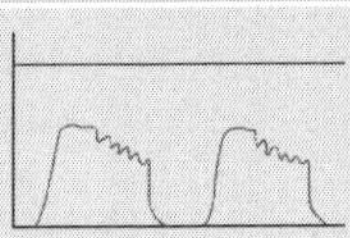	Small, regular, tooth-like humps at the end of the expiratory phase
Single lung transplantation Bronchial intubation Severe kyphoscoliosis	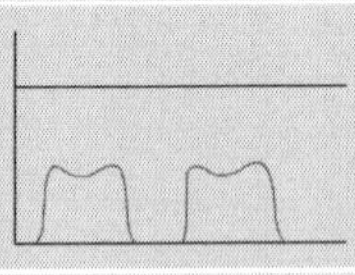	Capnogram with 2 peaks (bi-phasic capnogram)
Cardiac arrest	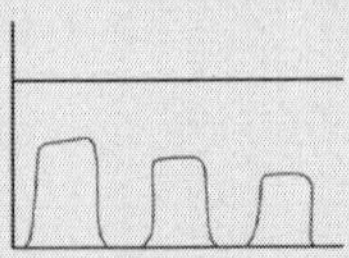	Fall in $EtCO_2$ proportional to the fall in cardiac output
Return of spontaneous circulation following CPR	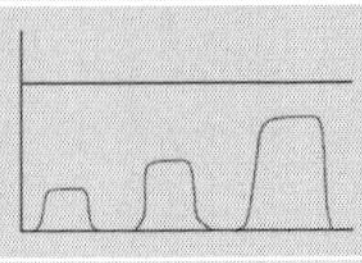	Gradual increase in $EtCO_2$
Bronchospasm	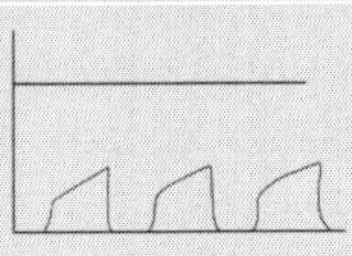	Upsloping plateau giving a 'shark fin' appearance
Ruptured ET cuff	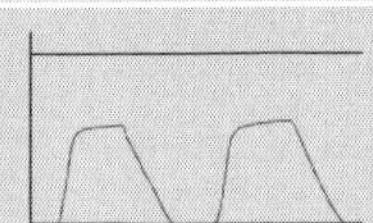	Gradual descent

Applications

The main application of $TcCO_2$ monitoring remains within the domains of neonatal intensive care. However, recent modifications and refinements in this technology have resulted in its use in the adult population as well. These include:

- Monitoring patients during mechanical ventilation in an intensive care or intra operative setting.
- It can be used in apnea testing for demonstration of brain death and helps negate the need for repeated ABG analysis.
- In the appropriate clinical setting, $TcCO_2$ measurements can reflect the pH and serum bicarbonate levels in our body. This can be of use in certain scenarios such as diabetic ketoacidosis where normalization of the $TcCO_2$ levels could indicate resolution of metabolic acidosis.
- $TcCO_2$ measurements can also be used to evaluate skin and tissue perfusion. This property is often utilized by vascular surgeons to assess skin graft vascularization.
- It is be used for monitoring patients during sleep studies and during procedural sedation.

Advantages over $TcCO_2$

Even though TcO_2 monitoring is less widely used compared to $EtCO_2$; there are certain scenarios where it scores over its counterpart. These include:

- Monitoring patients while using high frequency oscillatory ventilation.
- Utility in apnea testing.
- Monitoring patients on non-invasive ventilation without the need for specialized nasal cannula.
- Better accuracy in patient with congenital heart disease and right to left extrapulmonary shunting or ventilation perfusion inequalities.

However, unlike $EtCO_2$; $TcCO_2$ cannot be used to confirm the intratracheal position of the endotracheal tube or as a disconnect alarm in intubated patients. Thus, an ideal setup should implement the joint use of both these modalities to monitor patients particularly in critically ill pediatric patients.

CONCLUSION

Alterations in blood gas values and acid base disturbances lead to sudden and life-threatening changes in all the systems and hence a thorough understanding of blood gas derangement is mandatory for any treating physician. Disorders of acid-base balance can create complications in many disease states, and occasionally the abnormality may be severe so as to become a life-threatening event. Accurate results for a blood gas measurement depend on the proper collection, handling, and analysis of the specimen. BGA is particularly vulnerable to procedural errors. The procedure followed for blood gas analysis is by collecting arterial samples by puncturing an easily accessible artery. Continuous artery cannulation for frequent sampling in ICU is also practiced. Rarely venous samples are analyzed and results extrapolated to corresponding arterial values. Analysis and interpretation is also painstaking especially when it comes to mixed and complex acid base disorders.

Even though the direct measurement of blood gases would remain the gold standard in patient monitoring, it only provides a single measurement of a dynamic and rapidly changing clinical picture. Hence there is a necessity for continuous, non-invasive monitoring of blood gases. Few non-invasive methods are used to assess blood gas levels, especially in patients who need continuous monitoring.

SUGGESTED READING

1. Asif M, Sarkar PK. Three-digit Allen's Test. Ann Thorac Surg. 2007;84 (2):686–7. [Medline].
2. Bobbia X, Grandpierre RG, Claret PG, Moreau A, Pommet S, Bonnec JM, et al. Ultrasound guidance for radial arterial puncture: A randomized controlled trial. Am J Emerg Med. 2013;31(5):810–5. [Medline].
3. Brzezinski M, Luisetti T, London MJ. Radial artery cannulation: A comprehensive review of recent anatomic and physiologic investigations. Anesth Analg. 2009;109 (6):1763–81. [Medline].
4. Chan ED, Chan MM, Chan MM. Pulse oximetry: Understanding its basic principles facilitates appreciation of its limitations. Respir Med [Internet]. 2013;107(6):789–99. Available from: http://dx.doi.org/10.1016/j.rmed.2013.02.004.
5. Gilbert HC, Vender JS. Arterial blood gas monitoring. Crit Care Clin. 1995;11(1):233–48. [Medline].

6. Huch R, Lubbers DW, Huch A. Quantitiative continuous measurement of partial oxygen pressure on the skin of adults and new-born babies. Pflugers Arch. 1972; 337:185–98.
7. Peabody JL, Willis MM, Gregory GA, Tooley WH, Lucey JF. Clinical Limitations and advantages of transcutaneous oxygen electrodes. Acta Anaesthesiol Scand. 1978; 22:76–82.
8. Raffin TA. Indications for arterial blood gas analysis. Ann Intern Med. 1986;105 (3):390–8. [Medline].
9. Rang L, Murray H, Wells G, et al. Can peripheral venous blood gases replace arterial blood gases in emergency department patients? CJEM 2002; 4:7–15.
10. Severinghaus J. Transcutaneous blood gas analysis. Respir Care. 1982; 27:152–9.
11. Tremper KK, WC S, CR S. Transcutaneous PCO_2 monitoring on adult patients in the ICU and the operating room. Crit Care Med. 1981; 9:1752–59.
12. Zimmerman JL, Dellinger RP. Blood gas monitoring. Crit Care Clin. 1996; 12 (4):865–74. [Medline].

Chapter 8

Hypoxia and Hypoxemia

SK Jindal

Hypoxia and hypoxemia are commonly used interchangeably to describe deficiency of oxygen. The two terms, however, have different meanings. Hypoxia is defined as a condition characterized by lack or insufficient oxygen supply at the tissue level. On the other hand, hypoxemia is an alternate term which refers specifically to low arterial oxygen content and therefore low arterial oxygen supply to a particular tissue. Hypoxia can be further classified as generalized when the whole body is affected and localized when there is low oxygen supply to a particular region. Complete deprivation of oxygen is referred to as anoxia.

- **Local hypoxia:** Deficient blood supply to a particular region, such as due to arterial blockade causes local ischemia and oxygen deficiency. An ischemic organ appears pale which on surface feels cold and cyanosed. Severe hypoxia or anoxia will result in gangrene of the affected tissue.
- **Generalized hypoxia:** Hypoxia results when the oxygen available for use by the tissues is adequate. It is broadly classified into hypoxemic (in the presence of low PaO_2 and normoxemic (in the presence of normal PaO_2).

HYPOXEMIC HYPOXIA

A decrease in arterial PaO_2 can occur from either a decreased oxygen intake (i.e. low fraction of inspired oxygen [FiO_2]) or due to hypoventilation, ventilation - perfusion mismatching, right to left shunting of blood or impaired diffusion. Hypoxemic hypoxia can result from one or more of the following causes.

Decreased Oxygen Intake (FiO_2)

Total barometric pressure and partial pressure of oxygen are low at high altitude. Therefore, both alveolar and arterial PO_2 are also low.

Pathological lowering of FiO_2 occurs when oxygen in the inspired air is diluted/replaced by some other gas, e.g., carbon dioxide, carbon monoxide or methane in a smoke filled room or a mine. Oxygen intake also falls when oxygen from the atmospheric air gets consumed by fire. These pathological situations are acute and often fatal. In those who survive, the effect on blood gases is rarely ever demonstrated. By the time the blood sample is obtained, the subject is inhaling either room air or oxygen, administered therapeutically.

Hypoventilation

Hypoventilation implies a fall in total minute ventilation. If adequate air (therefore oxygen) is not inhaled, the oxygen uptake and carbon-dioxide removal from pulmonary capillary blood is impaired resulting in a fall of PaO_2 and a rise in $PaCO_2$. Relationship between alveolar ventilation and $PaCO_2$ is defined by the following equation:

$$PaCO_2 = K \times VCO_2/V_A \qquad (K = \text{Constant})$$

It is implied that if V_A is halved, the $PaCO_2$ doubles provided the VCO_2 (i.e. carbon dioxide produced) is unaltered. In other words, in pure hypoventilation, the arterial PO_2 and PCO_2 shall change in opposite directions by nearly the same amount.

Example: In a 40-year-old man, $PaCO_2$ of 60 mm Hg and $PaCO_2$ of 70 mm Hg indicate a change of 30 mm Hg on either side—a decrease in PaO_2 (from 90 mm Hg) and an increase in $PaCO_2$ (over 40 mm Hg). If the change is not the same, it indicates the additional presence of either a V/Q abnormality or shunt. This distinction is important in view of its therapeutic significance.

Pure hypoventilation shall occur when either the respiratory center is depressed due to anesthetic or sedative drugs or there is failure of neuromuscular control of respiration. In the presence of a parenchymal lung disease, hypoventilation is often accompanied by other disorders of gas exchange, i.e., V/Q mismatch or right to left shunting of blood.

Ventilation-Perfusion Mismatching

Some degree of V/Q abnormality is present in most lung diseases. An increase in the ratio, implying "wasted ventilation", is the most common cause of hypoxia. This is clinically encountered in chronic obstructive pulmonary diseases and pulmonary thromboembolism. The V/Q abnormality can be detected by calculating alveolo-arterial oxygen gradient (PAO_2-PaO_2). This can be done by determining PaO_2 from arterial blood sample and PAO_2 from FiO_2, atmospheric pressure and $PaCO_2$.

This can be easily understood by imagining lung as a two compartments (A and B) model **(Table 8.1)**. We can take example of normal lung (model I) in which both compartments receive equal and normal amount of ventilation and perfusion, and the other example (model II) in which compartments receives less (or inadequate) V_A. Although the total V_A in model II is the same as in model I, the ratio of distribution of ventilation in the two compartments A and B in model II is 2.3: 1. Since the blood flow (perfusion) is equal, the V/Q ratios are different, i.e., 1.16 and 0.5 in the two compartments. The alveolar and hence arterial oxygen and carbon dioxide tensions will be different in the two units. A difference in PAO_2-PaO_2 occurs because the relative hyperventilation of one compartment (A) does not fully compensate for the hypoventilation of the other compartment (B). This is more so for oxygen (than CO_2) because of the sigmoid shape of oxygen dissociation curve. While increased ventilation of unit A may help to normalize the "hypercapnia" resulting from hypoventilation of unit B, the hypoxia of hypoventilation (unit B) is not corrected by hyperventilation of unit A. This causes a lowering of PaO_2 compared to PAO_2 resulting in an $P_{A-a}O_2$ gradient.

Table 8.1: Change in relative ventilation of two compartments and its effects on arterial blood gases and $P_{A-a}O_2$.

	Model I Normal lung			*Model II V/Q abnormality*		
	A	*B*	*Total*	*A*	*B*	*Total*
Ventilation	2.5	2.5	5.0	3.5	1.5	5.0
Perfusion	3.0	3.0	6.0`	3.0	3.0	6.0
V/Q ratio	0.83	0.83	0.83	1.16	0.5	0.83
Arterial PCO_2	40	40	40	35	45	40
AlevelorPO_2	100	100	100	110	80	105
Arterial PO_2	100	100	100	110	80	90
PA-aO_2	0	0	0	0	0	15

(In both models FiO_2 is 0.21, mixed venous PO_2 and PCO_2 are presumed to be normal, i.e., venous PO_2 and PCO_2 of 40 mm Hg and 46 mm Hg respectively).

In a true clinical condition, the arterial PO_2 and PCO_2 are affected by the increasing V/Q inequality. The PO_2 falls continuously and rapidly while the PCO_2 rises gradually at first and more markedly afterwards, as the inequality increases. Therefore, when V/Q inequality is marked, PCO_2 is also increased. In fact, V/Q shunt more than 30% behaves clinically as right to left shunt.

Right to Left Shunt

Mixing of blood from the right with that of the left heart, without getting oxygenated in the lungs can occur either in the presence of a true right to left shunt or a V/Q inequality. The V/Q defect involves the presence of areas in the lung which are perfused but not ventilated, e.g., consolidations due to pneumonia or pulmonary edema. The gas exchange in the normal areas of the lung is unaffected, or may be slightly increased than the normal. But there is nil or inadequate gas exchange in the blood passing through the unventilated (or hypo-ventilated) areas, i.e., shunting of venous (or un oxygenated) blood. Mixing of the unoxygenated blood with that from the normal areas results in a net lowering of PaO_2. Often, there is no increase in $PaCO_2$ because the normal areas are able to eliminate the excess CO_2 in the blood from non-ventilated areas.

Hypoxia of V/Q inequality is corrected by administration of 100% O_2 while that due to shunt effect is not corrected. This principle is used to identify the mechanism of hypoxia by measuring the PO_2 before and after administering 100% O_2. In the presence of venous admixture (shunt effect), the $P_{A-a}O_2$ difference increases after inhalation of 100% O_2. The quantity of shunt as a percent of cardiac output can be determined with the help of shunt equation:

Qs/Qt = Cc' – Ca/Cc' – Cv

QS = cardiac output, QT= shunted blood, CC', Ca and CV' are oxygen contents of capillary, arterial and mixed venous blood respectively).

On rough estimate, the $P_{A-a}O_2$ of 15 mm Hg on breathing 100% O_2 indicates a shunt of about 1% of cardiac output.

A shunt of 2–3% of cardiac output is normally present on breathing 100% O_2. This occurs from the admixture of un oxygenated blood from bronchial and mediastinal veins which empty directly into the pulmonary and thebesian veins emptying into the left ventricle **(Fig. 8.1)**.

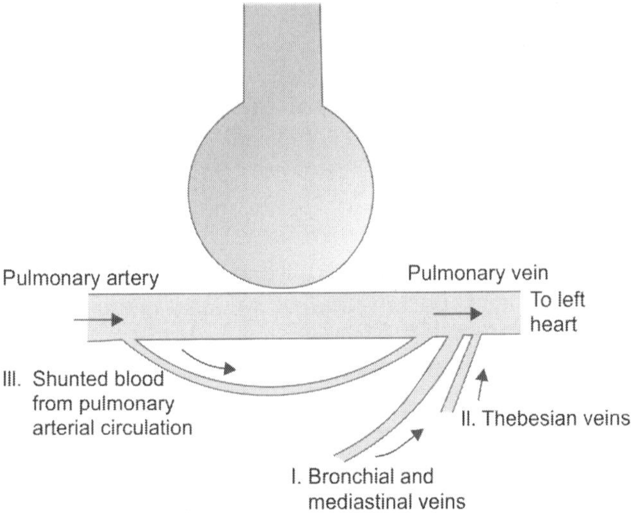

Fig. 8.1: Schematic representation to show venous admixture in pulmonary circulation: I and II, normal admixture from bronchial, mediastinal, thebesian and other systemic veins; III, pathological admixture due to shunted blood from pulmonary arterial circulation.

Both the causes and the treatment approaches are different for different types of hypoxemia **(Table 8.2)**. The effect of oxygen therapy is also different. It is therefore, important to identify the mechanism of hypoxemia in an individual patient.

Diffusion Defect

Diffusion of O_2 is impaired when the alveolo-capillary membrane is involved in either interstitial lung diseases or emphysema. In clinical practice however, impaired diffusion is not an important cause of hypoxemia. This is explained by the fact that the red blood cell takes about 0.75 second (transit time) to traverse the pulmonary capillary while it gets oxygenated (at rest) within the first 0.25 second **(Fig. 8.2)**. For the RBC to remain unoxygenated, the blood velocity should increase by more than three times (during exercise) to reduce the transit time to less than 0.25 second. Therefore, hypoxemia due to diffusion defect gets manifest only on exercise unless the disease is far advanced when oxygenation takes longer time and the blood velocity is also rapid. This occurs when the capillary bed volume is reduced due to progressive obliteration and destruction. The previously

Table 8.2: Clinical examples, identification and therapeutic approach to different causes of hypoxemia.

Cause	*Clinical condition*	*Identification criteria*	*Treatment approach*	*General response to oxygen therapy*
1. Decreased FiO_2	High altitude	Low P_{Atm}	Supportive	Rapid
	Fires, smoke	History	Supportive	Rapid
2. Hypo-ventilation	Neuromuscular failure; CNS depression	Almost similar increase in $PaCO_2$	Ventilatory support	Initial response good; later-variable
3. V/Q imbalance	COPD	Increased PAO_2–PaO_2	Bronchial hygiene	Moderately rapid
		Corrected by 100% O_2	Broncho-dilators	
4. R to L shunt	Pneumonia Atelectasis Edema	Not corrected by 100% O	Antibiotics Diuretics PEEP	Variable
5. Diffusion defect	Interstitial disease	Low VC, Low DLCO	Cortico-steroids	Moderately rapid

(PAO_2: alveolar partial pressure of O_2; PaO_2: arterial partial pressure of O_2; $PaCO_2$: arterial partial pressure of carbon dioxide; VC: vital capacity; DLCO: diffusing capacity of the lungs for carbon monoxide; PEEP: positive end-expiratory pressure)

non-perfused capillaries are recruited, the blood flow velocity in the remaining vessels increases, i.e., the transit time is reduced and not sufficient enough for uptake of oxygen by the red blood cells. This is the mechanism for exercise-induced hypoxemia observed in patients with interstitial lung diseases (ILDs).

NORMOXEMIC HYPOXIA

Tissue hypoxia occurring in the presence of normal PaO_2 is referred to as normoxemic hypoxia. It is difficult to measure in quantitative terms but diagnosed by clinical signs, symptoms and indirect laboratory parameters. It develops when the tissue demands for the oxygen are not supplied by the available oxygen stores. It is also difficult to define the tissue PO_2 below which the hypoxic damage may occur.

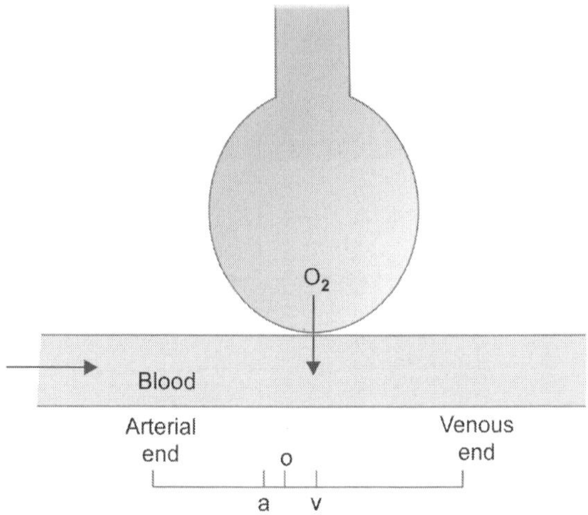

Fig. 8.2: Schematic representation to show transit time of pulmonary capillary circulation from arterial (a) to venous (v) end-about 0.75 sec; at rest, the blood gets fully oxygenated in about one-third of transit time (o).

Causes of Normoxemic Hypoxia

Tissue hypoxia is classified into one of the following types depending upon the pathophysiology.

Circulatory (Stagnant) Hypoxia

There is inadequate supply of oxygenated blood to the tissues.

- **Decreased blood flow:** Cardiac failure, intravascular volume depletion, hemorrhage, positive pressure ventilation, cardiac tamponade, pulmonary embolism, vasoactive states and drugs.
- **Altered blood flow:** Seen in the presence of excess positive end-expiratory pressure during mechanical ventilation, sepsis, abnormal body temperature, drugs, thyroid dysfunction etc.

The characteristic finding in these patients is the low central venous PO_2. Oxygen therapy does not help except when administered under hyperbaric conditions in the presence of tissue ischemia.

Cellular (Histotoxic) Hypoxia

Hypoxia may result from failure of cellular metabolism or energy generation due to inhibition of intracellular enzymes. This can occur in following circumstances:

- **Poisoning:** Toxic agents such as hydrogen sulfide, cyanide or carbon monoxide bind up cytochrome oxidase enzymes; salicylates and dinitrophenol causes uncoupling of oxidative phosphorylation and iron steals electrons and O_2 away from ATP producing reactions—all resulting in histotoxicity and hypoxia.
- **Altered oxygen diffusion:** Decreased mitochondrial oxygen consumption, edema, tissue ischemia and sepsis may lead to decrease PO_2 gradient.
- Endotoxemia and septic shock.
- **Deficiencies:** Thiamine deficiency impairs Kreb's cycle; phosphate deficiency causes decreased ATP while copper deficiency impairs cytochrome oxidase a_1 and a_3.
- **Miscellaneous:** Tissue hypoxia may also result from abnormal body temperature, thyroid dysfunction, ragged red cell disease and liver disease.

Anemic Hypoxia

Hypoxia due to deficiency of hemoglobin or altered affinity of Hb to oxygen is called anemic hypoxia. This may occur in the following conditions:

- Hemorrhage and anemia
- Altered P50, i.e., decreased O_2 Hb affinity secondary to low levels of 2,3 DPG in red blood cells, changes of pH and body temperature, carbon monoxide poisoning and hemoglobinopathies.
- Loss of Hb binding sites, e.g., carbon monoxide or cyanide poisoning; methemoglobinemia.

Demand Hypoxia

Hypoxia may also result where there is increased demand or utilization of O_2 by the tissues even though the O_2 delivery is normal (or even more). This may occur during conditions of excessive stress such as marked hyperpyrexia, excessive exercise or thyrotoxicosis. Cardiac output is increased but the mixed central venous PO_2 is decreased due to excessive tissue "extraction" (consumption) of oxygen.

Hypoxia and Respiratory Failure

Hypoxia indicates the presence of respiratory failure, i.e., failure of the respiratory system to efficiently perform one or both of its gas exchange functions: uptake of oxygen and removal of carbon dioxide.

Respiratory failure can be therefore classified as either hypoxemic (type I) or hypercapnic (type II). In type I respiratory failure, the arterial oxygen tension (PaO_2) is lower than 60 mm Hg with a normal or low arterial carbon dioxide tension ($PaCO_2$). On the other hand, type II failure is characterized by hypoxia and $PaCO_2$ higher than 50 mm Hg. Respiratory failure may also be classified as acute or chronic based on the duration of the underlying disease and onset of failure. Acute respiratory failure may often be characterized with life-threatening abnormalities of arterial blood gases and acid-base status. Chronic respiratory failure occurs in patients with chronic and protracted illnesses with gradual onset and relatively poorly distinguished clinical features.

The primary goal for oxygen therapy is to correct alveolar and/or tissue hypoxia. Therefore, any disorder causing hypoxia is a potential indication for oxygen administration. But the tissue oxygen delivery depends upon an adequate function of cardiovascular (cardiac output and blood flow), hematological (Hb and its affinity for oxygen) and the respiratory (arterial oxygen pressure) systems. Therefore, tissue hypoxia is not relieved only by oxygen therapy—functioning of all the three organ systems need to be improved.

To summarize oxygen is indicated whenever there is hypoxia with or without hypoxemia. Hypoxemic hypoxia, demonstrable on blood gas analysis results most often from diffuse pulmonary diseases. Oxygen is clearly indicated in all such disorders. On the other hand the presence of hypoxia in the absence of hypoxemia is difficult to document. Most such situations occur in sick patients suffering from non-pulmonary illnesses in whom, uses and indications for oxygen therapy should be carefully assessed.

SUGGESTED READING

1. Bates DV, Macklem PT, Christie RV. Respiratory function in disease. 1971. WB Saunders, Philadelphia.
2. Calzia E Rader, Macher P. Alveolar ventilation and pulmonary blood flow: Their V/Q concept. Intensive Care Med. 2003; 29:1229-32.
3. Campos JH, Feider A. Hypoxia during one-lung ventilation: A review and update. Cardiothorac Vasc Anesth. 2018; 32(5):2330-38.
4. Henig NR, Pierson DJ. Mechanisms of hypoxemia. Respir Care Clin N Am. 2000; 6(4):501-21.
5. MacIntyre NR. Tissue hypoxia: Implications for the respiratory clinician. Respir Care. 2014; 59(10):1590-6.

6. Pierson D. Normal and abnormal oxygenation: Physiology and clinical syndromes. Respir Care. 1993; 38:587.
7. Squara P. Matching total body oxygen consumption and delivery: A crucial objective? Intensive Care Med. 2004; 30:2170–79.
8. Swensen EW, Finley TN, Guzman SV. Unilateral hypoventilation in man during temporary occlusion of one pulmonary artery. J Clin Invest. 1961; 40:828.

Chapter 9

Clinical Prescription of Oxygen

Sahajal Dhooria, Puneet Saxena

Oxygen is not a drug, but a replacement or supplement to room air. However, it should be viewed just like a drug when one prescribes it. Despite growing evidence on the benefits and harms of oxygen therapy and the importance of implementing precision in oxygen therapy, the attitude of medical and paramedical personnel towards the prescription and administration of this vital substance remains unsatisfactory.

A physician may need to prescribe oxygen therapy to patients in three major clinical settings. One, for acute cardiorespiratory illness, including emergency situations. Two, for a patient being discharged after recovering from an acute illness, who may require oxygen for a short time at home. In some of these patients, the requirement may be for an indefinite time; how long the patient would require domiciliary oxygen might be unknown at the time of discharge. The third scenario is the prescription of long-term oxygen therapy (LTOT). There are several differences in the prescription of oxygen in the three settings that will be highlighted in the following subsections.

THE TRIGGER FOR OXYGEN THERAPY AND THE TARGET SATURATION

Oxygen is used to treat hypoxemia. It is not a drug for breathlessness. In the acute setting, the threshold of hypoxemia at which oxygen therapy should be initiated remains controversial. For most patients, a capillary oxygen saturation, measured by pulse oximetry, less than 90% is a definite trigger for administering oxygen. The range between 90–94% is contentious. There is some evidence that a liberal administration of oxygen might increase mortality (oxygen-ICU trial), but it has not been confirmed in other large studies. However, there is no convincing evidence till date, that not administering oxygen therapy to patients having an oxygen saturation in the range

90–94% is detrimental. One randomized study stopped early (the $LOCO_2$ trial), showed increased risk of intestinal ischemia and death in the conservative oxygen therapy group. A later randomized study published in 2021 (the HOT-ICU trial) did not find such a risk. Therefore, in general, we recommend a trigger of an oxygen saturation <90% to initiate oxygen therapy.

The recommendations on the target oxygen saturation during oxygen therapy are also not unanimous. The ranges suggested by different guidelines vary between 90–94% to 94–98%. In concordance with the trigger mentioned above, we suggest using a target of 90–94%, in general. In some situations, for example, in hypoxemic pregnant patients, a goal of 94–98% may be adopted to prevent fetal hypoxia. Having a lower target is advantageous in two ways. One, it reduces the potential harm of liberal oxygen therapy found in some studies. Albeit, the HOT-ICU trial found no difference in the safety of liberal or conservative oxygenation targets. Second, in the lower oxygen saturation range of 90–94%, the patient's oxygenation is in the steeper part of the oxygen dissociation curve. Thus, small changes in the partial pressure of oxygen in arterial blood (PaO_2) can be identified more easily, thus triggering the evaluation of potential causes of acute worsening. If at the same inspired oxygen concentration (FiO_2), there is a sustained drop in resting awake saturation by 3% or more, or if a sustained increase in the oxygen flow rate by 1 L/min or more is required to maintain the same target saturation, an assessment for the potential causes must be performed. Such an increase should be regarded as an 'event' and the nursing personnel should be instructed to inform the physician about it. It is not uncommon to hear that a patient, who was requiring low flow oxygen during the rounds the previous evening is found to be receiving high flow oxygen by the next morning without the physician being informed of the 'event' of a sustained increase in oxygen requirement. In such a case, an event such as pulmonary embolism might have occurred at night and 'missed.'

For patients having hypercapnic respiratory failure or a risk for the same (e.g., chronic obstructive pulmonary disease [COPD], bronchiectasis, morbid obesity, neuromuscular weakness, chest wall deformities), a lower oxygen saturation target of 88-92% should be used.

The above goals are not applicable when oxygen is prescribed for carbon monoxide poisoning, cluster headaches, sickle-cell crisis, pneumocephalus or pneumothorax. In these conditions, saturation goals are higher, approaching 100%.

Long-term oxygen therapy is prescribed to patients with chronic hypoxemic respiratory failure. The two groups of patients for whom, such therapy is most prescribed in clinical pulmonology practice are advanced cases of COPD and other obstructive airway disorders, and interstitial lung diseases (ILD). For patients with COPD, the trigger for prescribing LTOT is PaO_2 of 55 mm Hg or less or a SpO_2 88% or less documented twice over 3 weeks. In a patient with COPD, who also has pulmonary hypertension, chronic congestive failure or polycythemia, a higher PaO_2 threshold of 60 mm Hg is used for prescribing oxygen therapy. For patients with ILD, oxygen therapy may be prescribed if the resting PaO_2 is 90% or less. The target oxygen saturation range must be 88–92% for patients with COPD or those who have risk factors for hypercapnic respiratory failure, such as those with morbid obesity. For patients with ILD, a target of 90–94% may be prescribed.

Short term domiciliary oxygen might be required in patients who have improved after hospitalization for an acute respiratory illness but are mildly hypoxemic at discharge. Such conditions include pneumonia, acute exacerbations of an underlying chronic respiratory disorder such as COPD or ILD, and others. For such patients, similar thresholds, as used during hospitalization can be used. Several such patients will recover over the ensuing few weeks and would no longer remain hypoxemic. These patients must be reassessed after a period of 4 weeks to determine the need for LTOT.

SOURCE

The source of oxygen varies with the setting. During transportation of an acutely sick patient and in smaller healthcare set-ups such as small clinics and hospitals, the source is invariably compressed oxygen in a cylinder. In larger hospitals, the wall oxygen outlets are available supplied from a central source, the central oxygen manifold unit.

In the domiciliary setting, either oxygen cylinder or an oxygen concentrator can be used as a source. While oxygen cylinders contain 100% oxygen, the oxygen concentrators generally deliver a lower concentration of oxygen (about 93%). The concentrators may deliver oxygen either continuously or in pulses (pulse-dose oxygen). The numerical setting of pulse-dose concentrators does not correlate well to the L/min setting used with other devices. Small and light, battery-operated portable oxygen concentrators can be used to deliver oxygen during ambulation. For indoor ambulation, a longer connecting tube can also be used with the same source as for stationary use. Patients with COPD generally require lower flows and oxygen concentrators are sufficient for the purpose. Patients with progressive ILDs such as idiopathic pulmonary fibrosis might require higher flows, especially during activity and may mandatorily need an oxygen cylinder as the source. For post-hospital discharge short term oxygen therapy, oxygen cylinders are more cost-effective, especially when available on a rental basis.

DELIVERY DEVICE

When only oxygen is required to be delivered without artificial positive pressure respiratory support, masks or cannulae are used as delivery devices, by directly connecting to the oxygen source through a tubing. In case, additional respiratory support is needed, high flow nasal oxygen (HFNO) devices, continuous or bilevel positive airway pressure (CPAP or BPAP) devices or ventilators are used. Masks include simple face masks, reservoir masks (partial rebreathing mask or non-rebreather mask), and venturi masks. In emergency rooms, a reservoir mask (with an oxygen flow of 15 L/min) should be used at the first instance for an acutely hypoxemic patients, until the flow rate or FiO_2 required to maintain target saturation becomes clear. A simple face mask can then generally be substituted with flow rates of 5–10 L/min. If the oxygen requirement is even lower, nasal cannulae can be used at flow rates of 1–6 L/min. Venturi masks offer a more controlled delivery of the FiO_2 and are preferred when the oxygen saturation is required to be maintained in a narrow target range.

In the domiciliary setting, the nasal cannulae are the preferred device, as they allow the patient to eat and speak freely. Sometimes, simple masks may be required for patients requiring higher flow rates or those not tolerating nasal cannulae.

HUMIDIFICATION

At high flow rates, oxygen should be humidified. At low flow rates delivered through face mask or cannulae, the significance of humidification is unclear. When humidification is required, an appropriate humidification device should be used. Bubble bottles that allow a stream of oxygen to pass through a water container are not recommended.

DURATION

During acute illness, oxygen therapy needs to be administered continuously. However, chronically hypoxemic patients tolerate hypoxemia well. They are prescribed domiciliary oxygen with an aim to relieve hypoxemia, reduce dyspnea, and reduce the incidence of complications of chronic hypoxemia, such as cor pulmonale and polycythemia. To prevent these complications, a daily duration of oxygen therapy for a minimum duration of 15 hours in a day is essential; only nocturnal oxygen therapy is not enough. In patients with only exertional hypoxemia without resting hypoxemia, the use of oxygen only during ambulation has been found to be somewhat beneficial in patients with ILD (AmbOx trial), but not in those with COPD.

WEANING AND DISCONTINUATION

Patients admitted for acute illness are generally weaned from oxygen when the target saturation can be maintained with progressively lower FiO_2 delivery. This generally happens when the cause of hypoxemia has been adequately treated. The delivery device should be switched according to the FiO_2 requirement. If the patient's oxygen saturation can be maintained in the target range for 5–10 minutes on the new device and flow rate, the lower oxygen delivery method can be continued. The final device is generally nasal cannulae at low flow rates of oxygen (0.5–2 L/min). Finally, if the patient can maintain oxygen in the target range on breathing ambient air, oxygen therapy can be discontinued. However, a close monitoring of the oxygen saturation may be required for 24–48 hours after the discontinuation of oxygen therapy in order to identify any recurrence of hypoxemia.

MONITORING

Oxygen therapy should be monitored by trained personnel. If trained personnel are not available, the person monitoring the patient must be instructed clearly about the need for the continuous delivery of oxygen, the target saturation, and the general precautions such as checking for any disconnections in the case of a fall in saturation. The caregivers of the patients should be instructed that in patients with significant hypoxemia, oxygen cannot be discontinued for activities such as using the toilet, changing clothes, etc.

Pulse oximetry is used to monitor the patient's capillary oxygen saturation. The oxygen delivery should be aimed at maintaining the target range. Continuous pulse oximetry is desirable, however, patients getting weaned off during recovery, who require oxygen at flow rates of 2 L/min or less might be monitored once every 4 hours. Pulse oximetry may be unreliable in certain instances like hypotension, hypothermia or the presence of an abnormal hemoglobin. Assessment of PaO_2 is used to monitor oxygen therapy in such cases. For patients who have or are at a risk of hypercapnic respiratory failure, an arterial blood gas should be obtained at the initiation of therapy and whenever there is any increase in the FiO_2 requirement. Not exceeding the target range of 88–92% is crucial, and the same should also be clearly conveyed to the patient and his/her caregivers.

PRESCRIPTION OF OXYGEN

A clinical prescription of oxygen should contain all the components described above, such as the source, delivery device, target saturation range and the requirement for humidification. A fixed format for prescribing can be printed in one corner of the hospital's standard patient chart to ensure uniformity and adherence to prescription guidelines. A sample format is shown in **Box 9.1**. The additional notes item can be used to mention details such as humidification. A similar format can be used to prescribe domiciliary oxygen also.

Box 9.1: Sample format for prescribing oxygen therapy.

Oxygen supplementation using (Tick appropriate)

O Nasal cannulae   O Simple face mask   O Venturi mask

O Reservoir mask   O High-flow nasal cannulae

At a flow rate _______ L/min, or FiO_2 _________

To maintain a target saturation range of

O 88–92%   O 90–94%

O 94–98%   O Other, specify

Oxygen source: Wall socket/cylinder/oxygen concentrator

Inform physician if saturation falls by 3% or more, or oxygen flow requirement increases by 1 L/min or more

Additional notes: ____

In conclusion, the prescription of oxygen should involve the same degree of seriousness and precision as exercised for prescribing pharmacological agents. The paramedical staff and the caregivers of the patients should be adequately trained and instructed regarding the details of oxygen therapy.

SUGGESTED READING

1. Albert RK, Au DH, Blackford AL, et al. A randomized trial of long-term oxygen for COPD with moderate desaturation. N Engl J Med. 2016;375(17):1617–27. (In eng). DOI: 10.1056/NEJMoa1604344.
2. Barrot L, Asfar P, Mauny F, et al. Liberal or conservative oxygen therapy for acute respiratory distress syndrome. N Engl J Med. 2020;382(11): 999-1008. (In eng). DOI: 10.1056/NEJMoa1916431.
3. Continuous or nocturnal oxygen therapy in hypoxemic chronic obstructive lung disease: A clinical trial. Nocturnal oxygen therapy trial group. Ann Intern Med 1980;93(3):391-8. (In eng). DOI: 10.7326/0003-4819-93-3-391.
4. Girardis M, Busani S, Damiani E, et al. Effect of Conservative vs conventional oxygen therapy on mortality among patients in an intensive care unit: The oxygen-ICU randomized clinical trial. JAMA. 2016;316(15):1583-89. (In eng). DOI: 10.1001/jama.2016.11993.
5. Global strategy for the diagnosis, management, and prevention of Chronic Obstructive Pulmonary Disease (2022 Report). Global initiative for chronic obstructive lung disease. URL:https://goldcopd.org/2022-gold-reports/(accessed on 16 March 2022).
6. Long-term domiciliary oxygen therapy in chronic hypoxic cor pulmonale complicating chronic bronchitis and emphysema. Report of the Medical Research Council Working Party. Lancet. 1981;1(8222):681–6. (In eng).
7. Mackle D, Bellomo R, Bailey M, et al. Conservative oxygen therapy during mechanical ventilation in the ICU. N Engl J Med. 2020;382(11): 989-98. (In eng). DOI: 10.1056/NEJMoa1903297.
8. O'Driscoll BR, Howard LS, Earis J, Mak V. BTS Guideline for oxygen use in adults in healthcare and emergency settings. Thorax. 2017;72 (Suppl 1): ii1-ii90. (In eng). DOI: 10.1136/thoraxjnl-2016-209729.
9. Schjorring OL, Klitgaard TL, Perner A, et al. Lower or higher oxygenation targets for acute hypoxemic respiratory failure. N Engl J Med. 2021;384(14):1301–11. (In eng). DOI: 10.1056/NEJMoa2032510.
10. Siemieniuk RAC, Chu DK, Kim LH, et al. Oxygen therapy for acutely ill medical patients: A clinical practice guideline. BMJ 2018;363:k4169. (In eng). DOI: 10.1136/bmj.k4169.
11. Visca D, Mori L, Tsipouri V, et al. Effect of ambulatory oxygen on quality of life for patients with fibrotic lung disease (AmbOx): A prospective, open-label, mixed-method, crossover randomised controlled trial. Lancet Respir Med. 2018;6(10):759–70. (In eng). DOI: 10.1016/s2213-2600(18) 30289-3.

Chapter 10

Oxygen Therapy for Pulmonary Disorders

Anant Mohan, Tejas M Suri

An optimal supply of oxygen is indispensable for the survival of living tissues. Oxidative cellular respiration is the major source of energy for bodily processes. The oxygen present in the atmosphere needs to be delivered to the tissues for these functions. The lungs serve as the portal of entry of atmospheric oxygen into the blood which carries it to all parts of the body. Hence, any pulmonary disease which impairs this process of oxygenation of blood can be hazardous to the human body. In this chapter, we elucidate the mechanisms of impaired oxygenation in pulmonary diseases. We provide the basis for the use of supplemental oxygen to compensate for the impaired oxygenation. We emphasize that oxygen is akin to a drug which needs to be prescribed at an accurate dose, via the appropriate route for the optimal duration. We enumerate the pitfalls and adverse effects of oxygen therapy. We discuss the current evidence for the use of oxygen therapy in a few common pulmonary disorders, namely chronic obstructive pulmonary disease (COPD), interstitial lung disease (ILD) and acute respiratory distress syndrome (ARDS). Finally, we highlight the indications and practical considerations of oxygen therapy in pulmonary disorders.

INTRODUCTION: THE PATHOPHYSIOLOGICAL BASIS OF OXYGEN THERAPY IN PULMONARY DISORDERS

Oxygen is essential for oxidative cellular respiration and generation of energy to carry out various bodily processes. The atmospheric oxygen reaches the lungs on breathing. The lung then acts as a portal of entry for oxygen into the bloodstream by the process of diffusion from the alveoli into the pulmonary capillaries across the alveolar membrane. In blood, the dissolved oxygen rapidly binds with the hemoglobin protein with high affinity. The oxygenated pulmonary venous blood then reaches the left heart, from where it is pumped to the entire body.

Hypoxia refers to the lack of oxygen in the whole or part of the body; it can be rapidly fatal. Hypoxia may occur in one of the following four ways:

- Hypoxemic hypoxia: Reduced oxygen content in the blood due to impaired oxygenation by atmospheric air in the lungs (e.g., pulmonary disease, reduced atmospheric oxygen).
- Hypemic hypoxia: Reduced oxygen carrying capacity of blood (e.g., anemia, carbon monoxide poisoning, blood loss).
- Stagnant hypoxia: Decrease in flow of oxygenated blood to peripheral tissues, i.e., "low-flow" states (e.g., cardiac arrest, shock, peripheral vascular disease).
- Histotoxic hypoxia: Inability of cells to perform oxidative respiration despite adequate supply of oxygenated blood (e.g., cyanide toxicity inhibits cytochrome oxidase enzyme).

This chapter deals with hypoxemic hypoxia in the context of pulmonary disorders. At the outset, it is important to distinguish the term "hypoxemia" from hypoxia. Hypoxemia refers to reduced oxygen level in blood. Oxygen level in blood can be expressed in the following ways:

- **Partial pressure of oxygen in arterial blood (PaO_2):** It is the pressure of oxygen dissolved in arterial blood. It is measured using arterial blood gas (ABG) analysis. Normally, PaO_2 is greater than 80 mm Hg.
- **Oxygen saturation (SaO_2):** It is the percentage of hemoglobin in arterial blood which is saturated with oxygen. It is measured from the ABG. Alternatively, it can be estimated noninvasively using pulse oximetry (i.e., SpO_2). The normal SaO_2 is > 95%.

Most of the oxygen in the blood is carried in combination with hemoglobin (1 g of hemoglobin can combine with 1.34 mL of O_2), whereas a minority is dissolved in blood. Accordingly, the content of oxygen in the arterial blood (CaO_2) can be estimated as follows:

$$CaO_2 = [SaO_2 \times \text{Hb (g/dL)} \times 1.34] + [PaO_2 \times 0.00031] \text{ mL/dL}$$

Due to the high affinity of oxygen for hemoglobin, the oxygen dissociation curve is sigmoid shape. As PaO_2 increases above 60 mm Hg, the SaO_2 levels become greater than 90% and rise further to 100% slowly. However, at PaO_2 levels <60 mm Hg, the SaO_2 levels fall steeply leading to marked hypoxemia. It is noteworthy that there is no described fixed cutoff of hypoxemia level (SaO_2 or PaO_2) below which tissue hypoxia occurs.

To understand the mechanisms by which pulmonary diseases lead to hypoxemia, it is useful to know about the concept of alveolar-arterial (A-a) gradient: a measure of the oxygenation process in the lungs. The A-a gradient is the difference in the oxygen pressures in the alveolus and the arterial blood. The arterial oxygen pressure (PaO_2) is obtained by ABG whereas the alveolar oxygen pressure (PAO_2) is calculated using the alveolar gas equation:

$$PAO_2 = [FiO_2 \times (P_{atm} - P_{H_2O})] - [PaCO_2/R]$$

where, P_{atm} is the atmospheric pressure (760 mm Hg at sea level), P_{H_2O} is the partial pressure of water (usually 47 mm Hg), $PaCO_2$ is arterial partial pressure of carbon dioxide (roughly equivalent to $PACO_2$) and R is the respiratory quotient (normally, R = 0.8, although levels depend on relative metabolism of carbohydrates, proteins and fats). From this equation, it is evident that alveolar oxygen content increases with high FiO_2 (due to supplemental oxygen therapy) and decreases at high altitude (low P_{atm}) and with hypoventilation (high $PaCO_2$). Higher A-a gradient ($PAO_2 - PaO_2$) denotes impaired efficiency of oxygen transfer from lungs to the blood. The normal A-a gradient is age dependent according to the following equation:

Normal A-a gradient = (Age + 10)/4

Broadly, different pulmonary diseases cause hypoxemia by five mechanisms, which are summarized in **Table 10.1** and briefly described as follows:

Hypoventilation

A decrease in the ventilation of the lungs leads to impairment of carbon dioxide excretion. This results in a buildup of carbon dioxide partial pressure in the alveolus ($PACO_2$). As the net pressure of the constituent gases of the alveoli remains constant, and $PACO_2$ increases, this results in a fall in the PAO_2. Consequently, there is a fall in the PaO_2 leading to hypoxemia. There is no impairment in the process of gas exchange between the alveolus and pulmonary capillary, hence the A-a gradient remains normal. Furthermore, small amounts of supplemental oxygen can augment the PAO_2 and correct the hypoxemia.

Table 10.1: Mechanisms of hypoxemia.

Mechanism	*Examples*	*A-a gradient*	*$PaCO_2$ level*	*Improvement with supplemental O_2*
Hypoventilation	• Central nervous system depression (opioid, stroke, tumor) • Neuromuscular weakness (amyotrophic lateral sclerosis, myasthenia gravis, muscular dystrophy) • Chest wall deformity (kyphoscoliosis)	Normal	↑	++
Ventilation perfusion (VQ) mismatch	Interstitial lung disease, asthma, chronic obstructive pulmonary disease, pulmonary embolism, pulmonary hypertension	↑	Normal (or ↑)*	+
Shunt	Pneumonia, acute respiratory distress syndrome	↑	Normal	±
Diffusion limitation	Pulmonary hypertension, interstitial lung disease	↑	Normal	+
Low inspired pressure of O_2	High altitude	Normal	↓	+

*Although $PaCO_2$ levels are usually normal in VQ mismatch (and shunt), they may be elevated in advanced disease due to extensive areas with low VQ ratio, relative hypoventilation arising from respiratory muscle impairment (e.g. due to hyperinflation in COPD) or respiratory muscle fatigue (e.g. due to hyperventilation in acute respiratory failure).

Pure hypoventilation usually occurs due to extrapulmonary causes, including depressed central respiratory drive and neuromuscular causes. A component of relative hypoventilation may exist in patients with respiratory disease with other mechanisms of hypoxemia, and an inability to compensate appropriately by hyperventilating.

Ventilation-Perfusion (VQ) Mismatch

Normal human lungs are not uniformly ventilated or perfused with blood. Both ventilation and perfusion are maximum at the bases and minimum at the apices. However, the gradient for perfusion is steeper than that for ventilation. Hence, there is relative excess of ventilation compared with perfusion at the apices and vice versa at the bases. Regions of the lung with excess ventilation have low $PACO_2$, whereas those with low ventilation have high $PACO_2$ and low PAO_2. This physiological VQ mismatch is responsible for the normally occurring A-a gradient.

In various pulmonary diseases, parenchymal or vascular pathology results in exaggerated VQ mismatch leading to hypoxemia accompanied by elevated A-a gradient. Examples include interstitial lung disease (ILD), chronic obstructive pulmonary disease (COPD) and pulmonary embolism. Supplemental oxygen improves hypoxemia in some cases of VQ mismatch by improving oxygenation of areas with reduced ventilation.

Right-to-Left Shunt

In this condition, a portion of the deoxygenated blood from the right heart reaches the left heart without getting oxygenated in the lungs. Shunt may be anatomic or physiologic. Anatomic right-to-left shunt occurs when the blood bypasses the pulmonary capillaries altogether. It can be intracardiac (e.g., congenital heart disease) or extracardiac (e.g., pulmonary arteriovenous malformation). Physiologic shunt occurs when the blood passes through capillaries perfusing unventilated regions of the lungs (e.g. consolidation or collapse). Hence, shunt may occur in patients with pneumonia and acute respiratory distress syndrome (ARDS). Shunts cannot be corrected by supplemental oxygen alone.

Diffusion Limitation

Under normal circumstances, blood traverses the pulmonary capillaries in approximately 0.75 seconds, but it is fully oxygenated (i.e., all hemoglobin molecules saturated with oxygen) in just 0.25 seconds. During exercise, there is increase in the turnover of pulmonary blood flow. The increased demands are met by recruitment of additional pulmonary capillary beds. However, some pulmonary diseases may impair diffusion of oxygen across the alveolar-capillary membrane (e.g., pulmonary hypertension, ILD). This may result in hypoxemia, particularly with exercise. Administration of supplemental oxygen increases the diffusion gradient for oxygen across the alveolar-capillary membrane and may improve hypoxemia.

Low Partial Pressure of Inspired Oxygen

Although this is a mechanism of hypoxemia, it is not encountered in patients with pulmonary disease. This is usually seen at high altitude, where there is reduced ambient atmospheric pressure. Increasing the fraction of oxygen in the inspired air (FiO_2) by administering supplemental oxygen can overcome hypoxemia in these patients.

OXYGEN AS A DRUG—DEVICES, DOSAGE AND ADVERSE EFFECTS

Supplemental oxygen is a life saving therapy when used appropriately. However, it must be emphasized that oxygen is not a benign entity. When used in therapeutics, it must be treated akin to a pharmacological agent which needs to be administered by the correct device (route) at the optimal dose, failing which it may be associated with adverse effect.

Devices and Dosage

A detailed description of devices of oxygen delivery is available in dedicated texts. Briefly, supplemental oxygen can be delivered via low-flow and high-flow systems **(Fig. 10.1)**.

Low-flow Systems

These devices provide supplemental oxygen at flow rates < the patient's inspiratory flow rate. Hence, the deficit in the requisite flow rate is met by entraining environmental air. Patients with respiratory failure may have high minute ventilation with increased inspiratory flow rates. This leads to further entrainment of environmental air which dilutes the supplemental oxygen. Hence, the low-flow devices

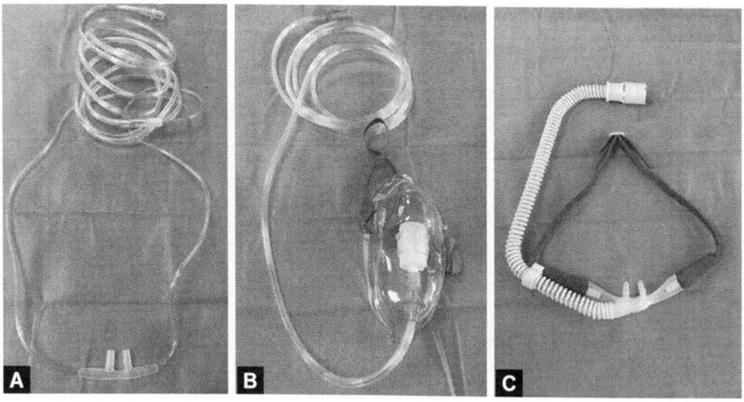

Fig. 10.1A to C: Oxygen delivery devices: (A) Nasal cannula is a low-flow device which is used to deliver up to 5 L/min oxygen; (B) Face mask is another low-flow device which is used to deliver between 5 to 15 L/min oxygen; (C) High flow nasal cannula is used to deliver high flow nasal oxygen at flow rates up to 60 L/min.

do not reliably deliver a desired FiO_2. Examples include nasal cannula (used for up to 5 L/min), face mask (up to 15 L/min), non-rebreather face mask, etc.

High-flow Systems

These devices provide supplemental oxygen at precise FiO_2 by either regulating the entrainment of environmental air (e.g. Venturi masks) or providing flow rates greater than the inspiratory flow rate of the patient [e.g. high-flow nasal cannula (HFNC)].

In addition, when oxygen is supplemented in the context of mechanical ventilation, an exact FiO_2 level can be delivered by the ventilator.

The Dosage of Oxygen

This is usually expressed as the FiO_2 which may range from 0.21 (environmental air—21% oxygen) to 1.0 (100% oxygen). The desired FiO_2 can be delivered with high precision using high-flow systems. For instance, the FiO_2 can be set directly while using HFNC. However, while using low flow devices, the FiO_2 cannot be set and is dependent on the set flow rate and the patient's inspiratory flow. Hence, the FiO_2 delivered is unpredictable. Although one can roughly estimate the delivered FiO_2 using nasal cannula (1–5 L/min) to be between 21% and

40%, such estimations are imprecise and are affected by changes in patient's minute ventilation.

Even though the exact FiO_2 delivered is not always measurable, the oxygen delivered can be titrated according to target oxygen levels in the blood. In most conditions, oxygen is supplemented to achieve an SpO_2 between 92% and 96%. However, in patients with COPD or obesity hypoventilation syndrome (OHS), the target SpO_2 is between 88% and 92%. The reason for lower SpO_2 target in COPD patients is discussed in the next section.

Adverse Effects of Oxygen

Injudicious oxygen supplementation may be associated with several adverse events. A few important adverse effects of oxygen are described below.

Absorptive Atelectasis

When supplemental oxygen is given at a high FiO_2 (e.g., greater than 0.6), it may increase the proportion of oxygen in alveoli by washing out the inert nitrogen. This oxygen readily diffuses across the alveolar-capillary membrane into the bloodstream. The resultant decrease in the intra-alveolar volume predisposes to alveolar collapse. Absorptive atelectasis may be more significant in regions with low VQ ratio (e.g., lung bases) where oxygen is rapidly absorbed and in conditions with increased oxygen uptake due to metabolic demands. To prevent absorptive atelectasis, it is essential to use the lowest FiO_2 possible to reach oxygenation targets for the minimum duration feasible. The use of positive end-expiratory pressure (PEEP) during mechanical ventilation may also be protective.

Worsening of Hypercapnia

Supplemental oxygen may result in carbon dioxide retention and worsening hypercapnic respiratory failure, particularly among patients with COPD. There are multiple mechanisms which contribute to this.

Worsening of VQ Mismatch

Application of supplemental oxygen increases the PAO_2 of the alveolar units which are relatively hypoventilating, without correcting the underlying hypoventilation. This reverses the hypoxic vasoconstriction of pulmonary capillaries serving such units. Hence blood is diverted from better ventilating alveoli to relatively hypoventilating ones, leading to impairment of carbon dioxide excretion.

Haldane Effect

Oxygenation of blood shifts the carbon dioxide-hemoglobin dissociation curve to the right. In other words, as oxygen saturates the hemoglobin molecule, carbon dioxide dissociates from hemoglobin. Hence applying supplemental oxygen increases the proportion of carbon dioxide in the dissolved state in blood leading to increased $PaCO_2$.

Loss of Hypoxemic Respiratory Drive

In patients with chronic hypercapnic respiratory failure, there is desensitization of the metabolic respiratory response to hypercapnia. These patients become dependent on the accompanying hypoxemia as a potent stimulant for respiration. Hence, correction of hypoxemia without correcting the underlying cause of hypercapnic respiratory failure leads to relative hypoventilation, thereby further worsening the hypercapnia.

Due to the particular vulnerability of patients with COPD and hypoventilation syndromes (e.g. OHS) to develop hypercapnic respiratory failure during oxygen therapy, lower SpO_2 targets (88 to 92%) are propagated for such patients.

Oxygen Toxicity

Oxygen may be directly toxic to cells due to generation of reactive oxygen species (superoxide anion, hydrogen peroxide and hydroxyl anion). These free radicals damage cellular components leading to cellular death. This oxidative process culminates in tissue injury and inflammation. Since the respiratory epithelium and alveoli are directly exposed to the effects of supplemental oxygen, they are particularly vulnerable to this oxygen toxicity. This may clinically manifest as tracheobronchitis and diffuse alveolar damage. It is difficult to distinguish oxygen toxicity from worsening of ARDS, superadded infection, or pulmonary edema.

Airway Burns

Oxygen is a combustible agent. Hence, the use of supplemental oxygen near an open flame (e.g., kitchen, prayer room, fireworks) or electrical sparking may result in fire in the patient's airways. The use of supplemental oxygen in active smokers can be hazardous. Patients who are being initiated on LTOT must be counseled regarding safe use of oxygen.

OXYGEN THERAPY IN SPECIFIC CONDITIONS—EVIDENCE, INDICATIONS AND PRACTICAL CONSIDERATIONS

In this section, we will summarize the evidence which supports supplemental oxygen in a few common pulmonary disorders and discuss the practical applications of the same.

CHRONIC OBSTRUCTIVE PULMONARY DISEASE (COPD)

Supplemental oxygen therapy has been most extensively studied in randomized controlled trials in the context of COPD **(Table 10.2)**. The landmark trials of the early 1980s, the Medical Research Council (MRC) trial and the Nocturnal Oxygen Therapy Trial (NOTT) demonstrated that in COPD patients with hypoxemia (defined as $PaO_2 < 60$ mm Hg), long-term oxygen therapy (LTOT) greater than 15 hours a day improves survival. However, subsequent trials failed to replicate the success of LTOT in COPD patients with moderate resting desaturation (SpO_2 89 to 93%) and exercise-induced desaturation. Furthermore, nocturnal oxygen therapy has not shown mortality benefit in patients with sleep-related desaturation in COPD.

Nonetheless, LTOT is one of the few interventions which have provided a mortality benefit in selected patients of COPD. Based on the aforementioned studies, LTOT has been recommended in the following patient groups:

- $PaO_2 \leq 55$ mm Hg (7.32 kPa) or $SpO_2 \leq 88\%$ (when measured at rest on room air).
- $PaO_2 \leq 59$ mm Hg (7.85 kPa) or $SpO_2 \leq 89\%$ (when measured at rest on room air), accompanied by pulmonary hypertension, right heart failure or polycythemia (hematocrit > 55%).

These measurements of oxygen level by ABG or pulse oximetry should ideally be performed when the patient is in stable condition (i.e., not during or immediately after an exacerbation). When home oxygen is prescribed after an acute exacerbation of COPD, patients should be re-evaluated for LTOT requirement after 8 weeks.

Table 10.2: Randomized controlled trials of oxygen therapy in COPD.

Trial	*Patients*	*Interventions*	*Outcomes*
Medical Research Council (MRC) Trial, 1981	Hypoxemic patients with PaO_2 < 60 mm Hg (n = 87)	O_2 at 2 L/min to achieve PaO_2 > 60 mm Hg for > 15 hours/day	Over 5 years, 19 of 42 (45.2%) oxygen patients died compared with 30 of 45 (66.7%) controls
Nocturnal Oxygen Therapy Trial (NOTT), 1980	Hypoxemic patients with PaO_2 < 60 mm Hg (n = 203)	Continuous O_2 vs 12-hour nocturnal O_2 (at 1–4 L/min to achieve PaO_2 between 60 and 80 mm Hg)	Mortality in nocturnal oxygen group was 1.94 times that of continuous oxygen group ($p = 0.01$)
Górecka et al, 1997	Moderate hypoxemia (PaO_2 = 56–65 mm Hg) (n = 135)	Long term oxygen therapy (LTOT) vs control	No difference in survival between LTOT and control
Chaouat et al, 1999	Moderate hypoxemia (PaO_2 = 56–69 mm Hg) with nocturnal desaturation (n = 76)	Nocturnal oxygen (to keep SpO_2 > 90% in sleep) vs control	No difference in survival or pulmonary hemodynamics between O_2 and control
Long-term Oxygen Treatment (LOTT) Trial, 2016	Moderate resting (SpO_2 = 89–93%) or exercise-induced desaturation (n = 738)	Long-term oxygen (24 hours/day at 2 L/min to achieve SpO_2 > 90%) vs no oxygen	No difference in time to death or first hospitalization between LTOT and control
Lacasse et al (INOX trial), 2020	Nocturnal desaturation (SpO_2< 90% for 30% of recording)	Nocturnal O_2 (2–4 L/min to maintain SpO_2 > 90%) vs sham concentrator	No difference in mortality between nocturnal oxygen and sham concentrator

Currently, LTOT is not recommended in patients with moderate desaturation at rest (SpO_2 between 89% and 93%). Although LTOT has not been found to have survival benefit in patients with exercise-induced desaturation, the use of supplemental oxygen in such patients during activity has been found to reduce dyspnea and improve exercise tolerance and quality of life. Among patients with nocturnal desaturation, it is important to consider the possibility of obstructive sleep apnea and sleep-related hypoventilation, and patients should ideally be evaluated with an in-lab polysomnography rather than prescribing nocturnal oxygen therapy.

LTOT is usually delivered using a nasal cannula at 2 L/min. The flow rate may be titrated to achieve a target SpO_2 of 88 to 92%. The flow rate may have to be increased during exercise or sleep by 1 to 2 L/min to compensate for desaturations. The target oxygen saturation in COPD is lower than that in other pulmonary disorders as these patients are prone to develop hypercapnia in response to oxygen therapy (as discussed above). During LTOT, supplemental oxygen should be provided nearly continuously, but at least greater than 16 hours a day.

The available oxygen sources include oxygen cylinders and concentrators. Oxygen cylinders are bulky and require frequent replenishment. In contrast, oxygen concentrators capture and enrich the oxygen from environmental air, and thus can be used without replenishment. Concentrators are operated by either battery or electricity. Consequently, it is advisable to use the oxygen concentrator as the primary device with a cylinder as backup in case of failure of concentrator device. Additionally, portable oxygen devices including ambulatory cylinders (cheapest and bulkiest), liquid systems and portable concentrators (expensive) are available. The use of portable devices should be encouraged if the patient is mobile and committed to an active lifestyle.

Oxygen therapy is also used during acute exacerbations of COPD. However, the use of oxygen in this situation should be judicious. Indiscriminate oxygen use in the emergency department can worsen hypercapnia leading to further desaturation. Knee jerk increases in oxygen flow rates precipitate hypercapnic respiratory failure requiring invasive mechanical ventilation. Hence, patients with acute exacerbation of COPD must be carefully monitored and SpO_2 must not exceed the target range (88 to 92%). Furthermore, the use of non-invasive ventilation (NIV) may improve survival and reduce need for mechanical ventilation in acute exacerbation of COPD with respiratory acidosis (pH <7.35). Supplemental oxygen can be combined with NIV to achieve the target SpO_2.

INTERSTITIAL LUNG DISEASE (ILD)

Almost all patients with ILD develop hypoxemia as their illness progresses. Profound hypoxemia can develop in ILD consequent to a combination of VQ mismatch and diffusion limitation. However, there is a lack of good quality data regarding use of oxygen therapy in ILD. This is inevitable as it is virtually impossible to recruit patients with advanced lung disease and severe hypoxemia into clinical trials with a placebo arm, thereby denying them oxygen therapy. Hence, the evidence from the trials of LTOT in COPD (MRC and NOTT) are extrapolated to ILD and the recommendations for LTOT in ILD is identical to those for COPD mentioned above. In ILD with exercise-related desaturation, small studies have shown improvements in exercise capacity but not dyspnea using oxygen therapy during exercise.

ACUTE RESPIRATORY DISTRESS SYNDROME (ARDS)

ARDS is a form of acute hypoxemic respiratory failure characterized by lung injury in response to systemic or pulmonary illness. The patient develops a non-cardiogenic pulmonary edema with alveolar flooding. Large portions of the lungs are fluid-filled and not ventilating. Patients may develop profound hypoxemia due to physiologic shunting of blood. Consequentially, it is unsurprising that the hypoxemia often fails to improve with high flows of supplemental oxygen delivered via low-flow systems. To oxygenate these patients, it is necessary to open collapsed alveoli by application of PEEP. Hence, a large proportion of these patients require invasive mechanical ventilation.

The definition of ARDS depends on the measure of the PaO_2/FiO_2 (P/F) ratio. While the normal PF ratio is greater than 400, ARDS has PF ratio < 300 despite application of PEEP ≥ 5 cm H_2O. ARDS severity is classified as follows:

- Mild: 300 ≥ PF ratio > 200
- Moderate: 200 ≥ PF ratio > 100
- Severe: PF ratio ≤ 100

In contrast to oxygen supplementation via low-flow systems, high-flow nasal oxygen may have a role in management of mild and moderate ARDS. In a multicenter randomized trial of ARDS patients randomized to receive high-flow nasal oxygen, non-invasive ventilation or supplemental oxygen by mask, the intubation rate in the three groups were 38%, 50% and 47%, respectively. Although these differences were not statistically significant, among a pre-defined subgroup of patients with PF ratio ≤ 200, HFNC reduced the rate of intubation. Furthermore, HFNC was associated with reduced 90-day mortality. The benefit of HFNC in ARDS may be related to its ability to precisely deliver high FiO_2 as well as its ability to generate of modest PEEP (approximately 1 to 5 cm H_2O). HFNC is also more comfortable for the patient compared with noninvasive ventilation.

Among patients with ARDS who are intubated, mechanical ventilatory strategies should be optimized to ensure an SpO_2 between 88% to 95% with the minimum possible FiO_2 (preferably < 0.6) to prevent oxygen toxicity.

OTHER PULMONARY DISORDERS

The use of supplemental oxygen in other pulmonary disorders has not been studied in randomized controlled trials. Nonetheless, oxygen is routinely used for treating hypoxemia in both acute and chronic pulmonary diseases. The optimal targets of oxygen therapy remain uncertain.

In the setting of acute hypoxemic respiratory failure (e.g., asthma, community-acquired pneumonia, pulmonary embolism etc.), supplemental oxygen should be initiated if the patient's SpO_2 is < 90%. It is prudent to target SpO_2 between 92% and 96%. If oxygen flow requirements are high, HFNC may be considered. However, if such patients are not adequately oxygenated with supplemental oxygen, then mechanical ventilation should be initiated without delay. Intubation and invasive mechanical ventilation is also imperative if the patient has cardiorespiratory arrest, hemodynamic instability or altered mentation.

Although the targeted SpO_2 is < 96% in most conditions to prevent oxygen toxicity, a notable exception is pneumothorax. In patients with primary spontaneous or iatrogenic pneumothorax which is small (i.e., < 2 cm at hilum) and managed by observation, the use of supplemental oxygen at FiO_2 of 1.0 is associated with sixfold increased rate of resorption. As previously mentioned, oxygen displaces nitrogen from alveoli and hence creates a diffusion gradient for nitrogen from pleura to alveoli. In this situation, oxygen at high FiO_2 is usually given using nonrebreather mask. The use of HFNC should be avoided as the attendant PEEP can worsen the pneumothorax.

Among patients with chronic hypoxemic respiratory failure due to various pulmonary disorders (e.g., pulmonary hypertension, bronchiectasis etc.), the use of LTOT is based on extrapolation of evidence from its use in COPD. Hence, the indications for LTOT are identical to the ones listed for COPD above. It is unknown if supplemental oxygen prolongs survival in these conditions.

CONCLUSION

Hypoxemia is defined as reduced oxygen level in the blood. Pulmonary diseases can impair oxygenation of blood in the lungs leading to hypoxemia by various mechanisms. Hypoxemia due to hypoventilation, VQ mismatch or diffusion limitation is amenable to improvement with supplemental oxygen. Since hypoxemia can result in fatal tissue hypoxia, use of supplemental oxygen to correct hypoxemia can be lifesaving and life prolonging. However, supplemental oxygen is akin to a pharmacological agent with adverse events. Injudicious supplemental oxygen can result in absorptive atelectasis, worsening hypercapnia, or oxidant injury.

Current evidence suggests that the use of long-term oxygen therapy (LTOT) for greater than 16 hours a day in stable chronic obstructive pulmonary disease (COPD) patients with daytime resting hypoxemia is associated with increased survival. The recommendations for use of LTOT for other causes of chronic hypoxemic respiratory failure is extrapolated from the evidence of its benefit in COPD. Oxygen therapy should be titrated according to the oxygen saturation measured using pulse oximetry (SpO_2). The usual SpO_2 target in patients with COPD or coexistent hypercapnia is 88 to 92%. In contrast, for patients with hypoxemic respiratory failure without hypercapnia, the SpO_2 target is 92 to 96%. Supplemental oxygen must be used at the least dosage to achieve the desired SpO_2 target to prevent oxygen toxicity.

SUGGESTED READING

1. Bell EC, Cox NS, Goh N, Glaspole I, Westall GP, Watson A, Holland AE. Oxygen therapy for interstitial lung disease: A systematic review. Eur Respir Rev. 2017;26(143):160080.
2. Chaouat A, Weitzenblum E, Kessler R, Charpentier C, Enrhart M, Schott R, Levi-Valensi P, Zielinski J, Delaunois L, Cornudella R, Moutinho dos Santos J. A randomized trial of nocturnal oxygen therapy in chronic obstructive pulmonary disease patients. Eur Respir J. 1999;14(5):1002–8.

3. Continuous or nocturnal oxygen therapy in hypoxemic chronic obstructive lung disease: A clinical trial. Nocturnal Oxygen Therapy Trial Group. Ann Intern Med. 1980 Sep;93(3):391–8.
4. Dunn WF, Nelson SB, Hubmayr RD. Oxygen-induced hypercarbia in obstructive pulmonary disease. Am Rev Respir Dis. 1991;144 (3 Pt 1): 526–30.
5. Frat JP, Thille AW, Mercat A, Girault C, Ragot S, Perbet S, Prat G, Boulain T, Morawiec E, Cottereau A, Devaquet J, Nseir S, Razazi K, Mira JP, Argaud L, Chakarian JC, Ricard JD, Wittebole X, Chevalier S, Herbland A, Fartoukh M, Constantin JM, Tonnelier JM, Pierrot M, Mathonnet A, Béduneau G, Delétage-Métreau C, Richard JC, Brochard L, Robert R; FLORALI Study Group; REVA Network. High-flow Oxygen through Nasal Cannula in Acute Hypoxemic Respiratory Failure. N Engl J Med. 2015; 372(23):2185–96.
6. Gorecka D, Gorzelak K, Sliwinski P, Tobiasz M, Zielinski J. Effect of long-term oxygen therapy on survival in patients with chronic obstructive pulmonary disease with moderate hypoxaemia. Thorax. 1997 Aug;52(8):674–9.
7. Lacasse Y, Sériès F, Corbeil F, Baltzan M, Paradis B, Simão P, Abad Fernández A, Esteban C, Guimarães M, Bourbeau J, Aaron SD, Bernard S, Maltais F; INOX Trial Group. Randomized trial of nocturnal oxygen in chronic obstructive pulmonary disease. N Engl J Med. 2020 Sep 17;383(12):1129–38.
8. Long-term Oxygen Treatment Trial Research Group, Albert RK, Au DH, Blackford AL, Casaburi R, Cooper JA Jr, Criner GJ, Diaz P, Fuhlbrigge AL, Gay SE, Kanner RE, MacIntyre N, Martinez FJ, Panos RJ, Piantadosi S, Sciurba F, Shade D, Stibolt T, Stoller JK, Wise R, Yusen RD, Tonascia J, Sternberg AL, Bailey W. A randomized trial of long-term oxygen for COPD with moderate desaturation. N Engl J Med. 2016;375(17):1617–27.
9. Long-term domiciliary oxygen therapy in chronic hypoxic cor pulmonale complicating chronic bronchitis and emphysema. Report of the Medical Research Council Working Party. Lancet. 1981;1(8222):681–6.
10. O'Driscoll BR, Howard LS, Earis J, Mak V; British Thoracic Society Emergency Oxygen Guideline Group; BTS Emergency Oxygen Guideline Development Group. BTS guideline for oxygen use in adults in healthcare and emergency settings. Thorax. 2017;72(Suppl 1):ii1–ii90.
11. Rodríguez-Roisin R, Roca J. Mechanisms of hypoxemia. Intensive Care Med. 2005;31(8):1017–9.

Chapter 11

Oxygen for Non-pulmonary Conditions

Srinivas Rajagopala

Oxygen is a titratable drug used for treating hypoxemia. However, tissue oxygen consumption in various pathological states is the main variable of interest and may be affected by an independent process despite adequate oxygen content of the blood. Tissue consumption of oxygen is dependent on oxygen delivery and adequate oxygen extraction. Oxygen delivery is a function of the oxygen content of blood [determined by hemoglobin (Hb) and percentage Hb saturation] and cardiac output. Tissue oxygen extraction in the face of normal oxygen delivery is rarely limiting. However, it can be affected by thrombosis of the local microcirculatory bed, abnormal dissociation of oxygen bound to hemoglobin, and interstitial edema. Normal tissue oxygen extraction is typically 20% of the oxygen content of arterial blood and is not limited by oxygen delivery. In conditions of lowered blood delivery (and thereby oxygen delivery), tissues compensate by extracting more oxygen from the supplied amount, but this efficiency is typically limited at 67%. Demand at this point can solely be met by increasing supply, and this is called "supply dependency".

Clinically, there are several situations where oxygen extraction is abnormal in the absence of hypoxemia. In these situations, the rationale for using oxygen is to maximize oxygen content to offset the increased oxygen extraction occurring or offer a higher gradient to overcome the abnormal tissue extraction. However, there are several limitations of providing higher fraction of inspired oxygen (FiO_2) to achieve higher oxygenation in the face of normoxemia. Firstly, the oxygen-hemoglobin curve is sigmoidal. The use of a higher FiO_2 under normobaric conditions does not lead to higher oxygen delivery to tissues in the absence of hypoxemia as dissolved oxygen does not contribute much to oxygen delivery under these conditions. Second, the excess of supplied oxygen does not guarantee an excess extraction if this is the limiting factor. Thirdly, the COVID-19 pandemic has highlighted the fragility of oxygen supply in the country and the need to conserve oxygen utilization. Finally, hyperoxia occurs because of excess oxygen administration and has its complications. These include:

- Production of toxic oxygen species, especially in the lungs, retina, and central nervous system.
- Absorptive atelectasis (as oxygen, which is an absorbable gas replaces nitrogen which is not) and damage to the airways and lung parenchyma. Atelectasis also worsens hypoxemia.
- Worsening of hypercapnia due to several other mechanisms; atelectasis secondary to hyperoxia worsens ventilation-perfusion mismatch; hyperoxia reduces central ventilatory drive; hyperoxia causes a reduction of the affinity for carbon dioxide, leading to an increase in $PaCO_2$ (the Haldane effect).
- Hyperoxia has been independently associated with in-hospital death in ventilated stroke patients in the ICU than with either normoxemia or hypoxemia (Rincon F et al.). This is possibly due to increased free radical formation and endothelial dysfunction, vasoconstriction caused by hyperoxia in the coronary and cerebrovascular bed with further reduced oxygen delivery, and lowered cardiac output caused by peripheral arterial vasoconstriction due to hyperoxia leading to higher afterload. Acute changes after hyperoxemia involve a change in the activity of ion channels, whereas long-term changes involve global gene expression.
- Hyperoxia has now been shown to increase mortality in any critically ill patient population independently. Oxygen-ICU, a single-center trial published in 2016, was one of the first looking at a mixed ICU population while assessing the effects of a conservative oxygen delivery (SpO_2, 94–98%) strategy against a conventional (SpO_2, 97–100%) one (Girardis M et al.). The researchers noted a significant mortality difference favoring conservative oxygen therapy, particularly in intubated patients. The IOTA systematic review and meta-analysis of 16,037 patients showed an increased relative risk of death in-hospital with hyperoxia that persisted over a prolonged period while conferring no obvious advantages (Chu DK, et al.).
- Three well-designed randomized controlled trials (RCTs) have not clarified the appropriate oxygen targets but have raised pertinent questions and informed clinical practice. The results of these

trials clearly show the safety of conservative oxygen targets and do not show any advantage of higher targets. The ICU-ROX study was an RCT conducted by the ANZICS group that enrolled 1000 patients to conservative (SpO_2, 90–96%) versus liberal oxygen therapy. 30% of the cohort was postoperative, 41% were acute brain disease, and 18% had suspected hypoxic encephalopathy. The ICU-ROX trial did not show any increase in the duration of ventilator stay, intensive care length of stay, and mortality with conservative as opposed to liberal oxygen therapy in the overall patient population (Mackle D et al.). However, there were more ventilator-free days in the conservative oxygen therapy group in the pre-specified population with hypoxic encephalopathy. The $LOCO_2$-REVA research network (Barrot et al.) enrolled patients with acute respiratory distress syndrome to conservative oxygen targets ((SpO_2 88–92%, PaO_2 55–80 mm Hg) versus liberal targets. This trial was stopped after 205 patients for futility (planned 805 at a 38% absolute risk reduction effect size). There were five episodes of mesenteric ischemia, all in the conservative oxygen group. The HOT-ICU trial (Schorring et al.) enrolled 2,928 patients with early hypoxemic respiratory failure to either PaO_2 of 60 mm Hg or 90 mm Hg. The 90-day mortality was similar between the groups (42.9% vs. 42.4%, $p = 0.64$).

- A large 40,000 patient multinational, multicenter pragmatic registry RCT, the MEGA-ROX trial is ongoing and aims to detect a difference as low as 1.5%, if present, between conservative and liberal oxygen therapy with several nested pre-specified subgroups (CTG1920-01). This trial is expected to provide conclusive answers to appropriate oxygen targets in several sub-groups of patients.

It is also essential to consider that our ability to monitor PaO_2 continuously is limited, and the measured surrogate SpO_2 is limited by the poor fidelity of pulse oximetry, especially at lower saturation levels. Data from the ICU-ROX and $LOCO_2$-REVA trials also suggest that the acceptable upper range for SpO_2 is 96% and 90% should the lower acceptable saturation, especially in critically ill patients. Given the lack of clear evidence of the benefit and possible harms of hyperoxemia, considerable controversy surrounds the use of oxygen in the absence of hypoxemia. There is a clear rationale and some supporting evidence to avoid hyperoxemia. However, what defines the lower limit of hyperoxemia is unclear, and the patient sub-populations where prevention of hyperoxemia is crucial need to be better defined by further cohorts. Herein, we examine the use of oxygen for non-pulmonary conditions.

CONDITIONS CHARACTERIZED BY REDUCED CARDIAC OUTPUT (AND OXYGEN DELIVERY)

Acute decompensated heart failure (ADHF) is characterized by reduced oxygen delivery to the microcirculation. Peripheral tissues suffer from hypoperfusion and hypoxia even though there is no hypoxemia. Oxygen has traditionally been used for over a century in this setting, regardless of oxygen saturation. As indicated above, hyperoxemia due to excess oxygen administration can cause vasoconstriction in the coronary and cerebrovascular bed with further reduced oxygen delivery. There is the potential for perpetuating the underlying disease due to lowered cardiac output caused by peripheral arterial vasoconstriction and reflex bradycardia. There are no well-designed clinical trials to answer this clinical question at present, but most guidelines recommend against routine administration of oxygen in cardiac failure. Three small studies in HF with reduced ejection fraction (HFrEF) can help guide practice. Mak et al. showed that extreme hyperoxemia (FiO_2 100) was associated with impaired cardiac relaxation and increased left ventricular end-diastolic pressure in those with stable coronary artery disease ($n = 12$) and those in HF ($n = 16$). In the HF cohort, there was an increase in systemic vascular resistance and reduction in stroke volume, cardiac output, and coronary sinus blood flow. Park et al. showed similar findings except for changes in stroke volume at a lower FiO_2 of 0.4 compared to 0.21. Haque et al. showed a reduction in stroke volume and increase in pulmonary wedge pressure in ADHF (baseline spO_2 92.4%) that were seen even with FiO_2 of 24%. More data is needed from controlled trials in both HFrEF and HF with preserved ejection fraction (HFpEF). However, evidence suggests that restricted use of oxygen in those without hypoxemia is reasonable.

LOCAL MICROCIRCULATORY BED ABNORMALITIES

Myocardial Infarction

Traditionally, oxygen was administered to all patients with myocardial infarction. Besides potentially increasing oxygen supply, it also allays the sense of breathlessness. Recently, with the increasing recognition of the harms of hyperoxemia, guidelines advise against routine oxygen administration. Breathlessness can be allayed by morphine and controlled oxygen delivery devices to meet high ventilatory demands without causing hyperoxemia. The AVOID trial by Stub et al. randomized 638 patients with STEMI (ST-elevation myocardial infarction) and demonstrated no reduction in myocardial infarct size by giving oxygen to normoxemic patients with STEMI undergoing PCI. Interestingly, the oxygen therapy arm had a higher rate of recurrent myocardial infarction (5.5% versus 0.9%; P = 0.006) and an increased frequency of cardiac arrhythmia (40.4% versus 31.4%; P = 0.05). At six months, the oxygen group had an increase in myocardial infarct size on cardiac magnetic resonance (n = 139; 20.3 vs. 13.1 g; P = 0.04). The $DETO_2X$ trial by Hofmann et al. was a registry-based RCT that evaluated outcomes with the use of oxygen versus none in myocardial infarction. This trial enrolled 6,629 patients and showed no difference in one-year mortality between room air and oxygen therapy in normoxemic patients with suspected AMI. In summary, there is evidence for the harm of oxygen therapy in normoxemic patients with MI and no evidence of benefit. Hence, oxygen must be administered only to patients with hypoxemia.

Cerebrovascular Disorders

Eubaric hyperoxemia was shown to improve neurological and neuropathological outcomes in experimentally-induced cerebral infarction in rats. It was also shown that 100% oxygen administered within 30 minutes of experimentally-induced stroke in rats salvaged ischemic brain tissue, especially in the cerebral cortex. As indicated in the section on the complications of hyperoxemia, excess oxygen can worsen cerebral perfusion. In the prespecified subgroups of the ICU-ROX trial, patients with hypoxic-ischemic encephalopathy had poorer outcomes with higher oxygen targets. The UK-based SO_2S RCT allocated 8,003 adults after stroke to groups to continuous oxygen, night-time oxygen, or no routine oxygen (control) within 24 hours. Participants' oxygen levels were monitored four times a day. The average age of participants was 72 years, 55% were men, and 92% were living independently before their stroke. Oxygen was administered before hospital admission in 20% of people, and the average oxygen saturation was 96.6% at randomization. The diagnoses included ischemic stroke (82%), hemorrhagic stroke (7%), and others (11%). There was no difference in 90-day disability, mortality, proportion living independently, or adverse events between groups. These studies collectively indicate that there is no routine role for oxygen therapy after stroke.

There are several case reports on hyperbaric oxygen therapy (HBOT) for treating neurological diseases and cerebral stroke. HBOT is shown to reduce cerebral edema, intracranial tension and reduce the penumbra size. HBOT may decrease the extent of brain infarction by improving mitochondrial dysfunction. It also diminishes the neurological deficit and post-infarction sequelae. HBOT is also reported to accelerate neurological recovery after spinal cord injury. The US-FDA declared ischemic stroke as one of the 13 indications for HBOT in 2013. The evidence base for HBOT is not robust and HBOT is not widely available. More data on the choice of patients, time of administration, dose, and outcomes are needed before HBOT can be recommended for this indication.

Problems of Oxygen Transport

As discussed above, most of the oxygen in the blood is carried bound to hemoglobin. Dissolved oxygen does not contribute significant amounts in normobaric conditions. For example, even at a FiO_2 of 100%, dissolved oxygen contributes less than 7% of the total oxygen content of blood, assuming lungs are normal. Oxygen transport and delivery to the tissues will be inadequate whenever there are problems with the total blood volume or cardiac output.

Blood Volume

While acute blood loss may occur following an accident or massive bleeding, plasma is lost in conditions associated with dehydration or burns. Given a relatively small amount of oxygen carried in the dissolved form, loss of plasma does not cause any significant change in the oxygen content of the blood. However, due to the diminished volume and hypotension, oxygen delivery is significantly impaired. Administration of oxygen is of limited value in such conditions unless cardiac output is restored.

Cardiac Output

Cardiovascular diseases responsible for alteration in the heart rate, preload, afterload, and myocardial contractility adversely affect oxygen supply. The examples include hypovolemia, sepsis, myocardial dysfunction due to ischemia or myocarditis, and pulmonary thromboembolism. Oxygen therapy is useful as a supplement to the primary treatment of the disease and should be administered in a higher concentration of 60 to 100% for a few hours. Prolongation of oxygen therapy is likely to cause problems of oxygen toxicity without accruing significant benefits.

Anemia

Chronic anemias are well tolerated by most patients as time is available for acclimatization to reduced supply by enhancing extraction (this is indicated by low venous oxygen saturation). On the contrary, acute anemia resulting from massive bleeding or intravascular hemolysis is tolerated poorly. Administration of a high concentration of oxygen is used as a short-term measure while blood volume is being replaced. Oxygen is temporarily useful in acquired methemoglobinemia, especially when severe. Methemoglobinemia is generally seen following toxic exposure to drugs or chemicals such as nitrates, nitrites, sulfonamides, and chlorates. Oxygen is an integral part of therapy for acute sickle cell crises as hypoxia (and acidosis) aggravates sickling crises. A critical form of histotoxic hypoxemia where oxygen is of definite help is acute carbon monoxide poisoning caused by carboxyhemoglobinemia (COHb). Given the higher affinity of carbon monoxide compared to oxygen to hemoglobin (× 210) and the reversible nature of the binding, 100% oxygen is used to displace carbon monoxide. Oxygen reduces the half-life of COHb from about 320 minutes to 60 to 80 minutes. HBOT reduces the half-life of COHb to 20 to 25 minutes and is an indication for HBOT.

Other Indications

Cluster Headache

Oxygen has been found helpful in the treatment of cluster headaches. It is administered at 7 to 8 liters/minute for about 10–15 minutes via a face mask. Significant relief is demonstrable in about 75% of patients. The effect is attributed to cerebral vasoconstriction due to oxygen administration.

Palliative Care

Patients with terminal illnesses and advanced cancers have breathlessness as a common symptom. Dyspnea is due to pulmonary involvement by cancer, worsening of concurrent cardiopulmonary disease, pulmonary embolism, anemia, and physical deconditioning. Oxygen is frequently used to reduce breathlessness. Oxygen is commonly observed to diminish the anxiety and discomfort associated with respiratory distress. There are few RCTs on the palliative role of domiciliary oxygen. In a study of 38 patients with primary or secondary lung cancer, oxygen and air were shown to ease the symptom of dyspnea regardless of the patient's arterial oxygen saturation, suggesting that it is more important to meet the patient's heightened minute ventilation. It was suggested that a trial of 15-minute oxygen therapy at 4 liters/min should be given to identify patients who are likely to benefit from the treatment. It was also suggested that opioids and benzodiazepines might potentiate the effect of oxygen. The palliative role of oxygen for breathlessness of advanced COPD, heart failure, and cancer was examined by the Working Party of the Association of Palliative Medicine Science Committee. The Committee suggested the need to tailor the oxygen use to the individual and a formal assessment of its efficacy to reduce breathlessness and improve the quality of life for that individual patient. In India in particular, it is also comforting for the near and dear ones of a dying patient to see that oxygen is being provided before the final death, and this is especially important where palliative care services are limited, and morphine and benzodiazepines are seldom used.

Surgical Indications for Oxygen Therapy

Abnormalities of gas exchange in surgical patients are present in those with lung diseases and in others, both during the surgical procedure and in the postoperative period.

Intraoperative

Oxygen is routinely administered during anesthesia and surgery. Oxygen administration is also employed during endoscopic and interventional procedures, even in the absence of anesthesia, especially in patients with a history of respiratory disease. Pre-oxygenation helps to reduce the anxiety of surgery, besides the improvements in oxygen reserves.

Postoperative

Pulmonary complications, especially infection, atelectasis, and thromboembolism, are frequent in postoperative patients. The complications are encountered in smokers, obese, age > 60 years, and pre-existing lung disease. Mild to moderate hypoxemia is expected in the first few hours after general anesthesia, especially when abdominal or thoracic surgery has been done, attributed to ventilation-perfusion mismatch. Central and peripheral ventilatory depression due to residual effects of anesthetic and pain-relieving drugs, shivering after anesthesia, and some degree of diffusion defect may also contribute to hypoxemia. The effects of this hypoxemia are likely to be serious in the presence of pre-existing risk factors or preoperative low arterial oxygen tension. Such patients would require oxygen therapy for several hours depending upon the levels of PaO_2 until fully awake and vital signs are normal and stable. Most patients require only small increases in FiO_2 administered with nasal cannulae at flow rates of 5 to 6 L/min.

In patients undergoing peripheral surgery, oxygen is generally not required unless complications occur.

SUGGESTED READING

1. Al-Waili NS, Butler GJ, Beale J, Abdullah MS, Hamilton RW, Lee BY, Lucus P, Allen MW, Petrillo RL, Carrey Z, Finkelstein M. Hyperbaric oxygen in the treatment of patients with cerebral stroke, brain trauma, and neurologic disease. Adv Ther. 2005;22:659–78.
2. Barrot L, Asfar P, Mauny F, Winiszewski H, Montini F, Badie J, et al; LOCO2 Investigators and REVA Research Network. Liberal or conservative oxygen therapy for acute respiratory distress syndrome. N Engl J Med. 2020;382(11):999-1008
3. Belda FJ, Aguilera L, deLaAsunicion JG, et al. Supplemental perioperative oxygen and the risk of surgical wound infection. A randomized controlled Trial. JAMA. 2005; 294:2035–42.
4. Bennett M, Jepson N, Lehm J. Hyperbaric oxygen therapy for acute coronary syndrome. Cochrane Database Syst Rev. 2005;18:CD004818.
5. Bennett MH, Wasiak J, Schnabel A, Kranke P, French C. Hyperbaric oxygen therapy for acute ischemic stroke. Cochrane Database Syst Rev. 2005;20:CD004954.
6. Booth S, Kelly MJ, Cox NP, Adams L, Guz A. Does oxygen help dyspnea in patients with cancer? Am J Respir Crit Care Med. 1996;153:1515–18.
7. Booth S, Wade R, Johnson M, Kite S, Swannick M, Anderson H. The use of oxygen in the palliation of breathlessness. A Report of the Expert Working

Group of the Scientific Committee of the Association of Palliative Medicine. Respir Med. 2004; 98:66–77.

8. Brostrom A, Hubbert L, Jakobsson P, Johansson P, Fridlung B, Dahlstrom U. Effects of long-term nocturnal oxygen treatment in patients with severe heart failure. J Cardiovasc Nurs. 2005; 20:385–96.
9. Carson S, McDonagh M, Russman B, Helfand M. Hyperbaric oxygen therapy for stroke: A systematic review of the evidence. Clin Rehabil. 2005;19:819–33.
10. Chu DK, Kim LH, Young PJ, Zamiri N, Almenawer SA, Jaeschke R, Szczeklik W, Schünemann HJ, Neary JD, Alhazzani W. Mortality and morbidity in acutely ill adults treated with liberal versus conservative oxygen therapy (IOTA): A systematic review and meta-analysis. Lancet. 2018;391 (10131):1693–1705.
11. De La Morandiere KP, Walter D. Oxygen therapy in acute stroke. Emerg Med J. 2003; 20:547.
12. Ding Z, Tong WC, Lu XX, Peng HP. Hyperbaric oxygen therapy in acute ischemic stroke: A review. Interv Neurol. 2014;2(4):201–11.
13. Emerman CL. Treatment of the acute decompensation of heart failure: Efficacy and pharmacoeconomics of early initiation of therapy in the emergency department. Rev Cardiovasc Med. 2003;4 Suppl 7:S13-20.
14. Fairley HB. Oxygen therapy for surgical patients. Am Rev Respir Dis. 1980; 122:37–44.
15. Fawole B, Hofmeyr GJ. Maternal oxygen administration for fetal distress. Cochrane Database Syst Rev. 2003; (4):CD000136.
16. Fillmore SJ, Shapiro M, Killip T. Arterial oxygen tension in acute myocardial infarction: Serial analysis of clinical state and blood gas changes. Am Heart J. 1970;79:620–29.
17. Flynn EP, Auer RN. Eubaric hyperoxemia and experimental cerebral infarction. Ann Neurol. 2002; 52:566–72.
18. Fulmer JD, Snider GL. American College of Chest Physicians—National Heart, Lung and Blood Institute Conference on Oxygen Therapy. Arch Intern Med. 1984; 144:1645–55.
19. Garcia-Botello SA, Garcia-Granero E, Lillo R, Lopez-Mozos F, Millan M, Lledo S. Randomized clinical trial to evaluate the effects of perioperative supplemental oxygen administration on the colorectal anastomosis. Br J Surg. 2006; 93:698–706.
20. Girardis M, Busani S, Damiani E, Donati A, Rinaldi L, Marudi A, et al. Effect of conservative vs conventional oxygen therapy on mortality among patients in an intensive care unit: The oxygen-ICU randomized clinical trial. JAMA. 2016;316(15):1583–89.
21. Helms AK, Whelan HT, Torbey MT. Hyperbaric oxygen therapy of cerebral ischemia. Cerebrovasc Dis. 2005; 20:417–26.
22. Hofmann R, James SK, Svensson L, Witt N, Frick M, Lindahl B, Östlund O, Ekelund U, Erlinge D, Herlitz J, Jernberg T. Determination of the role

of oxygen in suspected acute myocardial infarction trial. Am Heart J. 2014;167(3):322–8.

23. JH Park, S Balmain, C Berry, JJ Morton, JJ McMurray. Potentially detrimental cardiovascular effects of oxygen in patients with chronic left ventricular systolic dysfunction. Heart. 2010; 96: 533–38.
24. Kabon B, Kurz A. Optimal perioprative oxygen administration. Curr Opin Anesthesiol. 2006; 19:11–8.
25. Kudrow L. Response of cluster headaches to oxygen inhalation. Headache. 1981; 21:1.
26. Leigh JM. Postoperative oxygen administration. Br J Anesth 1975; 47:108.
27. Mackle D, Bellomo R, Bailey M, Beasley R, Deane A, Eastwood G, et al; ICU-ROX Investigators the Australian and New Zealand Intensive Care Society Clinical Trials Group. Conservative oxygen therapy during mechanical ventilation in the ICU. N Engl J Med. 2020;382(11):989–98.
28. Madias JE, Madias NE, Hood WB Jr. Precordial ST segment mapping: II. Effects of oxygen inhalation on ischemic injury in patients with acute myocardial infarction. Circulation. 1976; 53:411–17.
29. Mak S, Azevedo ER, Liu PP, Newton GE. Effect of hyperoxia on left ventricular function and filling pressures in patients with and without congestive heart failure. Chest. 2001;120(2):467–73.
30. Maroko PR, Radvany P, Braunwald E. Reduction of infarct size by oxygen inhalation following acute coronary occlusion. Circulation. 1975; 52:360–8.
31. Nicholson C. A Systematic review of the effectiveness of oxygen in reducing acute myocardial ischemia. J Clin Nurs. 2004; 13:996–1007.
32. Pancioli AM, Bullard MJ, Grulee ME, Jauch EC, Perkis DF. Supplemental oxygen use in ischemic stroke patients: Does utilization correspond to need for oxygen therapy? Arch Intern Med. 2002; 162;49–52.
33. Rawles JM, Kenmure ACF. Controlled trial of oxygen in uncomplicated myocardial infarction. Br Med J. 1976; 1:1121–4.
34. Rehder K. Anesthesia and respiratory system. Can Anesth Soc J. 1979; 26:451–62.
35. Rincon F, Kang J, Maltenfort M, Vibbert M, Urtecho J, Athar MK et al. Association between hyperoxia and mortality after stroke: A multicenter cohort study. Crit Care Med. 2014;42(2):387–96.
36. Roffe C, Nevatte T, Sim J, Bishop J, Ives N, Ferdinand P, Gray R; Stroke Oxygen Study Investigators and the Stroke OxygenStudy Collaborative Group. Effect of Routine Low-Dose Oxygen Supplementation on Death and Disability in Adults with Acute Stroke: The Stroke Oxygen Study Randomized Clinical Trial. JAMA. 2017;26;318(12):1125–35.
37. Ronning OM, Guldvag B. Should stroke victims routinely receive supplemental oxygen? A quasi-randomized controlled trial. Stroke. 1999; 30:2033–37.

38. Rotsztain A, Shugoll GI, Lloyd RA. Hypoxemia in acute myocardial infarction and in coronary insufficiency. Am J Med Sci. 1973; 266:253–60.
39. Sakakibara M, Sakata Y, Usui K, Hayama Y, Kanda S, Wada N, Matsui Y, Suto Y, Shimura S, Tanabe T. Effectiveness of short-term treatment with nocturnal oxygen therapy for central sleep apnea in patients with congestive heart failure. J Cardiol 2005; 46:53–61.
40. Sasayama S, Izumi T, Seino Y, Ueshima K, Asanoi H. Effects of nocturnal oxygen therapy on outcome measures in patients with chronic heart failure and cheyne-stokes respiration. Circ J 2006; 70:1–7.
41. Schjorring OL, Klitgaard TL, Perner A, Wetterslev J, Lange T, Siegemund M, et al; HOT-ICU Investigators. Lower or higher oxygenation targets for acute hypoxemic respiratory failure. N Engl J Med. 2021;384(14): 1301–11.
42. Singhal AB, Benner T, Roccatagliata L, Koroshetz WJ, Schaefer PW, Lo EH, Buonanno FS, Gonzalez RG, Sorensen AG. A pilot study of normobaric oxygen therapy in acute ischemic stroke. Stroke. 2005; 36:797–802.
43. Singhal AB, Dijkhuizen RM, Rosen BR, Lo EH. Normobaric hyperoxia reduces mri diffusion abnormalities and infarct size in experimental stroke. Neurology. 2002; 58:945–52.
44. Snider GL, Rinaldo JE. Oxygen therapy in medical patients outside the intensive care unit. Am Rev Respir Dis. 1980; 122:29–36.
45. Stringer E, McParland C, Hernandez P. Physician practices for prescribing supplemental oxygen in the palliative care setting. J Palliat Care. 2004; 20:303–7.
46. Stub D, Smith K, Bernard S, Bray JE, Stephenson M, Cameron P, Meredith I, Kaye DM; AVOID Study. A randomized controlled trial of oxygen therapy in acute myocardial infarction: Air Verses Oxygen in Myocar Dial Infarction Study (AVOID Study). Am Heart J. 2012;163(3):339–45.
47. Tallach RE, Ball DR. Routine pre-oxygenation. Anesthesia. 2004; 59: 943–5.
48. Valencia A, Burgess JH. Arterial hypoxemia following acute myocardial infarction. Circulation. 1969; 40:641.
49. WA Haque, J Boehmer, BS Clemson, UA Leuenberger, DH Silber, LI Sinoway. Hemodynamic effects of supplemental oxygen administration in congestive heart failure. J Am Coll Cardiol. 1996; 27: 353–57.

Chapter 12

Oxygen Therapy for COVID-19 Infection

Aditya Jindal

INTRODUCTION

Since the end of the year 2019, the world has been devastated by the novel coronavirus pandemic. Originating in Wuhan, China the novel coronavirus or COVID-19 spread all over the world in a matter of months. It led to weeks of lockdowns and unprecedented scenes of hospitals and national health care systems being overwhelmed by the mass of patients involved at the same time. Oxygen supplementation has emerged as the major lifeline, so to speak, for these patients.

CLINICAL CHARACTERISTICS

COVID-19 is an enveloped, positive stranded RNA virus, belonging to the *betacoronoviridae* genera of coronaviruses. It enters the cell by binding to the ACE 2 (angiotensin converting enzyme) receptor. These receptors are most common in the lungs, gastrointestinal tract and the kidneys, so these organs are the most commonly involved in this disease. The virus binds to the S1 spike protein of the receptor and enters the cell by endocytosis. After entering the cytoplasm of the cell the virus starts replicating and produces structural, non-structural and accessory proteins. The new virus particles are enveloped and then released into the extracellular space to infect other cells.

The clinical features of COVID-19 infection follow a biphasic pattern. The initial phase of illness consists of viral replication and lasts for approximately 1 week. During this phase the virus replicates in host cells and leads to the initial symptoms of fever, cough, sore throat, nasal congestion, fatigue, loss of smell and taste, etc. Most of the time this stage leads to clinical resolution as the host immune response clears the virus from the body and the patient recovers with minor symptoms. Some patients will develop viral pneumonitis and experience breathlessness and hypoxia, corresponding to the appearance of ground glass opacities on chest imaging.

However, in a few patients, persistent viral replication triggers off a sustained immune response, which becomes dysfunctional and leads to the severe effects of COVID. This phase, which is known by various names such as cytokine storm, hyper-inflammatory phase, etc., is the mainly responsible for the morbidity and mortality of COVID, and is characterized by the development of hypoxia, acute respiratory distress syndrome (ARDS), respiratory failure, thromboembolism, shock, etc.

ARDS is a clinical syndrome characterized by the presence of bilateral pulmonary infiltrates on chest imaging not explained by cardiac disease or fluid overload, acute onset of symptoms and hypoxia. There is a breach of the alveolar capillary barrier associated with acute inflammation in the lungs, increased vascular permeability, reduced compliance and ventilation perfusion mismatch resulting in increased work of breathing and hypoxia. Pathologically, there is a diffuse alveolar damage, with destruction of the alveolar capillary membrane, increased vascular permeability, formation of hyaline membranes in the alveoli, intra-capillary thrombosis, alveolar flooding and collapse.

COVID-19 is also characterized by the increased occurrence of thromboembolism, both arterial and venous. COVID-19 is associated not only with increased chances of conventional thromboembolism but also with increased pulmonary capillary micro thrombosis and angiogenesis. Patients with COVID have elevated level of d-dimers; the systemic proinflammatory state also contributes to the high chances of thromboembolism.

PATHOPHYSIOLOGY

When the virus binds the ACE-2 receptor and enters the host cells, a sequence of events is set in motion, involving the recruitment of inflammatory cells, production of proinflammatory cytokines and chemical mediators. Although protective in most cases, in certain individuals this host response may turn hyper-inflammatory, leading to further worsening.

Viral replication leads to the development of an immune response, with the recruitment of monocytes, activated macrophages and neutrophils. Monocytes release inflammatory cytokines such as tumor necrosis factor alpha (TNF-α) and interferons, leading to pneumocyte apoptosis. Activated macrophages release chemokines responsible for increased capillary permeability and neutrophil degranulation. Excess neutrophil degranulation leads to damage to both the respiratory epithelium and the capillary endothelium, leading to breach of the alveolar capillary barrier. Breach of the alveolar capillary barrier leads to flooding of the alveolar space with serum proteins, formation of hyaline membranes, alveolar and interstitial edema, culminating in ARDS.

Pathology

The pathology of COVID-19 follows that of conventional respiratory pathogens with certain peculiarities. The pathological picture is that of a diffuse alveolar damage. The first or exudative phase of illness—corresponding to the stage of viremia—is characterized by disruption of the alveolar capillary barrier leading to the extravasation of serum proteins and red blood cells into the alveolus. Alongside there is leakage of tissue fluid into the interstitium, and intense intra-alveolar inflammatory cell infiltrate. All this leads to the formation of intra-alveolar hyaline membranes. Radiologically, this corresponds to the presence of circumscribed areas of ground glass opacities and crazy paving.

The second or proliferative phase is characterized by intense activation of myofibroblasts and fibroblast proliferation and activation leading to the formation of either organizing pneumonia or acute fibrinous organizing pneumonia. This is manifested as worsening of ground glassing and development of widespread patches of consolidation. Subsequently, further progression leads to the third or fibrotic phase where there is deposition of extracellular matrix and subsequent pulmonary fibrosis. Radiologically, this manifests as traction bronchiectasis and fibrosis and is known clinically as post COVID fibrosis.

These phases do not occur uniformly throughout the lungs but may occur simultaneously in different areas. So, some areas of the lung may have active viral pneumonitis while some may have organizing pneumonia while others may show some amount of fibrotic changes. This correlates to the presence of ground glass opacities, consolidation and traction bronchiectasis in the same CT (computed tomography) scan. However, it can be said that there is a rough temporal sequence of causes of hypoxia seen in different clinical manifestations of COVID-19 which can be traced chronologically **(Table 12.1)**.

Table 12.1: Causes of hypoxia in COVID-19 depending upon different clinico-pathological manifestations.
1. Viral pneumonitis
2. ARDS
3. Cytokine storm syndrome
4. Pulmonary embolism
5. Pulmonary intracapillary microthrombosis
6. Pulmonary fibrosis

In addition, extensive intracapillary microthrombosis and conventional pulmonary embolism may also occur. Intracapillary microthrombosis is predisposed to by the formation of neutrophil extracellular traps or NETs which are formed when activated neutrophils degranulate and dump pro-inflammatory chemokines in the extracellular space. Some studies have described pulmonary microthrombi in vessels of 1–2 mm diameter in the pulmonary capillary circulation in 50–60% of patients. Elevated levels of d-dimers and the general pro-inflammatory and pro-coagulant state further exacerbates this problem and predisposes to conventional large vessel pulmonary thromboembolism.

Tricompartmental Model

A tricompartmental model to explain the high incidence of pulmonary infarction and hypoxia has recently been proposed. In the normal lung the oxygen supply to the lung tissue is from three sources—the pulmonary arteries, the bronchial arteries and directly from the alveolus through inspired air. The pulmonary arteries carry 100% of the cardiac output to the lungs but carry deoxygenated blood. On the other hand, the bronchial arteries, which arise from the aorta, carry only 1% of the cardiac output to the lungs but carry oxygenated blood. They serve as a major source of oxygen to the lung parenchyma. The pulmonary and bronchial arteries have an extensive anastomotic network at the pre-capillary, alveolar capillary and the post capillary level. The bronchial veins also anastomose with the pulmonary veins and drain directly into the left atrium.

Conventional pulmonary embolism involves mainly large sized pulmonary arteries. The incidence of infarction and hypoxia is less because the bronchial arteries, which carry oxygenated blood to the lungs, are not involved. However, in case of COVID-19, all the three compartments of the oxygen supply to the lungs are involved, i.e., the pulmonary arterioles, the bronchial arteries and the alveolus. So the oxygen supply to the lung parenchyma is critically reduced in COVID-19, which leads to a high index of pulmonary infarction and hypoxia.

Happy Hypoxia

It has been noticed that patients suffering from COVID-19 infection present with low oxygen saturation levels in the absence of or with minimal dyspnea or discomfort. This condition has been termed happy hypoxia or silent hypoxia and one might see this situation in many patients whose oxygen saturation is in the 80s or even 70s and who are sitting comfortably without any major discomfort!

Many theories and physiological explanations have been put forward to explain this phenomenon. These are as follows:

- Hypoxia is sensed mainly by the carotid bodies from afferent signals are transmitted upto the medulla oblongata in the brain. From here, efferent signals are transmitted by the phrenic nerves to the diaphragm, which leads to increased minute ventilation. However, the increased minute ventilation itself is not enough to cause dyspnea or discomfort in breathing, which is a subjective and not objective sensation. Fibers projecting to the cerebral cortex from the medulla oblongata are transmit any heightened activity to the cortex and it this increased cortical activity which is responsible for dyspnea. This might be different in COVID.
- The co-existence of hypercapnia strongly influences the development of dyspnea. In COVID patients the carbon dioxide levels are mostly low or in the normal range. This might be an additional factor why patients with COVID are not dyspneic.
- A large number of patients with COVID are elderly and have diabetes mellitus. Both these conditions blunt the response to hypoxia.
- The oxygen dissociation curve shifts to the right in patients with fever. So, febrile patients would have higher levels of PaO_2 (partial pressure of oxygen in blood) at similar levels of oxygen saturation as compared to non-febrile ones. Dyspnea and increased minute ventilation is mainly a response to low PaO_2 levels rather than to low oxygen saturation. So this can be another factor why these patients are less dyspneic.

- Most of these patients are managed by oxygen saturation which requires a simple percutaneous probe rather than with PaO_2 levels, which require arterial blood sampling and measurement. In patients with critical illness the probe may be less reliable at picking up saturation levels. There may be a difference of almost 4% between blood measurements and probe ones.
- There is also a putative idiosyncratic effect of the virus on the respiratory control system which is responsible for the development of silent hypoxia.

TREATMENT

Most of the patients in this pandemic have been mildly symptomatic and did not need any treatment. However, a significant number ranging from 5–15% were sicker and required only supplemental oxygen therapy or non-invasive ventilation; mechanical ventilation was required in a minority. Oxygen has literally been lifesaving and is used in different phases of the illness, from prophylactic use at homes to high flow oxygen in the admitted patient and ling term used in patients with permanent lung damage.

There is an acute need to identify patients at need for supplemental oxygen. While it may be painfully obvious in a patient with frank respiratory failure and distress, the indication for prescription of oxygen may be difficult in cases who have mild or moderate symptoms. These patients may or may not deteriorate further and need to be followed up regularly, which may be extremely difficult because of logistical, medical, social, financial and/or other issues.

Some studies have described clinical and biochemical biomarkers for initiating oxygen therapy in less symptomatic individuals whose oxygen levels are fluctuating or borderline. A retrospective observational study of over eight hundred patients noted that the presence of respiratory failure associated symptoms such as fever, increased respiratory rate, respiratory distress and dyspnea were associated were predictive of and increased need of oxygen during the course of illness. Also, biochemical markers like low albumin and globulin were also associated with a higher odds ratio of requirement of supplemental oxygen.

Pulse oximetry has been used extensively in the pandemic for both domiciliary and hospital based monitoring of oxygen saturation. Criteria based on oxygen saturation use have been widely disseminated among the general public and medical professionals for identifying clinical deterioration. However, along with oxygen levels, other parameters provided by the oximeter are also useful in identifying patients at risk of deterioration. Increased respiratory efforts in hypoxemic patients leading to wide swings in pleural pressure have been associated with self inflicted lung injury. Quantification and monitoring of these pressure swings generally requires a pleural or esophageal probe, which is not feasible in routine clinical settings, either outpatient or inpatient. However, these pressure swings are also reflected in the pulse oximetry waveform, where the term 'pulsus paradoxus' has been used to describe them. Sufficiently large changes can also be identified by simple physical examination. An index of pulse volume variability also known as the pleth variability index (PVI) can be calculated and used to approximate respiratory efforts and the need for further treatment.

Acute Care

Prophylactic Oxygen

Patients with early COVID infection may have elevated levels of hypoxia inducible factor 1α (HIF-1α). High levels of this factor lead to the development of an inflammatory cascade and has been proposed to be involved in the development of the cytokine storm syndrome and hypercoagulable state in the second phase of COVID. Thus, it has been proposed that early and prophylactic initiation of oxygen therapy can prevent this stage from happening. Also, it has been proposed that prophylactic use of oxygen might inhibit viral replication by improving the body's immune responses. Nocturnal oxygen therapy has been proposed to be used in the early phases of COVID infection. However, this has remained a speculation and no proof is yet available as to its efficacy.

Therapeutic Oxygen

Respiratory disease due to COVID-19 is treated like any other respiratory illness, with fluid management, monitoring, other supportive care and oxygen administration. Oxygen can be given by conventional methods like nasal cannulae, venturi masks or non-rebreathing masks or by newer techniques like high frequency nasal cannula (HFNC). The flow and rate of oxygen administration depends upon the severity of the disease and is titrated according to standard principles and guidelines.

HFNC

HFNC consists of delivering high flow heated and humidified oxygen to the patient though a nasal cannula. Extremely high flow rates (40–60 L/min on average) and high concentration of inspired oxygen can be achieved with this device. It consists of a flow meter attached to a piped oxygen supply capable of supplying high flow rates of oxygen. An air blender further mixes the oxygen with air according to the settings and a humidifier heats and humidifies the mixture. The oxygen-air mixture (with fraction of inspired oxygen going up to 1) is delivered through a nasal cannula as mentioned earlier.

The advantage of this system are manifold. First, need for invasive mechanical ventilation is reduced. Second, as the inspired air flow and oxygen concentration can be matched up with the patient demand, it is more physiological and better tolerated. Thirdly, because pre-heated and humidified oxygen is delivered there is preservation of the muco-ciliary mechanism and less chances of drying of airway secretions, atelectasis and infections. Fourth, the high flow rate generates positive end-expiratory pressure, which is helpful in maintaining alveolar collapse and atelectasis.

There has been concern that the high flow rates associated with HFNC may lead to aerosolization of coronavirus particles and secondary infections in health care workers. Contradictory reports are available regarding this issue and no satisfactory conclusion can be drawn at present. Simple techniques like putting surgical masks over the nasal cannulae have shown significant reduction in aerosolization. However, till further data is available, health care workers in the critical care units caring for patients on HFNC should wear complete personal protective equipment.

Comparison with Non-invasive Ventilation (NIV)

There have concerns about the use and effectiveness of HFNC in COVID patients despite its widespread use. The concerns include potential delay in invasive mechanical ventilation, spread of infection to health care workers and doubts about efficacy as compared to NIV, i.e., continuous positive airway pressure and bilevel positive airway pressure. Till further data is available, it would be the treating physicians personal choice based on availability, feasibility, expense, expertise and other such factors which would decide choice of treatment modality.

Prone Positioning

Use of prone positioning was one of the features of the COVID pandemic. Prone posture was used during all stages of acute illness, from patients with mild illness to those with severe ARDS (acute respiratory distress syndrome). In ARDS, proning has been recommended for upto 16 hours per day while the duration in less severe illness has not yet been formalized.

Prone positioning has been postulated to produce a multitude of physiological changes which benefit oxygenation. Change to the prone position redistributes blood flow to allow for better ventilation perfusion matching and hence better oxygenation. It also results in a more uniform pleural pressure gradient leading to a more uniform alveolar size. The prone position also leads to relief of compression of the left lung by the heart, better systemic hemodynamics and better secretion clearance.

Other than steroid use in indicated cases, prone positioning was the only modality shown to improve indices of oxygenation and mortality rates in COVID.

Ozone therapy: Ozone has been tried in respiratory disease for a long time, with no solid data to back its use. The putative mechanism of action in COVID is cytotoxic effects through free radical generation and also by immune-modulation of the cell mediated immune system. This should be considered experimental.

Chronic Care

Patients who have recovered from the acute phase of COVID can still be left with significant lung damage or fibrosis. This was common enough in the pandemic to merit a name of its own—'post COVID lung fibrosis.' Commonly, the basal and peripheral areas of the lung are involved, corresponding to the earlier ground glass opacities. However, some patients may present with extensive lung fibrosis. Interestingly, the distribution of fibrosis is different from that in conventional (non-COVID) ARDS survivors where the fibrosis is predominantly anterior.

Various theories have been put forward regarding post COVID fibrosis, comparing the pathophysiology with that of idiopathic lung fibrosis (IPF) and progressive fibrosing interstitial lung diseases (PF-ILD). Similar to the use of antifibrotics in these conditions, they have also been tried in post COVID fibrosis with limited success.

Domiciliary oxygen use for these patients is the only option other than lung transplantation. Oxygen can be provided by oxygen concentrators or cylinders, depending upon availability and resources. Guidelines for oxygen use follow that meant for any chronic lung disease. It should be mentioned that it is important not to label these patients as chronic as a significant number would improve over time and be oxygen independent despite the amount of fibrosis visible on chest imaging at outset!

AFTERWORD

The COVID pandemic was marked by the large volume of cases worldwide, leading to overwhelmed healthcare systems. In this scenario, understanding of basic physiological principles and of simple measures like oxygen support and prone positioning helped in significantly reducing the morbidity and mortality.

SUGGESTED READING

1. Batah SS, Fabro AT. Pulmonary pathology of ARDS in COVID-19: A pathological review for clinicians. Respir Med. 2021;176:106239. doi: 10.1016/j.rmed.2020.106239. Epub 2020 Nov 19. PMID: 33246294; PMCID: PMC7674971.
2. Chalmers JD, Crichton ML, Goeminne PC, Cao B, Humbert M, Shteinberg M, Antoniou KM, Ulrik CS, Parks H, Wang C, Vandendriessche T, Qu J, Stolz D, Brightling C, Welte T, Aliberti S, Simonds AK, Tonia T, Roche N. Management of hospitalised adults with coronavirus disease 2019 (COVID-19): A European Respiratory Society living guideline. Eur Respir J. 2021;57(4):2100048. doi: 10.1183/13993003.00048-2021. PMID: 33692120; PMCID: PMC7947358.
3. Johnson NJ, Luks AM, Glenny RW. Gas exchange in the prone posture. Respir care. 2017;62(8):1097–1110. doi: 10.4187/respcare.05512. Epub 2017 May 30. PMID: 28559471.
4. McGonagle D, Bridgewood C, Meaney JFM. A tricompartmental model of lung oxygenation disruption to explain pulmonary and systemic pathology in severe COVID-19. Lancet Respir Med. 2021;9(6): 665–72. doi: 10.1016/S2213-2600(21)00213-7. Epub 2021 May 14. PMID: 34000237; PMCID: PMC8121498.
5. Michard F, Shelley K, L'Her E. COVID-19: Pulse oximeters in the spotlight. J Clin Monit Comput. 2021;35(1):11–14. doi: 10.1007/s10877-020-00550-7. Epub 2020 Jun 23. Erratum in: J Clin Monit Comput. 2020;PMID: 32578070; PMCID: PMC7308445.

6. Ni Y-N, Wang T, Liang B-m, Liang Z-A. The independent factors associated with oxygen therapy in COVID-19 patients under 65 years old. PLoS ONE 16(1): e0245690.
7. Procopio G, Cancelliere A, Trecarichi EM, Mazzitelli M, Arrighi E, Perri G, Serapide F, Pelaia C, Lio E, Busceti MT, Pelle MC, Ricchio M, Scaglione V, Davoli C, Fusco P, La Gamba V, Torti C, Pelaia G. Oxygen therapy via high flow nasal cannula in severe respiratory failure caused by sars-Cov-2 infection: A real-life observational study. Ther Adv Respir Dis. 2020 Jan-Dec;14:1753466620963016. doi: 10.1177/1753466620963016. PMID: 33070706; PMCID: PMC7580191.
8. Rali AS, Nunna KR, Howard C, Herlihy JP, Guntupalli KK. High-flow nasal cannula oxygenation revisited in COVID-19. Card Fail Rev. 2020;6:e08. doi: 10.15420/cfr.2020.06. PMID: 32377387; PMCID: PMC7199186.
9. Tobin MJ, Laghi F, Jubran A. Why COVID-19 silent hypoxemia is baffling to physicians. Am J Respir Crit Care Med. 2020;202(3):356-360. doi: 10.1164/rccm.202006-2157CP. PMID: 32539537; PMCID: PMC7397783.

Chapter 13

Long-term Oxygen Therapy

Ritesh Agarwal, SK Jindal

Long-term oxygen therapy (LTOT) is used for managing chronic respiratory failure (CRF) secondary to various respiratory disorders. When first introduced, domiciliary LTOT was limited mainly to patients with chronic obstructive pulmonary disease (COPD) and CRF. Subsequently, the indications have expanded to include any chronic respiratory disease characterized by hypoxic organ damage, including interstitial lung disease, bronchiectasis, cystic fibrosis, kyphoscoliosis, sleep apnea syndrome, severe cardiac failure, and others. Domiciliary oxygen has also been tried in patients with breathing disorders who experience hypoxemia only during sleep or exercise but not when alert and awake. We believe that the selection criteria required for LTOT are more important than the underlying disease.

SELECTION OF PATIENTS

All patients with CRF are potential candidates for LTOT. The following guidelines are helpful in selecting patients for LTOT:

- A definitive documented diagnosis of the respiratory disease responsible for chronic hypoxemia.
- Optimal medical treatment in place.
- Patients in a stable condition without any exacerbation of the underlying disease.
- Oxygen administration showing improvement in hypoxemia and clinical status.

The guide to prescribing LTOT is not $PaO_2 \leq 55$ mm Hg alone but the presence of a chronic hypoxemic pulmonary disease. LTOT will not benefit patients with dyspnea who are not hypoxemic. Healthy people living at an altitude of 10,000 feet or more do not require oxygen and can acclimatize to even severe degrees of hypoxemia. In fact, man has survived without oxygen, even at the summit of Mount

Everest (altitude 29,028 feet). The lack of ability to adapt to hypoxemia encountered in chronic pulmonary disease defines the need for LTOT.

BENEFITS

Long-term oxygen therapy is shown to benefit patients with COPD and CRF. There is limited experience with other chronic pulmonary hypoxemic diseases. In COPD, LTOT improves survival, exercise tolerance, cognitive mental function, and quality of life. There was an appreciable reduction in pulmonary hypertension and right ventricular failure attributable to supplemental domiciliary oxygen therapy when added to the optimal medical regimen.

LTOT IN PATIENTS WITH SIGNIFICANT ($PaO_2 \leq 55$ mm Hg) DAYTIME RESTING HYPOXEMIA

Two landmark studies, namely the Medical Research Council (MRC) trial and the nocturnal oxygen therapy trial (NOTT) have shown that continuous LTOT can improve survival in patients with COPD and resting daytime hypoxemia (**Fig. 13.1**).

The results of both the randomized controlled trials (RCTs) are summarized below:

Nocturnal Oxygen Therapy Trial (NOTT)

The NOTT was an open-label RCT that randomized 122 and 101 hypoxemic COPD patients to nocturnal and continuous oxygen therapy, respectively. The oxygen source was either an oxygen concentrator, liquid oxygen, or compressed gas (flow 1–4 liters/minute). The mean age was about 66 years, and most patients were men. The mean PaO_2, $PaCO_2$, and FEV_1 were 51 mm Hg, 43 mm Hg, and 29%, respectively, and were not different between the two groups. In the NOT group, 82% used oxygen for 13 hours or less, while 56% used oxygen for 19 hours or more in the continuous oxygen therapy group. There was a significant improvement in survival in the continuous oxygen therapy group. The overall mortality in the NOT group was 1.94 times that of the continuous oxygen therapy group. The continuous oxygen therapy group also showed improvement in stroke volume index, pulmonary vascular resistance, and pulmonary artery pressure than the NOT group.

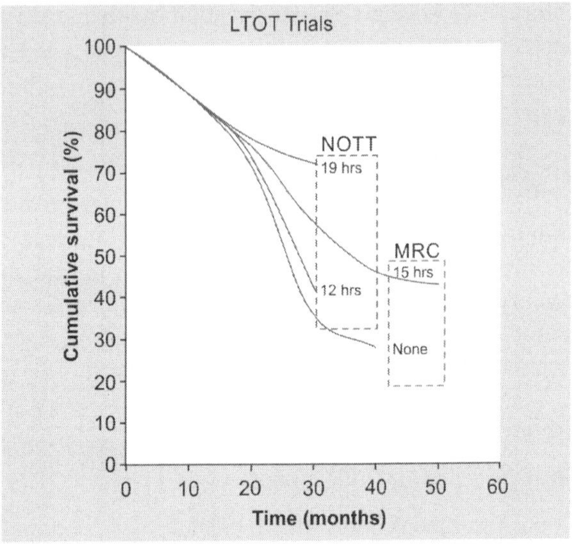

Fig. 13.1: Kaplan-Meier curve showing time to survival (in months) in subjects of the Nocturnal Oxygen Therapy Trial (NOTT) and the Medical Research Council (MRC) trials on long-term oxygen therapy (LTOT). There was increased time to survival in patients receiving LTOT (See the text for further details).

Medical Research Council (MRC) Oxygen Therapy Trial

Eighty-seven patients with a diagnosis of hypoxemic COPD (PaO_2 40–60 mm Hg) and right heart failure were randomized to receive continuous oxygen therapy (at least 15 hours a day at a flow of 2 liters/minute) or no oxygen. The study was not blinded. The mean age, FEV_1, PaO_2, and $PaCO_2$ were around 58 years, 0.7 liters, 50 mm Hg, and 54 mm Hg, respectively. There was an improvement in survival in the group receiving oxygen therapy (Peto odds ratio 0.42, 95% confidence intervals, 0.18–0.98) but only beyond 500 days of treatment. Although the total pulmonary resistance and the pulmonary artery pressure increased in the control group, this was not statistically significant.

Data from these two trials suggest a survival benefit with continuous oxygen therapy but not with NOT alone. Recent studies have also shown that LTOT can decrease hospitalization in patients with COPD. Importantly, oxygen should be taken for as long as possible, as hypoxemia-related pulmonary vascular changes could occur rapidly. The current indications for LTOT in COPD are summarized below **(Box 13.1)**.

Box 13.1: Indications for long-term oxygen therapy in patients with chronic obstructive pulmonary disease.

- PaO_2 ≤55 mm Hg (or SpO_2 <88%) at rest, in non-recumbent position.
- PaO_2 56–59 mm Hg (or SpO_2 89–92%) with demonstrable hypoxic organ dysfunction such as pulmonary hypertension or hematocrit ≥55% or CNS dysfunction.
- Demonstrable fall in PaO_2 <55 mm Hg during sleep associated with disturbed sleep pattern, cardiac arrhythmias, or pulmonary hypertension. These patients may benefit from nocturnal oxygen therapy.

LTOT IN PATIENTS WITH MILD DAYTIME RESTING HYPOXEMIA OR EXERCISE-INDUCED DESATURATION

Currently, there is no evidence for prescribing LTOT in patients with mild hypoxemia (PaO_2, 56-65 mm Hg). In one study, 135 patients with COPD, severe airflow limitation (FEV1 <1L), and PaO_2 of 56-65 mm Hg were randomly allocated to the control (n = 67) or LTOT (n = 68) group. The patients were followed every three months for at least three years or until death. There was neither any improvement in survival in patients treated with LTOT nor did more prolonged oxygen use (over 15 hours per day) improve the outcome. In the largest RCT on LTOT (LOTT trial), 738 patients with stable COPD and resting SpO_2 of 89-93% or moderate exercise-induced desaturation (SpO_2 ≥80% for ≥5 minutes and <90% for ≥10 seconds during a 6-minute walk test) were enrolled. Patients were randomly assigned to receive LTOT or no LTOT. In the LTOT group, patients with resting desaturation were prescribed 24-hour oxygen and those with exercise desaturation only during exercise and sleep. There was no significant difference in the time to death or first hospitalization, rates of all hospitalization, COPD exacerbations, COPD-related hospitalizations, quality of life, lung function, the 6-minute walk distance between the two groups. Thus, LTOT in COPD patients with mild daytime hypoxemia (56-60 mm Hg) should currently be considered only in those with hypercapnia, polycythemia, and evidence of pulmonary hypertension.

There is little evidence to show improved exercise tolerance in patients who use intermittent oxygen therapy prior to exercise. In the absence of any definite data, intermittent oxygen may be prescribed in individual patients where the benefits (dyspnea, exercise capacity) have been shown by exercise testing, especially in those awaiting lung transplantation or lung volume reduction surgery, to maintain an increased level of fitness before surgery. We also consider intermittent oxygen therapy in those with severe exercise-induced desaturation (SpO_2 <80% for more than one minute on exercise).

LTOT IN PATIENTS WITHOUT DAYTIME RESTING HYPOXEMIA BUT HYPOXEMIA DURING SLEEP

Patients with COPD can experience prolonged episodes of oxygen desaturation during rapid eye movement sleep. Studies indicate that nocturnal hypoxemia can exacerbate pulmonary hypertension in patients with COPD. However, in a recent large RCT of 243 patients (INOX trial), 39% (48/123) and 42% (50/119) assigned to nocturnal oxygen and placebo, respectively, met the criteria for LTOT or had died at 3 years of follow-up, and was not significantly different. Thus, there appears to be no role of LTOT in patients with nocturnal hypoxemia without daytime hypoxemia.

In patients with nocturnal hypoxemia without daytime hypoxemia, our practice is to exclude concomitant obstructive sleep apnea and intensify medical management (smoking cessation, long-acting beta-2 agonists, and antimuscarinic agents, inhaled corticosteroids, pulmonary rehabilitation). We prescribe LTOT if the patient has evidence of chronic hypoxia-related sequelae like polycythemia or pulmonary hypertension or if the SpO_2 repeatedly falls below 88% for more than one-third of the night.

INITIATION AND REASSESSMENT OF LTOT

Patients with COPD and FEV_1 <40% or pulmonary hypertension should be routinely screened for LTOT. Before prescribing LTOT, the indication should be confirmed on at least two occasions two to three weeks apart with a resting arterial blood gas analysis performed on room air. Patients should be stable on maximal and optimal medical therapy. It is vital to ensure that the patient is compliant with the medical treatment, including smoking cessation. Continued smoking aggravates the underlying disease, decreases the benefits of oxygen therapy, and poses a grave risk of accidental fires while on LTOT. We set the oxygen flow rate to maintain a PaO_2 >60 mm Hg (or SpO_2 >92%) during rest. Usually, 1-2 liters/minute through nasal prongs would suffice. Higher flow rates are required for those with other chronic respiratory diseases, especially ILD. The oxygen flow rate should be increased by 1 liter/minute during sleep, exertion, and air travel. Patients with AE-COPD who are prescribed supplemental oxygen at discharge from the hospital should be reassessed for LTOT after 4-6 weeks. The goal of LTOT should be confirmed by performing an arterial blood gas analysis after 1-2 months of initiating oxygen therapy and documenting a PaO_2 >60 mm Hg. A repeat blood gas analysis also helps in the assessment of the hypercapnic response to oxygen therapy. Patients with significant hypercapnia during LTOT may also require domiciliary noninvasive pressure support ventilation.

SUPPLY SOURCES

There are three main types of systems commercially available for oxygen supply at home, namely compressed gas cylinders, liquid oxygen, and oxygen concentrators.

Compressed Gas Cylinder

The commonly used gaseous system in the home consists of H or K cylinders (7,842 liters) containing compressed oxygen. A pressure regulator and a flow meter are required to adjust the amount delivered to the patient. When continuously used at 2 liters/minute, each cylinder will last about two-and-a-half days necessitating frequent fillings. They are also heavy, giving an unsightly look to the room. Moreover, regulation of pressure and flow requires some effort and additional help.

Nevertheless, compressed gas cylinders are most often used for domiciliary use in India because of their lower cost, lack of requirement for electricity, and easy availability compared to the other systems. Gas cylinders also form a good backup facility in case of a failure of other systems. Portable D and E cylinders are available for ambulatory use. Aluminum cylinders are better suited for portability as these are lighter in weight than the cast-iron cylinders; however, they are expensive.

Liquid Oxygen System

Liquid oxygen system (LOX) is a smaller version of the bulk liquid system used in the hospitals. The reservoir (stationary) unit contains about 70 to 90 pounds of liquid oxygen at –273°F. The oxygen lasts for

4 to 10 days at a continuous flow rate of 2 liters/minute. The vessel is about 3 to 4 feet tall and about 18 inches in diameter. The internal pressure is about 22 to 50 psi which can generate flow rates of 0.25 to 15 L/min. Besides the stationary unit, a lightweight, portable unit can be carried by the patient for ambulatory and outdoor activities. The portable units are designed to be safely filled from the stationary reservoir unit. There is a loss of gaseous oxygen from the liquid gas units at a rate of about 1 lb/day. Therefore, the units should not be stored in a small and closed space to avoid gaseous accumulation posing a fire hazard. A liquid gas system is more practical but expensive. Moreover, it is not readily available in India.

Oxygen Concentrator

It is an electrical device that provides oxygen from the atmospheric air. It employs a molecular sieve (zeolite) that filters out the nitrogen molecules, water vapor, and other trace gases. The concentrator can deliver 90% oxygen at flow rates of up to 5 liters/minute. The polymeric membrane concentrators can deliver 30% to 40% oxygen at flow rates of up to 10 liters/minute. A concentrator is ideal for use at home as it obviates the need for regular filling of the oxygen cylinders. Although the initial cost is high, the running cost is negligible. Proper maintenance of equipment and replacement of filters is required. A backup source of oxygen supply (e.g., compressed oxygen cylinder) is necessary in case of power failure. There is a generation of some noise and heat that some patients may find bothersome. This issue can be avoided by placing the concentrator in an adjacent room and using a longer oxygen tube. However, the longer tubing increases the backpressure necessitating a pressure compensated flow meter to assure accurate oxygen flow.

DELIVERY DEVICES

The devices used to deliver LTOT include nasal cannula and masks. Those are essentially the same as used in the hospitals (for details, see Chapter 21). Nasal cannulae are preferred because of cosmetic reasons. It is easy to conceal oxygen tubing by applying it to ordinary thick-rimmed frames of eyeglasses ("Oxyspecs"). Different kinds of "oxyspecs" and other devices are now commercially available for this purpose. There is no difference in the type of delivery devices used with different types of oxygen sources. Humidification is not essential at flow rates less than 4 liters/minute unless the patient complains of dryness of the nose or mouth, nasal irritation, or crusting. A humidifier is a potential source of infection and needs regular cleaning and disinfection. While disposable humidifiers are available, they significantly increase the cost.

OXYGEN-CONSERVING DEVICES

LTOT is a costly proposition. Many patients tend to conserve oxygen by reducing the flow as well as the duration of administration. Notably, the standard oxygen supply devices allow the flow of oxygen both during inspiration and expiration. Only 15 to 20% of the respiratory cycle is inspiration that delivers oxygen to the alveoli, indicating significant wastage of oxygen in the surroundings. Several methods have been devised to conserve oxygen in recent years. It is possible to save up to 50% oxygen with some of these methods. There are three types of devices commercially available for this purpose. The most used are the reservoir oxygen delivery devices. Other methods include electromechanical pulse devices and transtracheal catheters. In reservoir devices, oxygen is stored during exhalation in a reservoir (approximately 20 mL), which subsequently becomes available at the beginning of inhalation. There are two types of reservoir cannula:

Pendant Reservoir (Oxymizer Pendant)

The reservoir coupled to the nasal prongs consists of a collapsing chamber that hangs at the chest. It saves oxygen between 2: 1 to 4: 1 over continuous flow oxygen therapy.

Moustache Configured Oxymizer

The reservoir sits right on the face, thus being noticeable and cosmetically unsightly. Its efficiency is like that of a pendant reservoir.

Both the reservoirs provide equivalent oxygen saving at flow rates of 0.5 liters/min. However, the pendant reservoir can be operated at 0.25 liters/min to achieve oxygen saturation like those of a flow of 1 liter/minute with a steady flow delivery system. A pendant that allows pursed-lip breathing and oxygen saving mechanism increasing the efficiency of oxygen conservation to about 7: 1 compared with standard steady flow systems.

Electromechanical Pulsing Devices

The electromechanical demand devices deliver oxygen only during inhalation, thereby conserving oxygen delivery. It consists of a box-shaped unit attached to the outlet of the oxygen source and a solenoid valve which opens on sensing the decrease in pressure as the patient inhales. A "pulsed" volume of 15 to 35 mL of oxygen is delivered each time. Compared to a continuous flow system, the pulse device reduces the amount of oxygen usage by 35 to 75% producing a saving of about 7: 1. Electronic demand devices are also available for use with portable cylinders and piped-in oxygen systems in the hospitals. Some of the demand devices available in the Western market include Pulsair, DO_2 S, and Oxymatic. They add to the cost and produce a "clicking" sound at the bedside. Both these factors make it unacceptable to many patients.

Transtracheal Catheter

Transtracheal catheter is a narrow lumen catheter inserted directly into the trachea. Oxygen is delivered through tubing attached to a small fitting at the neck. Transtracheal catheter allows oxygen delivery ahead of the nasopharynx, bypassing some of the anatomical dead space. The upper airways serve as a reservoir towards the end of expiration, and the oxygen delivered is not diluted with atmospheric air before entering the respiratory tract. Transtracheal catheters are especially useful for patients receiving high oxygen flow as they save oxygen by an efficiency factor of 2:1 to 3:1. The efficiency can be further enhanced by combining it with pulsed oxygen delivery. An intratracheal catheter is more acceptable to the patient as it can be easily hidden beneath the collars and the look is not unsightly.

Moreover, there is no nasal or auricular irritation, and the catheter does not get dislodged during sleep. There is a small risk of infection and subcutaneous emphysema when the catheter is introduced. The catheter gets plugged with mucus and secretions and should be cleaned daily. Some of the transtracheal catheters available commercially are Heimlich Microtrach, the SCOOP catheter, and the intratracheal oxygen catheter (ITOC). The preferred method for inserting a transtracheal catheter is the Lipkin method, where the surgical tract matures in 7–10 days rather than the Seldinger technique that requires 6–8 weeks. The ITOC is implanted through a subcutaneous tunnel from the chest wall to the trachea and is of more permanent nature. Patients with transtracheal catheters should have conventional cannulae at home for use in an emergency when the transtracheal catheter gets blocked due to kinking or plugging.

RISKS OF LTOT

There are three types of risks associated with long-term use of oxygen, namely physical, functional, and cytotoxic.

Physical Risks

Since oxygen supports combustion, the tanks are potential risks of fire hazard and tank explosion, although these risks are relatively small. Patients should be strictly advised to stop smoking. The supply source (such as a cylinder) should not be kept in a small, closed room to avoid the accumulation of the vented gas. The other minor risks of oxygen therapy include injury to the nose and face from catheters and masks. Dryness and crusting may occur from dry, non-humidified gas.

Functional Risks

Oxygen therapy may accentuate hypoventilation in patients with COPD, which may induce hypercapnia and carbon dioxide narcosis. As the risk is small, chronic carbon dioxide retention is not considered a contraindication LTOT. It has been suggested that arterial pH is a better guide to monitoring therapy than $PaCO_2$. Patients with carbon dioxide retention also tolerate and benefit from long-term oxygen if arterial blood gas does not show acidemia.

Cytotoxic Damage

LTOT can cause structural damage to the lungs. Both proliferative and fibrotic changes of oxygen toxicity have been shown at autopsy on COPD patients treated with long-term oxygen. However, the histologic changes do not affect the clinical course or survival of these patients. Most of the structural damage attributable to hyperoxia results from high FiO_2 administration in acute conditions.

OXYGEN THERAPY FOR COPD DURING AIR-TRAVEL

Modern aircraft are pressurized to cabin altitudes up to 2,450 m (8000 ft), although this limit may be breached in emergencies. At 2,450 m (8000 ft), the PaO_2 will be equivalent to breathing 15%

oxygen at sea level. The PaO_2 at 2,450 m (8000 ft) will fall to about 53–64 mm Hg in a healthy individual. However, this low FiO_2 in the aircraft may exacerbate hypoxemia in COPD patients, especially those with resting hypoxemia. While there are several methods for determining the need for oxygen during air travel, the most used is a prediction equation derived from COPD patients who have had measurements of PaO_2 in a hypobaric chamber while breathing FiO_2 at 15%. The accuracy can be improved by the inclusion of FEV1 in the equation. These equations are reliable to establish upper and lower thresholds for "no in-flight oxygen required" (SpO_2 >95%) or "in-flight oxygen needed" (SpO_2 <92%). One commonly used prediction equation is: $PaO_2(Alt) = 0.519 \times PaO_2$ ground (mm Hg) + $11.855 \times$ FEV1 (L) - 1.760. Personal oxygen supply equipment is not allowed on aircrafts. Thus, oxygen requirements during travel must be communicated beforehand, and inquiries made about the available supply facilities (See Chapter 15).

SUGGESTED READING

1. AARC Clinical Practice Guideline: Oxygen therapy for adults in the acute care facility—2002 revision and update. Respir Care. 2002; 47: 717–20.
2. Albert RK, Au DH, Blackford AL, Casaburi R, Cooper JA, Jr., Criner GJ, Diaz P, Fuhlbrigge AL, Gay SE, Kanner RE, MacIntyre N, Martinez FJ, Panos RJ, Piantadosi S, Sciurba F, Shade D, Stibolt T, Stoller JK, Wise R, Yusen RD, Tonascia J, Sternberg AL, Bailey W. A randomized trial of long-term oxygen for copd with moderate desaturation. N Engl J Med. 2016; 375(17): 1617–27.
3. Balfour-Lynn IM, Primhak RA, Shaw BNJ. Home oxygen for children: who, how and when? Thorax. 2005; 60: 76–81.
4. Barach AL. Ambulatory oxygen therapy: Oxygen inhalation at home and out of doors. Chest. 1959; 35:229–41.
5. Bradley JM, Lasserson T, Elborn S, Macmahon J, O'Neill B. A systematic review of randomized controlled trials examining the short-term benefit of ambulatory oxygen in COPD. Chest. 2007; 131(1): 278–85.
6. British Thoracic Society recommendations: Managing passengers with respiratory disease planning air travel. Thorax. 2002; 57: 289-304.
7. Calverley PMA. Supplementary oxygen therapy in COPD: Is it really useful? Thorax 2000; 55: 537–38.
8. Chailleux E, Fauroux B, Binet F, Dautzenberg B, Polu JM. Predictors of survival in patients receiving domiciliary oxygen therapy or mechanical ventilation. A 10-year analysis of ANTADIR observatory. Chest. 1996; 109:741–9.

9. Christopher KL, Schwartz MD. Transtracheal oxygen therapy. Chest. 2011; 139(2): 435–40.
10. Crockett AJ, Cranston JM, Antic N. Domiciliary oxygen for interstitial lung disease. Cochrane Database Syst Rev. 2001; 3:CD002883.
11. Crockett AJ, Cranston JM, Moss JR, Alpers JH. Domiciliary oxygen for chronic obstructive pulmonary disease. Cochrane Database Syst Rev. 2000; Issue 4. CD001744.
12. Douglas WW, Ryu JH, Schroeder DR. Idiopathic pulmonary fibrosis: impact of oxygen and colchicines, prednisone, or no therapy on survival. Am J Respir Crit Care Med. 2000; 161:1172–8.
13. Dunne PJ. The clinical impact of new long-term oxygen therapy technology. Respir Care. 2009; 54(8): 1100–11.
14. Dupont M, Gacouin A, Lena H, Lavoue S, Brinchault G, Delaval P, Thomas R. Survival of patients with bronchiectasis after the first icu stay for respiratory failure. Chest. 2004; 125:1815–20.
15. Eaton T, Fergusson W, Kolbe J, Lewis CA, West T. Short-burst oxygen therapy for COPD patients: A 6-month randomized, controlled study. Eur Respir J. 2006; 27:697–704.
16. Eaton T, Lewis C, Young P, Kennedy Y, Garrett JE, Kolbe J. Long-term oxygen therapy improves health related quality of life. Respir Med. 2004; 98:285–93.
17. Eaton T, Lewis C, Young P, Kennedy Y, Garrett JE, Kolbe J. Long-term oxygen therapy improves health-related quality of life. Respir Med. 2004; 98:285–93.
18. Fauroux B, Sardet A, Foret D. Home treatment for chronic respiratory failure in children: A prospective study. Eur Respir J. 1995; 8:2062–66.
19. Fulmer JD, Snider GL. American College of Chest Physicians (ACCP)—National Heart Lung and Blood Institute (NHLBI) Conference on Oxygen Therapy. Arch Intern Med. 1984; 144:1645–55.
20. Global Initiative for Chronic Obstructive Lung Disease. Am J Respir Crit Care Med. 2001.
21. Gorecka D, Gorzelak K, Sliwinski P, et al. Effect of Long-term oxygen therapy on survival in patients with chronic obstructive pulmonary disease with moderate hypoxemia. Thorax. 1997; 52: 674–79.
22. Gottlieb DJ, Punjabi NM, Mehra R, Patel SR, Quan SF, Babineau DC, Tracy RP, Rueschman M, Blumenthal RS, Lewis EF, Bhatt DL, Redline S. CPAP versus oxygen in obstructive sleep apnea. N Engl J Med. 2014; 370(24): 2276–85.
23. Gould GA, Hayhurst MD, Scott W, Flenley DC. Technical and clinical assessment of oxygen concentrators. Thorax. 1985; 40:811–16.
24. Guleria R, Batra YK, Sharma BK, Jindal SK. Domiciliary mechanical ventilation in a patient with severe obstructive lung disease and respiratory failure. Ind J Chest Dis Allied Sci. 1992; 34:149–52.

25. Jindal SK, Agarwal R. Long-term oxygen therapy. Expert Rev Respir Med. 2012; 6(6): 639–49.
26. Jones DJ, Paul EA, Bell JH, Wedzicha JA. Ambulatory oxygen therapy in stable kyphoscoliosis. Eur Respir J. 1995; 8:819–23.
27. Kutty K. Sleep and chronic obstructive pulmonary disease. Curr Opin Pulm Med. 2004; 10:104–12.
28. Lacasse Y, Sériès F, Corbeil F, Baltzan M, Paradis B, Simão P, Abad Fernández A, Esteban C, Guimarães M, Bourbeau J, Aaron SD, Bernard S, Maltais F. Randomized trial of nocturnal oxygen in chronic obstructive pulmonary disease. N Engl J Med. 2020; 383(12): 1129–38.
29. Lacasse Y, Wong E, Guyatt GH, et al. Meta-analysis of respiratory rehabilitation in chronic obstructive pulmonary disease. Lancet. 1996; 348: 1115–19.
30. Landsberg R, Friedman M, Ascher-Landsberg J. Treatment of hypoxemia in obstructive sleep apnea. Am J Rhinol. 2001; 15:311–3.
31. Levi-Valensi P, Weitzenblum E, Pedinielli JL, Racineux JL, Duwoos H. Three-month follow-up of arterial blood gas determinations in candidates for long-term oxygen therapy: A Multicentric study. Am Rev Respir Dis. 1986; 133(4): 547–51.
32. McDonald CF, Crockett AJ, Young IH. Adult domiciliary oxygen therapy. Position Statement of the Thoracic Society of Australia and New Zealand. Med J Aust. 2005; 182: 621–26.
33. Meecham-Jones DJ, Paul EA, Bell JH, Wedzicha JA. Ambulatory oxygen therapy in stable kyphoscoliosis. Eur Respir J. 1995; 8:819–23.
34. Murphy R, Mackway-Jones K, Sammy I, et al. Emergency oxygen therapy for the breathless patient: Guidelines prepared by North West Oxygen Group. Emerg Med J. 2001; 18: 421–23.
35. O'Driscoll BR. Short burst oxygen therapy in patients with COPD. Monaldi Arch Chest Dis. 2008; 69(2): 70–4.
36. O'Reilly P, Bailey W. Long-term continuous oxygen treatment in chronic obstructive pulmonary disease: Proper use, benefits and unresolved issues. Curr Opin Pulm Med. 2007; 13:120–24.
37. Palange P, Crimi E, Pellegrino R, Brusasco V. Supplemental oxygen and heliox: 'New' tools for exercise training in chronic obstructive pulmonary disease. Curr Opin Pulm Med. 2005; 11: 145–48.
38. Petty TL. Home oxygen therapy. Mayo Clin Proc. 1987; 62:841–47.
39. Ram FSF, Wedzicha JA. Ambulatory oxygen for chronic obstructive pulmonary disease. Cochrane Database Syst Rev. 2002; Issue 1. CD000238.
40. Strom K, Boman G. Long-term oxygen therapy in parenchymal lung diseases: An analysis of survival. The Swedish Society of Chest Medicine. Eur Respir J. 1993;6:1264–1270.
41. Tiep B, Carter R, Zachariah F, Williams AC, Horak D, Barnett M, Dunham R. Oxygen for end-of-life lung cancer care: Managing dyspnea and hypoxemia. Expert Rev Respir Med. 2013; 7(5): 479–90.

42. Tiep B, Carter R. Oxygen conserving devices and methodologies. Chron Respir Dis. 2008; 5(2): 109–14.
43. Tiep BL, Lewis MI. Oxygen conservation and oxygen conserving devices in chronic lung disease. Chest. 1987; 92:263-72.
44. Wedzicha JA, Muir JF. Noninvasive ventilation in chronic obstructive pulmonary disease, bronchiectasis and cystic fibrosis. Eur Respir J. 2002; 20:777–84.
45. Wijkstra PJ, Guyatt GH, Ambrosino N, Celli BR, Guell R, Muir JF, Prefaut C, Mendes ES, Ferreira I, Austin P, Weaver B, Goldstein RS. International approaches to the prescription of long term oxygen therapy. Eur Respir J. 2001; 18:909–13.
46. Wijkstra PJ, Guyatt GH, Ambrosino N, Celli BR, Guell R, Muir JF, Prefaut C, Mendes ES, Ferreira I, Austin P, Weaver B, Goldstein RS. International approaches to the prescription of long term oxygen therapy. Eur Respir J. 2001; 18:909–13.
47. Zielinski J. A Nationwide System of Long-term oxygen therapy: The polish experience. Respir Care. 2000; 45:231–5.
48. Zielinski J. Effects of long-term oxygen therapy in patients with chronic obstructive pulmonary disease. Curr Opin Pulm Med. 1999; 5:81–87.

Chapter 14

Oxygen Therapy in the Intensive Care Unit

AN Aggarwal

Not all critically ill patients in an intensive care unit (ICU) require supplemental oxygen. The need for oxygen is determined through a multi-parameter assessment of clinical indicators and laboratory investigations. In patients admitted to the ICU, reliance on clinical features alone can be hazardous, as several clinical features of inadequate oxygenation are nonspecific and can be seen in several other medical conditions commonly encountered in critically ill patients. For instance, cyanosis could result from inadequate tissue perfusion due to hypotension, rather than hypoxemia per se. Similarly, other commonly described manifestations of inadequate oxygenation such as dyspnea, tachypnea, altered sensorium, arrhythmias, etc., are also otherwise commonly seen in critically ill patients. Such clinical information therefore needs to be interpreted in context of more objective measures.

ASSESSMENT OF NEED FOR SUPPLEMENTAL OXYGEN

Noninvasive monitoring of arterial oxygen saturation by pulse oximetry (SaO_2) and arterial blood gas (ABG) analysis are the two most common ways of objective evaluation for need for supplemental oxygen.

In contrast to other patients admitted to a health care facility, interpretation of pulse oximetry readings and/or ABG reports from critically ill patients is complicated by several disease and patient related factors peculiar to such patients. Pulse oximetry, although a simple and widely available technique, gives inconsistent results in patients with hemodynamic instability, especially in conditions associated with hypotension or low pulse volumes. The technique is also not of much use in patients with hemoglobin abnormalities (such as carbon monoxide poisoning, methemoglobinemia, etc.).

In chronically hypoxemic patients, compensatory mechanisms such as polycythemia, shift of oxygen-hemoglobin dissociation curve, and increased oxygen extraction allow relatively better tissue oxygenation even at lower levels of blood oxygenation, and this must be taken into consideration when deciding on oxygen therapy once these patients are admitted to the ICU with a disease exacerbation.

Measurements of both SaO_2 and PaO_2 can be normal despite substantial tissue hypoxia associated with anemia, low output cardiac states, and disorders resulting in failure of tissue to utilize oxygen. Under such circumstances, management should be guided by tissue oxygenation rather than blood oxygenation. Two independent procedures—measurement of mixed venous oxygen saturation ($ScvO_2$) and gastric tonometry—have been proposed as biomarkers of tissue oxygenation in critically ill patients. Gastric tonometry is an indirect method to assess adequacy of splanchnic perfusion and ischemia. $ScvO_2$ is measured invasively through a catheter placed in the superior vena cava and reflects the amount of oxygen left over in blood after body tissues have extracted whatever oxygen they need. A low $ScvO_2$ value suggests that the cardiac output and level of oxygenation are insufficient for meeting the metabolic demands of body tissues. Routine measurement of $ScvO_2$ has also been suggested as a component of the 'early goal directed therapy' in critically ill patients with severe sepsis.

INDICATION AND UTILITY OF OXYGEN IN CRITICALLY ILL PATIENTS

Oxygen, like any other drug used in the ICU, works best if administered only when necessary, and in the correct dosages. Failure to realize this, and considering supplemental oxygen as a universal panacea, is likely to lead to over-prescription of oxygen. This not only adds to the cost of ICU care, but also instills a false sense of security in the clinician's mind, without contributing anything substantial to patient outcome.

Before prescribing oxygen to an acutely ill patient, one should ensure that the airway is sufficiently patent to be able to deliver the oxygen to the lungs. This might require endotracheal intubation or tracheostomy before initiating oxygen supplementation. Oxygen should always be started and titrated based on an objective evaluation of patient's oxygenation status. In certain emergency situations (such as cardiac or respiratory arrest, or acute onset respiratory distress or hypotension) oxygen supplementation can be initiated empirically while more detailed clinical and physiological evaluation is being concurrently carried out. Even under such circumstances, ABG should be analyzed as quickly as possible, not only to assess level of hypoxemia, but also the acid-base status. In general, oxygen therapy is necessary for any patient in the ICU having documented arterial hypoxemia (PaO_2 below 60 mm Hg).

Hypoxemia results from several mechanisms in critically ill patients. Increasing the partial pressure of inspired oxygen (FiO_2) can ameliorate only some of these defects by raising the oxygen content in arterial blood. Oxygen therapy is the essential cornerstone of management of respiratory failure of several etiologies [such as acute respiratory distress syndrome, exacerbations of chronic obstructive pulmonary disease (COPD) or asthma, etc.]. When hypoxemia results from ventilation-perfusion mismatch related to consolidated, atelectatic, or otherwise diseased lung zones, oxygen supplementation is generally helpful, although the exact response is unpredictable and dependant on the quantum and distribution of mismatched areas. Similarly, in patients with alveolar hypoventilation, oxygen supplementation rapidly corrects hypoxemia, but the primary aim must be to correct the underlying cause. However, oxygen therapy is of lesser benefit if there is a problem with blood circulation (e.g. severe hypotension, pulmonary vascular blockade, large right-to-left shunt, etc.) or if hypoxia occurs at tissue level (e.g. severe anemia). Under such circumstances, oxygen therapy can at best provide some additional time to the clinician while the underlying disorders are being tackled.

Oxygen therapy is generally begun at high FiO_2 levels for most ICU patients. It is customary to start with 100% oxygen in patients who have sustained a cardio-respiratory arrest. Patients with acute hypoxemic respiratory failure generally require oxygen at an initial FiO_2 exceeding 0.50; this can then be titrated upward or downward depending on clinical and physiological response. For patients with hypercapnic respiratory failure (especially those with a preexisting component of chronic hypoventilation), it is advisable to begin with lower FiO_2 levels to avoid worsening CO_2 retention once the PaO_2 is normalized. However, one must never be overcautious in providing less than optimum FiO_2 to these patients, as hypoxemia is always more deleterious than hypercapnia.

OXYGEN DELIVERY IN THE ICU

There are three main components of oxygen administration in an ICU:

1. A control section that includes regulators and flowmeters between the source of high-pressure supply and the point of oxygen delivery to patient.
2. Blending of oxygen and air.
3. Actual oxygen delivery through patient interfaces such as masks, etc.

Almost all well-equipped ICUs have continuous pressurized oxygen and air supply available at each patient bed. The main advantage of such a supply mode is that both oxygen and air can simultaneously be fed into an oxygen blender and the final output FiO_2 actually delivered to the patient can be precisely controlled. The centralized hospital source of such supply could be variable, and these issues are discussed elsewhere in this book. In some resource-limited settings, oxygen cylinders are used to provide oxygen. Patients requiring oxygen through mask at low FiO_2 can also be managed through oxygen concentrators. Most ICUs have oxygen cylinders and/or concentrators as a backup in case of failure of central oxygen supply.

Oxygen can be delivered to patients either noninvasively through masks or cannulas, or as a component of assisted respiratory support, either though noninvasive positive pressure ventilation (NIPPV) or through conventional mechanical ventilation after endotracheal intubation. The choice of method of oxygen delivery depends entirely on the patient's clinical condition. Although the proportion of patients receiving oxygen as part of assisted respiratory support is much higher in an ICU as compared to other hospital areas, several patients can still be managed with noninvasive oxygen supplementation.

OXYGEN SUPPLEMENTATION THROUGH MASKS AND CANNULAE

The principles and utility of oxygen supplementation through masks and cannulae has been detailed elsewhere. A few important points however should be remembered in the ICU scenario. Since most patients in the ICU are quite sick with high ventilatory requirements, and have primarily been referred there because conventional therapy outside the ICU area proved ineffective, high flow systems are generally more useful. Several patients also require rather high FiO_2, and hence delivery systems designed for optimal use with low FiO_2 (such as nasal cannulas and simple face masks) are not as effective. These systems may, however, still have a role among patients requiring lesser or loosely controlled FiO_2.

The best systems for routine use are the Venturi masks, and they have several advantages. They allow a fairly tight control over the FiO_2 being delivered; this helps clinicians to monitor patients well and to precisely titrate amount of oxygen being supplemented. These masks are particularly useful for patients admitted with acute exacerbation of COPD, where controlled oxygen supplementation at a relatively lower FiO_2 is necessary to maintain oxygenation at slightly subnormal levels to prevent worsening of carbon-dioxide retention. However, Venturi masks must be used carefully, using oxygen flow rates recommended for the mask. It is a general tendency to increase the oxygen flow rate to higher than that recommended for a particular FiO_2, in hope of improving oxygen delivery to the patient. However, these masks work on the Venturi principle, and increasing oxygen flow without changing the entraining aperture size will lead to entrainment of more air, leading to more than expected dilution. The resulting FiO_2 reaching the patient is unpredictable and may even be less than the mask setting.

Oxygen delivery through a mask can be improved by adding a reservoir to the mask. Such a partial rebreathing circuit collects the initial portion of the exhaled air coming from the anatomic dead space into a reservoir and delivers it to the patient during the next inspiratory cycle. A high FiO_2 of up to 0.6 can be delivered through these masks.

More recently, an innovative high-flow nasal cannula (HFNC) system has been developed that delivers a very high flow (typically 30–60 L/min) of warm, humidified oxygen through nasal prongs, with precise FiO_2 titration. This is emerging as a popular and easily implementable strategy for critically ill patients whose high inspiratory flow demands cannot be met by more conventional oxygen delivery devices. HFNC use washes out anatomic dead space, reduces work of breathing, and also provides low level of positive airway pressure.

OXYGEN SUPPLEMENTATION DURING NIPPV

NIPPV is a useful technique to assist ventilation through a tight-fitting nasal or full-face mask in patients with acute respiratory failure associated with COPD or sleep-related breathing disorders, as well as during weaning from conventional mechanical ventilation. Several such patients will require supplemental oxygen along with ventilatory support. NIPPV can be delivered either through conventional mechanical ventilators or through portable systems. While the former can provide precisely controlled FiO_2 during conventional ventilation, they may not do so during in the presence of mask leaks, which invariably occur during NIPPV. The portable systems compensate for mask leaks better; however, most of them do not have an oxygen control mechanism.

Supplemental oxygen is delivered by simply adding it to the mask or circuit, and hence an accurately controlled FiO_2 cannot be achieved. The delivered FiO_2 using these systems is a complex interaction between several factors such as the site of addition of oxygen (whether into the mask or the circuit), position of exhalation port (whether in mask or the circuit), and the level of inspiratory and expiratory pressures used. When the exhalation port is located within the mask and oxygen is directly added into the mask, presumably much of the oxygen gets exhausted out through the exhalation port, because of the close proximity of the oxygen entrainment site and the leak port. Adding oxygen distally into the circuit allows more time for mixing than when the leak port is in the mask. The highest oxygen concentration of oxygen is generally achieved with oxygen added to the mask, with the leak port in the circuit, and with the lowest settings of inspiratory and expiratory pressures. However, the delivered FiO_2 still remains unpredictable. When a more precise oxygen delivery is needed, it is desirable to use a conventional ventilator with an integrated oxygen blender.

OXYGEN SUPPLEMENTATION THROUGH CONVENTIONAL MECHANICAL VENTILATORS

Most of the currently available mechanical ventilators can deliver tightly controlled and high levels of FiO_2 to intubated patients. These machines have integrated microprocessor-controlled gas blenders for precise mixing of compressed oxygen and compressed air, and allow delivery of a preset FiO_2 for continued and long periods. It is also possible to deliver high FiO_2 (up to even 1.0) through such systems; a feat that no noninvasive system can achieve in a sustained manner. It is no surprise that mechanical ventilation is the cornerstone of our efforts to improve oxygenation to a satisfactory level in patients with the most severe forms of respiratory failure admitted to ICUs.

DANGERS AND COMPLICATIONS OF OXYGEN THERAPY IN CRITICALLY ILL PATIENTS

Like any other pharmacologic agent, oxygen too is associated with toxicity if used in higher than needed doses. Application of high concentrations of oxygen for prolonged periods, which is often necessary to reverse acute hypoxemia in the critically ill patients, can lead to several physiologic and cellular alterations, and even lung injury. The pathogenesis is largely linked to production of cytotoxic free oxygen radicals that overwhelm the body's natural antioxidant defense mechanisms, resulting in accumulation of reactive oxygen intermediates. The mechanisms resulting in oxygen toxicity, and associated clinical manifestations, are detailed elsewhere in this book. The dangers of pulmonary toxicity due to oxygen, ranging from atelectasis to pro-inflammatory processes, and the risks of overzealous oxygen prescription for patients with COPD, are widely recognized. Despite this, physicians themselves are sometimes responsible for aggravating oxygen toxicity through their endeavor to try and normalize blood oxygenation. It is well known that arterial oxygen saturation at a PO_2 of 60 mm Hg is about 90%, and any additional increase in PO_2 beyond that (by increasing FiO_2 further) does not result in a proportionate improvement in oxygen saturation or tissue oxygen delivery. Since patients in ICUs are perceived to be critically ill and in need of oxygen, physicians often overprescribe oxygen.

Short term exposure to high oxygen concentrations is tolerated fairly well, and hence ICU patients needing short-term oxygen supplementation (24–36 hours) are unlikely to develop oxygen toxicity. Patients needing prolonged oxygen supplementation are definitely at risk. Since there is hardly any treatment for oxygen toxicity, the goal in an ICU setting should be to prevent this complication. Simple measures that are useful in the ICU setup include—(a) use of lowest possible FiO_2 (preferably less than 0.5-0.6) to achieve arterial PO_2 of 60-70 mm Hg, and (b) judicious upward titration of positive end-expiratory pressure (PEEP) in ventilated patients to reduce their overall FiO_2 requirement. In addition, regular monitoring for manifestations of oxygen toxicity should be undertaken. Several symptoms and signs of oxygen toxicity such as restlessness, nausea, dyspnea, cough, retrosternal discomfort, paresthesias, etc. are fairly nonspecific in any critically ill patient; nevertheless, oxygen toxicity should be a consideration if such features appear freshly in any patient otherwise improving on therapy. Worsening infiltrates on chest radiographs, or increasing FiO_2 and/or PEEP requirements, may also be a pointer to relatively severe pulmonary oxygen toxicity.

The other important issue with oxygen delivery systems in the ICU is related to nosocomial infection. Under normal circumstances, low-flow oxygen systems do not present clinically important risk of infection and need not be routinely replaced. High-flow systems that employ heated humidifiers and aerosol generators, particularly when applied to patients with artificial airways, can pose important risk of infection. In the absence of definitive studies to support change-out intervals, results of institution-specific and patient-specific surveillance measures should dictate the frequency with which such equipment is replaced.

MONITORING OXYGEN THERAPY IN ICU

Patients admitted to ICUs and requiring supplemental oxygen are usually quite sick, and are monitored frequently for their general condition, vital signs and level of dysfunction of various organ systems. Monitoring of oxygen therapy is an integrated component of this management paradigm.

It is important to regularly check patient's temperature, heart rate, respiratory rate and respiratory effort to be able to assess a patient's ventilatory requirement. This in turn, will help in selecting the oxygen delivery system and oxygen flow rate best suited for the patient. For instance, a patient using nasal prongs may need to be shifted to a high flow system if he starts hyperventilating after developing fever in the ICU. More importantly, it is necessary to periodically check the oxygenation status of these critically ill patients. This is best accomplished by continuous noninvasive monitoring through a pulse oximeter, supplemented by periodic ABG measurements.

It is important to obtain an arterial blood gas analysis before initiating oxygen supplementation. Once oxygen supplementation (with or without mechanical ventilation) is started, ABG should be repeated after about two hours (or earlier depending on clinical condition) to establish efficacy of oxygen therapy. Subsequent monitoring depends on patient's clinical condition and level of FiO_2. In general, patients on low FiO_2 need less frequent monitoring than patients on high FiO_2 or receiving mechanical ventilation. Patients with hypercapnic respiratory failure may also require more frequent monitoring. Once patients have stabilized, ABG analysis is perhaps needed only once a day, with intermittent or continuous monitoring with oximeter in between. The goal of all such monitoring is to try and keep FiO_2 levels in a safe range to prevent oxygen toxicity, and at the same time ensure a level of oxygenation that does not put the patient to risk due to hypoxia.

Some patients may also benefit from monitoring of adequacy of oxygen delivery to the tissues. Serum lactate, anion gap, base excess, and pH may be used to assess the severity of metabolic acidosis and shock. However, these are global measurements and are not sensitive to regional hypoperfusion. The adequacy of systemic or global oxygen delivery is most commonly assessed directly by measuring the oxygen content of arterial and mixed venous blood, estimating cardiac output, and then calculating oxygen delivery. Gastric tonometry, which measures gastric PCO_2 and calculates gastric intramucosal pH, was developed based on the principle that fluid in a hollow organ can be used to measure the gas tension of the surrounding tissue. This index is an indirect measure of splanchnic perfusion and oxygenation.

A recent advance in the initial management of critically ill patients with severe sepsis has been the concept of "early goal directed therapy". The protocol involves intensive monitoring of these patients using central venous oxygen saturation. This is an indirect marker for the quantum of tissue extraction of oxygen, and the goal is to eventually get a central venous oxygen saturation value exceeding 70% with supportive therapy (such as volume resuscitation, blood transfusion, inotropic support, etc.).

In addition to the patient, the oxygen delivery systems in the ICU also need to be monitored. This ensures that results of clinical and laboratory monitoring are interpreted in a correct perspective. All oxygen delivery systems should be checked at least once per day. Mechanical ventilators should be periodically calibrated with respect to oxygen blending and delivery.

DISCONTINUATION

Oxygen should be stopped once the critical illness leading to hypoxemia has considerably resolved, and when arterial oxygenation is adequate with the patient breathing room air (PO_2 60 mm Hg, $SaO_2 > 90\%$). In patients without arterial hypoxemia but at risk of tissue hypoxia, oxygen should be stopped when the acid-base state and clinical assessment of vital organ function are consistent with resolution of tissue hypoxia.

SUGGESTED READING

1. Bateman NT, Leach RM. ABC of oxygen: Acute oxygen therapy. BMJ. 1998;317:798–801.
2. Girardis M, Busani S, Damiani E, Donati A, Rinaldi LM, Morelli A, et al. Effect of conservative vs conventional oxygen therapy on mortality amongst patients in an intensive care unit. JAMA. 2016;316(15):1583–89.
3. Huang YC. Monitoring oxygen delivery in the critically ill. Chest. 2005;128(5 Suppl 2):554S–560S.
4. Kallstrom TJ. AARC clinical practice guideline: Oxygen therapy for adults in the acute care facility - 2002 Revision and Update. Respir Care. 2002;47:717–20.
5. Leach RM, Treacher DF. The pulmonary physician in critical care* 2: Oxygen delivery and consumption in the critically ill. Thorax. 2002;57:170–7.
6. Martin DS, Grocott MPW. Oxygen therapy in critical illness: Precise control of arterial oxygenation and permissive hypoxemia. Crit Care Med. 2013;41(2):423–32.
7. O'Driscoll BR, Dark P, Wijesinghe M, McAuley D. Oxygen use is becoming more conservative on intensive care units in the UK. Thorax. 2016;71(Suppl 3):A176.
8. O'Driscoll BR, Smith R. Oxygen use in critical illness. Respiratory Care. 2019, 64 (10) 1293–1307.
9. Rivers E, Nguyen B, Havstad S, Ressler J, Muzzin A, Knoblich B, et al. Early goal-directed therapy in the treatment of severe sepsis and septic shock. N Engl J Med. 2001;345:1368–77.
10. Schwartz AR, Kacmarek RM, Hess DR. Factors affecting oxygen delivery with bi-level positive airway pressure. Respir Care. 2004;49:270–5.
11. Siemieniuk RAC, Chu DK, Ha-Yeon Kim L, Guell-Rous MR, Alhazanni W, et al. Oxygen therapy for acutely ill medical patients: A clinical practice guideline. BMJ. 2018;363:k41069.

Chapter 15

Oxygen Therapy during Air Travel

Ajay Handa

INTRODUCTION

Air travel is a preferred mode of transportation due to the convenience and shorter travel time. Most people traveling by air are healthy individuals; however, approximately 5–10% have underlying illnesses, including chronic respiratory diseases. The prevalence of respiratory diseases is increasing worldwide, and most such patients would prefer air travel for convenience. In-flight medical emergencies are not only potentially life-threatening, but the diversion can also lead to economic losses and inconvenience to the co-passengers. Respiratory emergencies accounted for the third leading cause of diversions after cardiac and neurological diseases. This chapter discusses the concept of pre-flight assessment for 'fitness-to-fly' and the prescription of supplemental oxygen during flight to make air travel safe in patients with chronic respiratory illnesses.

PHYSIOLOGY AT ALTITUDE AND ITS EFFECTS

The knowledge of changes in pulmonary physiology with altitude and aviation is essential for physicians assessing 'fitness-to-fly' in chronic respiratory diseases. With increasing altitude, the atmospheric pressure declines logarithmically, while the temperature decreases linearly. The fall in PaO_2 with altitude can cause hypobaric hypoxia during air travel. Commercial aircraft fly at 10,000–13,000 meters above sea level (ASL), and cabin pressurization is maintained at about 2,450 meters ASL. For technical reasons, the cabin altitude cannot be maintained lower than 2,450 m. At this altitude, the ambient air contains 15.1% oxygen instead of 21.1% seen at sea level. Hence, the PaO_2 falls to 53–64 mm Hg (SpO_2, 85–91%) during flight. This decline in PaO_2 does not produce any symptoms in healthy subjects; however, it can cause significant hypoxemia and precipitate respiratory failure in patients with chronic lung disease. Therefore, patients with chronic respiratory illness need thorough pre-flight evaluation and optimization of medical treatment and supplemental in-flight oxygen in selected cases. Most guidelines recommend prescribing supplemental oxygen in-flight for patients who have $PaO_2 < 50$ mm Hg breathing room air.

Severe lung diseases complicated with pulmonary hypertension are at risk of worsening due to hypoxic pulmonary vasoconstriction, which may lead to arrhythmias, ischemia, and in some cases, right heart failure during flight. These problems are likely to be aggravated during long flights as there is not only prolonged exposure to hypoxemia, but sleep can also induce greater desaturation in such patients. Further, there are risks of immobility-related deep venous thrombosis during long-duration flights.

Another physical effect of ascent to altitude is the expansion of gases due to a decrease in the ambient pressure (Boyle's law). The gas within a non-communicating bulla can expand by 30% at 2,450 m ASL and can rupture to cause complications, including pneumothorax, pneumo-mediastinum, and rarely air embolism. COPD patients with large bullae are at increased risk and should be advised to avoid air travel due to the risk of tension pneumothorax.

The overall incidence of in-flight emergencies is reported to be 1 in 30,000 passengers. The emergency was found to be due to syncope, respiratory illness, cardiac stroke, and cardiac arrest in 37.4%, 12%, 7.7%, 2%, and 0.3%, respectively. Fortunately, the fatality rate is exceedingly low at one death per 3–10 million passengers. In about 65% of cases, the medical emergencies are related to previous medical conditions, emphasizing the need for pre-flight assessment as a good preventive strategy.

ASSESSMENT OF FITNESS FOR AIR TRAVEL

The aim of a comprehensive preflight assessment is to identify those persons who are at risk of developing significant hypoxemia during air travel. Those patients who using domiciliary oxygen therapy or ventilator, severe COPD (FEV_1 <30% predicted), severe ILD (FVC <30% predicted), recent acute respiratory illness within six weeks, significant symptoms during previous air travel, or presence of cardiac diseases should be assessed for fitness. Other respiratory diseases, including long-standing asthma, bronchiectasis, and bullous lung disease will also benefit from such assessment. Undrained pneumothorax is an absolute contraindication to air travel and needs treatment and observation for two weeks before air travel. Ongoing hemoptysis, lung malignancy with airway obstruction, and massive pleural effusion must be treated and observed for two weeks before air travel. Patients using long-term home oxygen therapy at rate ≥4 liters/minute are unfit to fly.

Pre-flight assessment should include a detailed history and physical examination, optimization of medical therapy, and counseling, followed by tests for assessing the propensity for developing hypoxemia. The methods used for evaluation for the need for oxygen supplementation include exercise test, blood gas analysis, spirometry, use of prediction equations, and the hypoxia challenge test (HCT).

Airline medical authorities traditionally have used the fifty-meter walk test for screening passengers. Those who can walk 50 m are considered fit to fly. The test is a very crude assessment of cardiopulmonary reserve and should preferably be replaced by the 6-minute walk test. The 6-minute walk test is increasingly used for the assessment of functional status and exercise capacity in chronic respiratory diseases. A resting SpO_2 >95% and SpO_2 >84% after a 6-minute walk test had a sensitivity and specificity of 100% and 80%, respectively, for 'fitness-to-fly.'

Arterial blood gas analysis is done if SpO_2 is <85% on room air and those with chronic lung diseases or other risk factors. Patients with room air PaO_2 >70 mm Hg are considered safe for air travel. Those with PaO_2 <70 mm Hg need assessment by a physician and further evaluation before fitness. Spirometry aids the assessment of disease severity and selection of cases for hypoxic challenge tests if a severe functional impairment is noted. However, lung functions failed to predict hypoxemia or complications during air travel in many studies. There are many prediction equations for estimating PaO_2 at altitude. he equations use blood gas parameters and spirometry data and have been developed from studies in COPD patients exposed to hypoxic environment **(Table 15.1)**. Due to the limited availability of HCT, prediction equations are most frequently used to assess 'fitness for flying.' If the predicted PaO_2 is <50 mm Hg, supplemental oxygen in-flight is advised. There are many drawbacks of the predicted PaO_2, including a poor agreement with altitude PaO_2 and overestimation of oxygen needs compared with HCT. More studies are required to find the best prediction model for patients with chronic lung diseases.

Table 15.1: Equations for calculating predicted PaO_2 at altitude.
PaO_2 altitude = 0.84 + 0.68 (PaO_2 sea level)
PaO_2 altitude = 0.295 (PaO_2 sea level) + 0.086 (FEV_1% predicted) + 23.211
PaO_2 altitude = 0.245 (PaO_2 sea level) + 0.171 (FEV_1/FVC% predicted) + 21.028

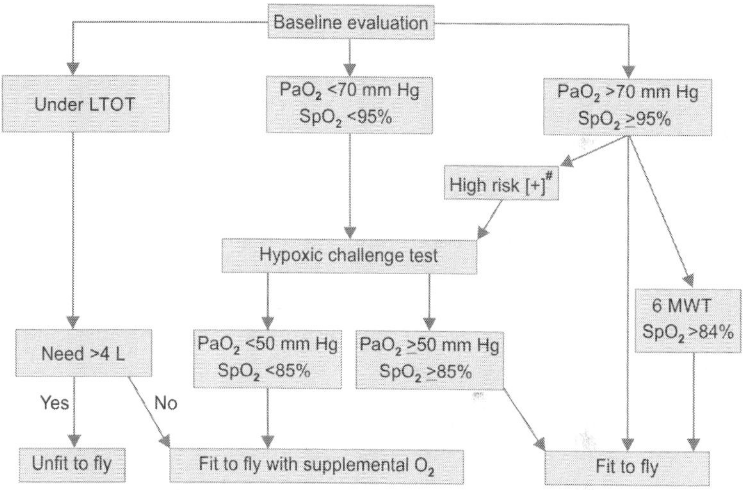

Fig. 15.1: Algorithm for assessment of fitness to fly in COPD patients [reproduced with permission from Dr Ergan B, et al.].

[#]Risk factors include pre-existing requirement of oxygen/ventilatory support, bullous lung disease, comorbid conditions that may worsen hypoxemia like cardiac disease and significant symptoms during previous air travel

(LTOT: long-term oxygen therapy)

HYPOXIA CHALLENGE TEST (HCT)

HCT (also called hypoxia altitude simulation test) remains the reference standard for pre-flight assessment. The patient breathes a gas mixture with 15% oxygen using a tight-fitting face mask. The test is performed with continuous pulse oximetry and electrocardiographic monitoring to monitor severe desaturation and cardiac arrhythmias. Arterial blood gas analysis is done at baseline and after 20 minutes of HCT. HCT is usually advised for those with room air SpO_2 92–95% and presence of risk factors for possible desaturation such as a previous episode of in-flight hypoxemia, FEV1 <30% predicted, bullous lung disease, and associated cardiac diseases. **Figure 15.1** describes algorithmic

Table 15.2: Recommendations based on hypoxic challenge test.

Blood gas analysis after HCT	*Recommendation*
PaO_2>50 mm Hg and SpO_2 ≥ 85%	In-flight oxygen not required
PaO_2<50 mm Hg and SpO_2< 85%	In-flight oxygen at 2 liters/minute required

approach for assessment of COPD for fitness to fly. Based on the ABG analysis after HCT, a person with PaO_2 >50 mm Hg (SpO_2 ≥85%) is 'fit-to-fly', and oxygen supplementation is not required. Whereas if PaO_2 <50 mm Hg (SpO_2< 85%), the individual needs supplemental oxygen in flight **(Table 15.2)**. The SpO_2 during flight compares well with SpO_2 obtained during the HCT. The limited availability and costs of HCT preclude its wider usage. Further research is recommended for the relevance of HCTs in resource-limited countries where the physician relies on clinical, blood gas analysis, spirometry, and 6-minute walk test for decision making.

PRESCRIBING IN-FLIGHT OXYGEN

Passengers with risk of hypoxemia during air travel based on physician's assessment, 6-minute walk test, prediction PaO_2 at altitude or HCT would be given a certificate of fitness to travel by air and prescribed medications and oxygen by the physician. Most commercial airlines will provide in-flight oxygen on advance request by the passenger based on a physician's prescription. Oxygen-dependent passengers must make additional arrangements for the use of supplemental oxygen not only during the flight but in the airports as well. The oxygen expenses are usually borne by the traveler rather than by the airlines or insurance firms.

The oxygen supply is usually provided from cylinders. The prescription must specify the rate of flow and duration, and mode of administration so that an adequate amount of oxygen is available during the journey. The flow rate of oxygen of 2 L/minute is suitable for most passengers. Those on long-term oxygen therapy (LTOT) are advised to increase the flow rate 2 L/minute above the usual flow rate during air travel.

Most airlines provide oxygen through simple face masks, and passengers are advised to carry their nasal prongs to prevent

Box 15.1: Guidelines for air travel with chronic lung diseases.

- Carry physicians' medical certificate of fitness to fly
- Carry prescription and all inhaled and oral medications in hand baggage
- Inform about oxygen requirement at the time of booking and 72 hours before the date of journey
- Inform about the need for wheelchair assistance and oxygen in waiting areas
- Preferably take a nonstop flight to destination
- Book aisle seat near the toilet to minimize walking
- Avoid alcohol and sedatives during flight
- Stay hydrated and keep moving the toes and ankles during flight

rebreathing. The oxygen and cabin air are devoid of moisture and can lead to drying of tracheobronchial mucosa and precipitation of bronchospasm. The airlines must be informed of humidified oxygen for patients with asthma and COPD. Also, the patients must be advised to stay hydrated and carry their medications and inhalers in their hand baggage for use during flight.

Passengers must remember that the airline does not provide oxygen during waiting periods and stop-overs. Some airports restrict oxygen use in the airport because of the risk of explosion. Patients on long-term oxygen therapy cannot use their cylinders or concentrators but may be able to take these items with them as baggage for use at their destination. It is also important for these patients to carry medical documents and extra supplies during the travel **(Box 15.1)**.

CONCLUSION

For most passengers, air travel is quick, safe, and comfortable. Those with significant respiratory diseases are at risk of significant hypoxemia during air travel and may develop complications needing emergency care on board or diversion of aircraft. Patients with chronic lung diseases need assessment for fitness to fly, optimization of medications, and in-flight oxygen supplementation for safe travel. There are limited facilities for hypoxic challenge test in resource-limited setting, and physicians must use clinical assessment, spirometry, and 6-minute walk test for deciding the 'fitness-to-fly'.

SUGGESTED READING

1. Ahmedzai S, Balfour-Lynn IM, Bewick T, et al. Managing passengers with stable respiratory disease planning air travel: British Thoracic Society Recommendations. Thorax. 2011; 66: i1ei30. doi:10.1136/thoraxjnl-2011-200295.
2. Berg BW, Dillard TA, Rajagopal KR, Mehm WJ. Oxygen supplementation during air travel in patients with chronic obstructive lung disease. Chest. 1992; 101:638–41.
3. British Thoracic Society Standards of Care Committee. Managing passengers with respiratory disease planning air travel: British Thoracic Society Recommendations. Thorax. 2002; 57: 289–304.
4. Celli BR. ATS standards for the optimal management of chronic obstructive pulmonary disease. Respirology. 1997; 2:S1–4.
5. Cramer D, Ward S, Geddes D. Assessment of oxygen supplementation during air travel. Thorax. 1996; 51:202–3.
6. Dillard TA, Berg BW, Rajagopal KR, et al. Hypoxaemia during air-travel in patients with COPD. Ann Intern Med. 1989; 111: 362–7.
7. Dillard TA, Moores LK, Bilello KL, et al. The pre-flight evaluation: A comparison of the hypoxia inhalation test with hypobaric exposure. Chest. 1995; 107: 352–7.
8. Ergan B, Akgun M, Pacilli, Stefano Nava AMG, et al. Should I stay or should I go? COPD and air travel. Eur Respir Rev. 2018; 27: 180030.
9. Gendreau MA, DeJohn C. Responding to medical events during commercial airline flights: Current concepts. N Engl J Med. 2002; 346: 1067–73.
10. Gong H, Tashkin DP, Lee EY, et al. Hypoxia-altitude simulation test. Am Rev Respir Dis. 1984; 130:980–6.
11. Johnson AOC. Chronic obstructive pulmonary disease: Fitness to fly with COPD. Thorax. 2003; 58: 729–32.
12. Khilnani GC, Bhatta N. Air travel and supplemental oxygen in patients with cardio-pulmonary diseases. J Assoc Physicians India. 2002;50: 811–15.
13. Lyznicki JM, Williams MA, Deitchman SD, Howe JP 3rd; Council on scientific affairs, American Medical Associate. Medical oxygen and air travel. Aviat Space Environ Med. 2000;71: 827–31.
14. Mills FJ, Harding RM. Fitness to travel by air. I: Physiological Considerations. BMJ. 1983;286: 1269–71.
15. Mills FJ, Harding RM. Fitness to travel by air. II: Special Medical Considerations. BMJ. 1983;286: 1240–41.
16. Stoller JK, Hoisington E, Auger G. A comparative analysis of arranging in-flight oxygen aboard commercial air carriers. Chest. 1999; 115: 991–5.
17. Vohra KP, Klocke RA. Detection and correction of hypoxemia associated with air travel. Am Rev Respir Dis. 1993; 148:1215–9.

Chapter 16

Oxygen Therapy and High-altitude Illness

Nazia Mehfooz, Parvaiz A Koul

Across the globe around 140 million people are permanently residing at an altitude >2500 m. Each year several mountaineers and trekkers visit many high-altitude destinations. Among them, the Himalayas with Mount Everest (8,848 m) being the highest elevation in the world. At high altitudes there is a direct relationship between partial pressure of inspired oxygen (PIO_2) and barometric pressure. However, the percentage of oxygen (fraction of inspired oxygen) remains constant at 21%. With increasing altitudes there is fall in barometric pressure which causes decrease in partial pressure of inspired oxygen (PIO_2) and arterial saturation (SO_2) **(Table 16.1)**.

This creates a hypobaric hypoxic environment which leads to a series of physiologic responses in human body. Based on the physiologic stresses the high altitudes are divided into three levels:

1. **High altitude (1500 to 3500 m):** Decreased in arterial PO_2 levels with maintained oxygen saturation of 90%.
2. **Very high altitude (3500 to 5500 m):** Oxygen saturation falls below 90% with hypoxemic episodes during exercise and sleep.

Table 16.1: Relationship of altitudes, barometric pressure, estimated PaO_2 and inspired PO_2.

Altitudes	*BP (mm Hg)*	*Estimated PaO_2 (mm Hg)*	*Inspired PO_2 (% of sea-level)*
Sea level	760	159	100%
2000	596	125	79%
3000	526	110	69%
4000	463	97	60%
5000	405	85	52%
8000	268	56	34%

3. **Extreme high altitude (> 5500 m):** Marked hypoxemia, hypocapnia and alkalosis are characteristic of extreme altitudes. Central sleep apnoea contributes to hypoxemia at this altitude.

At high altitude, due to decreased PaO_2, the transport of oxygen lies on the steep portion of oxygen dissociation curve to facilitate oxygen release from hemoglobin. Lowlanders upon ascent to high altitude develop hyperventilation which results in acute respiratory alkalosis. This consequently leads to a leftward shift in the oxygen-hemoglobin dissociation curve to optimize oxygenation in lungs. However, at the tissue level oxygen dissociation curve shift to right due to simultaneous increase in red cell 2,3 diphosphoglycerate (2-3,DPG) which to facilitate oxygen release from Hb and improves the oxygen uptake in the tissues.

High altitude syndromes (HAS) are the group of potentially fatal disorders involving multiple organs due to decreased availability of oxygen at altitude > 2500 m. Tseen Hanshoo first described high altitude illness as the "Great and Little Headache" mountains on the journey along the silk route around 2000 years ago.

GENETIC BASIS FOR HIGH ALTITUDES SYNDROMES (HAS)

Since the first description of the disease by Tseen Hanshoo, extensive research has been done in this area to explain the difference in the susceptibility of developing high altitude syndromes among lowlanders and natives. Recent research highlights the genetic factors and not only acclimatization as being responsible for these different adaptive phenotypes found at high altitude.

The Tibetans and Andeans are two major population that have well adapted to high altitude but with strikingly different phenotypes. This phenotypic difference is due to different variants of many genes which are responsible for their adaptation at high altitude. High-altitude adaptation has been proposed as one of the strongest instances of natural selection acting on humans.

One genetic pathway is hypoxia-inducible factor (HIF) pathway which is the major switch for molecular response to acute and chronic hypoxemic conditions and controls around 5% of human genes, including erythropoietin a hormone that causes increases RBC production which leads to an increased haematocrit and O_2-carrying capacity. There are two subunits of HIF transcription factors namely β and α (HIF-1α, -2α or -3α) responsible for gene expression in hypoxic conditions. In response to hypoxemia the concentration of HIF-1α increases which then combines with HIF-β and finally affects the hypoxia response component. HIF mainly help the cells to survive in an environment of hypobaric hypoxia which is found at high altitudes. The main genes belonging to the hypoxia-inducible factor (HIF) pathway are EGLN1, EPAS1, PPARA and PRKAA1. The EPAS1 gene encodes the HIF-2α subunit and EGLN1 gene encodes prolyl hydroxylase 2 (PHD2). Mutation of these two genes has been reported to be associated with anemia and polycythemia. EGLN1 gene and PPARA (peroxisome proliferator-activated receptor-α), are also associated with red blood cell production. Evolutionarily selected Tibetan prolyl hydroxylase-2 ($PHD2^{D4E;C127S}$) variant degrades the hypoxia-inducible factor (HIFα) more efficiently and protects these highlanders from hypoxia-triggered elevation in hemoglobin concentration. High altitude sickness is often accompanied by an inflammatory response and exposure to hypobaric hypoxia is presumed to be the principal causative agent. More recently we demonstrated that gain-of-function $PHD2^{D4E;C127S}$ variant can protect against inflammation elicited by hypobaric hypoxia. Augmentation of PHD2 activity therefore may be an important method to alleviate inflammatory response to inspired hypoxia. In this regard, alpha-ketoglutarate reduced the inflammation and might prove to be of therapeutic value in high altitude sickness.

HIGH ALTITUDE SYNDROMES

High altitude syndromes (HAS) are classified as:

1. **High-altitude diseases of lowlanders:** Which includes acute mountain sickness (AMS), high altitude pulmonary edema (HAPE), and high-altitude cerebral edema (HACE).
   Diagnosis of these condition is based on Lake Louise scoring system mentioned in **Box 16.1**.
2. **High-altitude diseases of long-term highlanders:** It includes chronic mountain sickness (CMS) which is also known as Monge's disease.

High-altitude Diseases of Lowlanders

Epidemiology

Prevalence of AMS varies with the rate of ascent to high altitude and susceptibility to develop high altitude illness in unacclimatised

Box 16.1: Lake Louis classification of high-altitude illnesses.

Acute mountain sickness (AMS)

In the setting of a recent gain in altitude, there is presence of headache and at least one of the following:

- Gastrointestinal (anorexia, nausea or vomiting)
- Fatigue or weakness
- Dizziness or light-headedness
- Difficulty sleeping

High-altitude cerebral edema (HACE)

Can be considered "end stage" or severe AMS. In the setting of a recent gain in altitude, there is either:

- Presence of a change in mental status and/ or ataxia in a person with AMS
- Or the presence of both mental status changes and ataxia in a person without AMS

High-altitude pulmonary edema (HAPE)

In the presence of a recent gain in altitude, the presence of the following:

At least two of the following symptoms:

- Dyspnea at rest—cough
- Weakness or decreased exercise performance
- Chest tightness or congestion

At least two of the following signs:

- Crackles or wheezing in at least one lung field
- Central cyanosis
- Tachypnea
- Tachycardia

lowlanders. It is around 25–40% with passive ascent to 3000–3500 m. The incidence of HAPE and HACE are less than 1% and 4% respectively. However, incidence of HAPE reported may get increased up to 15.5% with rapid ascent to altitude 5500 m as opposed to gradual trekking. A case series of 31 Amarnath Yatris from northern part of the country during the holy pilgrimage to the " Shri Amarnath Ji" cave/ shrine showed that all yatris satisfied the lake Louise criteria for HAPE with a median score of 7 (range of 4–14), whereas 10 had additional evidence of HACE. The unacclimatised people of lowlanders were more susceptible for developing high-altitude illness during their yatra to the "Shri Amarnath Ji" cave/shrine and there was a direct association with the rapidity of ascent.

Identification of risk factors responsible for developing HAS is essential for minimising these illnesses in mountaineers and trekkers. Rapid ascent to an altitude < 3500 m, low oxygen saturation (SPO_2), young age, obesity, and heavy exercises are found to be an independent risk factors in various studies.

Pathophysiology of High-altitude Sickness

The AMS, HAPE, and HACE are due to the effects of hypobaric hypoxemic environment in unacclimatised individuals at high altitude. Hypobaric hypoxemia at high altitude is caused by low barometric pressure which decreases partial oxygen pressure. This hypoxemic state causes vasodilatation, increased cerebral blood flow and intracranial hypertension and leads to headache in individuals with AMS. High-altitude cerebral and pulmonary edema developed due to increased hydrostatic capillary pressure, overperfusion of the microvascular beds and leakage in both the blood-brain barrier and blood-gas barrier in the lungs.

The factors responsible for HAPE are nonhomogeneous hypoxic pulmonary vasoconstriction which exposes the pulmonary capillaries to high pressure, consequently overdistension and damage to the capillaries walls leads to extravasation of edema fluid, blood cells and plasma proteins, into the interstitial and alveolar spaces. Another factor is decreased bioavailability of nitric oxide responsible for the elevated pulmonary artery pressure. Free oxygen radicals have also been incriminated in the pathogenesis of HAPE.

In HACE, damage due to hypoxia can either be vasogenic (extra-cellular, due to blood-brain barrier leakage), cytotoxic (intracellular, due to cellular swelling) or a combination of the both. Cytotoxic edema affects both gray and white matter whereas vasogenic edema preferentially spreads along white matter tracts.

Clinical Perspective

Acute Mountain Sickness (AMS)

The AMS is the most common form of high-altitude illness. It is a self-limiting illness usually manifested at an altitude more than 2500 m. The symptoms are non-specific in nature characterised by headache which is bitemporal and throbbing most severe after night stay at high altitude and is expected within 4 to 36 hours of high-altitude exposure.

The Lake-Louise self-scoring grading systems is commonly used to categorise the severity of AMS. According to this system each symptom in a set of four symptoms (headache, gastrointestinal symptoms, fatigue and/or weakness, dizziness/light headedness) is graded from 0–3. If the individual has at least 1 point for headache and at least 3 points in total of four symptoms and had no neurological findings then AMS can be diagnosed. AMS can be stratified on the basis of the total score as 3–5 mild, 6–9 moderate and 10–12 severe AMS. On physical examination heart rate and blood pressure are usually within the normal range. Arterial oxygen saturation are usually normal or sometime low for a given altitude.

High-altitude Pulmonary Edema (HAPE)

High-altitude pulmonary edema is defined as noncardiogenic (left ventricular function is preserved) pulmonary edema caused by pulmonary blood-gas barrier leak in the lung. This is the most mortal form of HAI. The earliest symptoms are decreased exercise performance and dry cough and as the HAPE progresses tachycardia, tachypnoea, lassitude, productive cough and cyanosis worsen and eventually coma develop. On physical examination, a prominent P2 and right ventricular heave may be appreciated with auscultation and palpation. Rales are often first appreciated in the right mid-lung field. In a minority of patients, rales absent at rest can be elicited after brief exertion. Chest radiographs typically show patchy lung infiltrates with normal heart size and absence of these infiltrates suggest alternative diagnosis.

Electrocardiography may reveal findings of right heart strain consistent with acute pulmonary hypertension. Arterial blood gas analysis reveals respiratory alkalosis with severe hypoxemia. Partial pressure of arterial oxygen is typically between 30 and 40 mm Hg.

High Altitude Cerebral Edema (HACE)

The HACE is considered as an extreme form of AMS and is thought to be a continuum of AMS representing the final encephalopathic, life-threatening stage of cerebral altitude effects. The diagnosis is based on the setting, symptoms, and findings. It is characterized by ataxia, hallucinations, confusion, vomiting, and decreased activity and is mostly but not necessarily accompanied by severe, unbearable headache. Ataxia is the key sign, manifested by a positive Romberg test.

Medical Society Practice Guidelines for the Prevention and Treatment of Acute Altitude Illness (2014 Update) defined HACE as worsening symptoms seen in moderate-severe AMS with any of following neurological findings; ataxia, severe lassitude, alter mental status and encephalopathy. Imaging studies and laboratory analysis are primarily used to rule out an alternative diagnosis.

Typical findings in HACE include normal cell counts and elevated CSF opening pressure. Values up to 220 cm water have been reported in the literature. Computed tomography of the head typically shows white matter signal attenuation with effacement of sulci and flattening of gyri. MRI findings include increased T2 signal observed in the splenium of the corpus callosum. Alternatively, MRI using susceptibility-weighted imaging can show hemosiderin deposition owing to microhemorrhage in the corpus callosum. HACE requires immediate treatment.

High-altitude Diseases of Long-term Highlanders [Chronic Mountain Sickness (CMS)]

This condition, also known as Monge's disease, was described in 1920s by Carlos Monge in high-altitude residents of the Andes who presented with polycythemia. It is characterized by a triad of polycythemia, hypoxemia and impaired mental function among long term residents (> 1 year). Beside the classical triad the other symptoms are bone and muscle pain, headaches, dizziness, dyspnea, insomnia, tinnitus, loss of appetite and even hallucinations. They have poor exercise tolerance; though exertional breathlessness is uncommon. They also have clubbing and cyanosis. The severity of the condition increases with advancing age. It is reversible upon descent from high altitudes.

These cases have extreme polycythemia, with Hb and hematocrit values as high as 23 g/dL and 83% respectively. The very high hematocrit increases the viscosity of the blood, and sometimes it is difficult to remove a venous blood sample. They have lower oxygen saturation and hypoxic ventilatory response with relative hypercapnia. They develop pulmonary hypertension and right ventricular enlargement. The pathogenesis of CMS is poorly understood but hypoxia is likely to be a major factor. Other possible factors include a low hypoxic ventilatory response, sleep-disordered breathing, increasing age, genetic factors, and possibly exposure to heavy metals such as cobalt. Poor understanding of pathogenesis raises the question as to why some individuals are susceptible to AMS and CMS while others are not, under the same hypoxic conditions. Tibetans may be one of the oldest high-altitude adapted ethnic groups in the world with origins from the neolithic period based on current genetic data. Tibetans have a lower incidence of CMS than Andeans, consistent with their lower hematocrit. CMS is a syndrome resulting from the loss of human adaptation to high altitude and can occur in permanent residents residing in this environment.

ROLE OF OXYGEN THERAPY IN HIGH-ALTITUDE DISEASES OF LOWLANDERS

The hypoxemic hypobaric environment at high altitude is mainly responsible for all forms of high altitude illnesses. Therefore descent to an altitude lower than where symptoms began is the treatment of choice.

Mild AMS is usually self-limiting and requires only symptomatic treatment. Moderate AMS requires low flow oxygen (0.5–1 L/min) to relieve persistent symptoms, e.g., headache and dizziness.

The HAPE requires oxygen administration as it is the therapy of choice leading to rapid improvement in patient's clinical status. Oxygen administration improves arterial saturation, heart rate and decreases pulmonary artery pressures. High flow rates of oxygen through face mask/nasal prongs should be titrated to maintain a targeted SpO_2 of 90 to 92%. In cases of nonavailability of oxygen rapid descent to an altitude at least 1000 m lower is effective .

The HACE is one of the medical emergencies at high altitude. Rapid descent is imperative and it should be upto at least 600 m. Oxygen should be administered at the rate of 2–4 L/min and drugs like acetazolamide and dexamethasone are recommended in severe cases of HACE. Hyperbaric therapy, using portable inflatable hyperbaric chambers like the Gamow bag, the CERTEC bag and the portable altitude chamber (PAC), is an effective alternative when oxygen is not available and descent is not possible. The apparatus consist of cylindrical bag that is capable of being pressurised by a foot driven pump. The patient is placed inside the bag lying flat and pressurized all around upto 2 psi. These hyperbaric chambers simulate benefits of 2000 feet to 5000 feet descent.

The nonpharmacological measures which are helpful in increasing oxygenation at high altitudes are application of positive airway pressure by facemask or helmet, oxygen enrichment of room air and pursed-lip breathing. The pharmacological measures should also be started simultaneously to hasten the recovery in HAI.

ROLE OF OXYGEN IN HIGH-ALTITUDE DISEASES OF LONG-TERM HIGHLANDERS

Oxygen supplementation has no role in the management of Monge's disease. It may temporarily relieve pulmonary artery hypertension. Descent to sea level is the definitive treatment as it is reversible upon descent from high altitudes.

Phlebotomy is beneficial for those who wish to remain at an altitude as it improves exercise performance and neuropsychological symptoms. However, recent data have questioned the role of repeated phlebotomies in conditions with high hematocrit like polycythemia vera and those that result in secondary polycythemia.

SUGGESTED READING

1. Aksela G, erem Çorbacıoglub SK, Özen C. High-altitude illness: Management approach. Turkish J Emerg Med. 2019;19:121-26.
2. Bhattacharya S, Shrimali NM, Mohammad G, Koul PA, Prchal JT, Guchhait P. Gain-of-function Tibetan PHD2D4E;C127S variant suppresses monocyte function: A lesson in inflammatory response to inspired hypoxia. EBioMedicine. 2021;68:103418.
3. Bigham AW. Genetics of human origin and evolution: High-altitude adaptations. Curr Opin Genet Dev. 2016;4:8-13.
4. Buroker NE, Xue-Han Ning XH, Zhou ZN, et al. EPAS1 and EGLN1 associations with high altitude sickness in Han and Tibetan Chinese at the Qinghai-Tibetan Plateau. Blood Cells, Mol. Dis. 2012;49: 67-73.
5. Davis C, Dimm DT, Hackett P. Advances in the prevention and treatment of high altitude illness. Emerg Med Clin N Am. 2017 ;35:241-60.
6. Davis PR, Pattinson KTS, Mason NP, et al. High altitude illness. J R Army Med Corps. 2005;151: 243-49.
7. Koul PA, Khan UH, Hussain T, Koul AN, Malik SU, Shah SU, Jan RA. High altitude pulmonary edema among "Amarnath Yatris". Lung India. 2013;30(3):193-98.
8. Lorenzo FR, Huff C, Myllymäki M et al. A genetic mechanism for Tibetan high-altitude adaptation. Nat Genetics. 2014;46(9): 951-56.
9. Luks AM, Swenson ER, Bärtsch P. Acute high-altitude sickness. Eur Respir Review. 2017; 26:160096.
10. Netzer N, Strohl K, Faulhaber M , et al. Hypoxia-related altitude illnesses. J Travel Med. 2013;20 (4): 247-55.
11. Paralikar SJ, Paralikar JH. High-altitude medicine. Ind J Occupat and Environ Med. 2010;14 (1):6-12.
12. Simonson TS, Huff CD, Witherspoon DJ, et al. Adaptive genetic changes related to hemoglobin concentration in native high-altitude Tibetans. Exp Physiol. 2015;100(11): 1263-68.
13. Taylor AT. High-altitude illnesses: Physiology, risk factors, prevention, and treatment. Rambam Maimonides Medical Journal. 2011; 2 (1): e0022.
14. West JB. Commuting to high altitude: Value of oxygen enrichment of room air. High Altitude Med Biol. 2002;3(2):223-35.
15. West JB. High-altitude medicine. Am J Resp Crit Care Med. 2012;186: 1229-37.

Chapter 17

Oxygen Use in Diving Medicine

PS Tampi

INTRODUCTION

Divers are entirely dependent on the oxygen carried in their lungs or their gas supply. Moreover, in diving, it is not always possible to breathe adequately and comfortably, and the diver's safety, work capacity and equipment are impaired to the extent that his breathing is limited. At higher atmospheric pressures (greater depth of diving) oxygen itself causes acute oxygen toxicity which can manifest with convulsions and can even kill the diver. Hence the diver in his underwater environment has a paradoxical problem with oxygen. To understand the diver's narrow knife-edge between fatal hypoxia and equally dangerous hyperoxia, calls for a thorough understanding of physical properties of gases at sea level and underwater.

PHYSIOLOGY

All organisms require oxygen for metabolism, but the oxygen in water is unavailable to mammals, which includes divers, whales and seals. The body obtains energy for life and activity from the internal chemical reactions of oxidative metabolism, basically comparable to combustion.The fuel for metabolism is provided by food and is readily stored, but oxygen must be supplied to the sites of metabolic reaction on a continuous basis matched to need. At the same time, carbon dioxide (CO_2) that is produced by this reaction must be eliminated. If delivery of O_2 or removal of CO_2 is impaired by environmental factors or the limitation of breathing apparatus, the divers capacity for exertion will, accordingly be limited. Life itself is threatened when exchange of O_2 and CO_2 is severely restricted.

PHYSICS

At sea level, the weight of the atmosphere exerts a pressure of 101.325 kilopascals (kPa), or 760 mm Hg which will support a column of water ten meters high; thus, ten meters under water the pressure on a diver is 200 kPa. According to Boyle's law, the volume of gas in a diving bell full of air at sea level is halved at 10 meters, at 20 m the pressure is 300 kPa absolute and the gas is compressed to one-third the volume. Also, since dry air is composed of roughly 21% oxygen, 78% nitrogen and 1% other gases, the partial pressure of oxygen at any depth will be 21% of the total pressure exerted by the air.

Gases dissolve in the liquid with which they are in contact. Among the various gases in the air, nitrogen is fat-soluble and there are several liters dissolved in our bodies at sea level. At 10 m depth by breathing air, the partial pressure of nitrogen is doubled. Consequently, once equilibration occurs there will be double the numbers of nitrogen molecules as at sea level. Since oxygen in our blood is largely bound to hemoglobin, and only partly dissolved in solution, doubling the inspired partial pressure of oxygen only doubles the dissolved component. The hemoglobin in arterial blood is virtually saturated at an inspired partial pressure of oxygen of 21 kPa; increasing the partial pressure of oxygen, therefore has little effect on the amount of oxygen bound to hemoglobin.

TYPES OF DIVING

Breath-hold Diving

An average healthy person can hold his/her breath for about half a minute. During the breath hold, the oxygen content of tissues progressively decreases, but the breath hold is broken as a result of carbon dioxide production from tissues and resulting acidosis which stimulates the respiratory centre. With practice and special training one can learn to resist the stimulus to breathe during breath holding. Hyperventilation immediately prior to breath holding can extend its duration.This is due to carbon dioxide washout resulting in starting with a higher cerebrospinal fluid pH. Here it is the hypoxic stimulus that triggers respiration before the pH of cerebrospinal fluid falls enough to do so. Hence, it follows that it may be possible to hold a breath for over 5 minutes by prior hyperventilation on

100% oxygen, which would increase the total oxygen content of blood considerably.

Hyperventilation before diving enables breath hold divers to stay down longer but is very dangerous. The diver starts with a low CO_2 content, a high pH, and a normal O_2 tension. During descent to say, 30 m, the pressure increases fourfold, compressing the airspaces to one-fourth their surface volume (from TLC of 6 liters to 1.5 liters, near residual volume). The partial pressures of O_2 and N_2 in the lungs also increase 4-fold and produce corresponding increase in arterial and tissue gas tensions. During diving, O_2 is consumed and CO_2 is produced. Due to preceding hyperventilation, the diver does not feel the need to breathe until the arterial O_2 tension has fallen to levels which stimulate the carotid chemoreceptors. As the diver ascends, hydrostatic pressure is reduced 4-fold with a 4-fold reduction in O_2 tensions in alveolar gas, arterial blood, and tissues. The rapidly falling cerebral O_2 pressure may be inadequate for consciousness to be maintained and the diver could drown during ascent. Even coming to the surface from the bottom of a two meter deep pool can reduce the O_2 pressure sufficient to cause loss of consciousness, and some fatalities have occurred this way.

Surface Oriented Diving

Refers to those diving operators where the diver travels between the surface and his worksite through the water column and without being protected within a closed diving bell. Thus he may swim, climb or be lowered in a basket or wet (or open) bell. The maximum depth of such operation is usually 165 ft (50 m) and air is normally the breathing gas (**Fig. 17.1**).

GASES USED IN UNDERWATER BREATHING

Air

This is the cheapest and most easily available gas to use for SCUBA (Self Contained Underwater Breathing Apparatus) or surface supplied diving. It can be compressed easily and is less likely to produce a fatal mixture than gas mixing but has several disadvantages. Nitrogen narcosis can result from high partial pressures at depth which can affect the function of cell membranes. At 30 meters, only mild impairment of intellectual function may occur, but this may progress to unconsciousness as the diver descends to depths near100 meters.

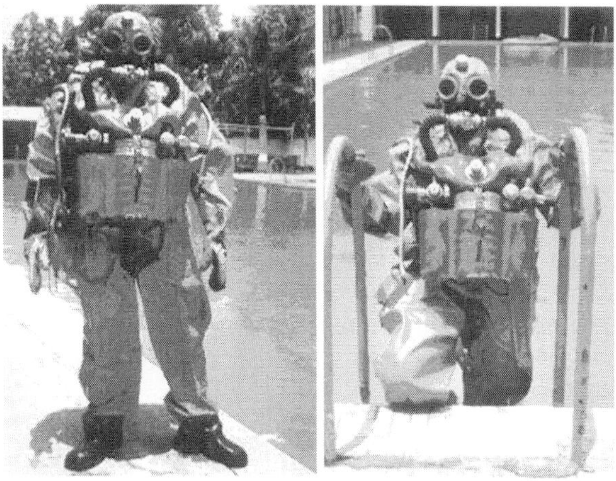

Fig. 17.1: Diver with suitably designed equipment.

During ascent or decompression, this large volume of highly soluble, dissolved nitrogen from the tissues is liberated. If the ascent/decompression is too rapid, large amounts of bubbles are liberated from the supersaturated tissues and this can lead to the well known "diver's bends" (Caisson's disease or decompression sickness). The recommended rate of ascent for most air dives is not more than 10–15 meters/min.

Nitrogen is a relatively dense gas and hence the work of breathing at 30 meter depth is twice as great as at the surface. A breathing system using air must liberate the exhaust gas (low in O_2 and high in CO_2 and N_2), though bubbles can be a problem in covert military operations and while defusing naval mines with acoustic sensors.

Oxygen

To overcome the problems of nitrogen, several alternatives were considered. Oxygen rebreathing systems allow divers to breathe 100% O_2 but CO_2 accumulation occurs and is removed by a CO_2 absorber. When pure O_2 is breathed, much smaller amounts of gas need to be carried and produces no bubbles. However, there can be problems which can even be fatal. The fraction of inspired nitrogen is zero in such a system. However, the diver's body contains several liters of dissolved nitrogen, which can as a consequence of the pressure gradient pass back to the lung and into the counter-lung.

O_2 is consumed, CO_2 is removed and nitrogen accumulates, gradually reducing the percentage of O_2 in the counter-lung. This can lead to unconsciousness. Flushing the system with pure O_2 periodically can overcome this problem. But high partial pressures of O_2 can increase blood pressure and reduce heart rate.

Pulmonary toxicity and eventually irreversible pulmonary fibrosis can result from prolonged breathing of a gas with $FiO_2 > 0.6$, though this may take many hours or days. Acute O_2 toxicity can occur within minutes causing convulsions when $PIO_2 > 160$ kPa, and if underwater, is usually fatal. Breathing air with 21% O_2 risks acute O_2 toxicity at depths > 66 m; breathing 100% O_2 there is a risk of convulsion at only 6 m.

Mixed Gas Diving

This is synonymous with bell diving and in systems used for diving beyond 165 feet (50 m) but may also be used at shallower depths. It is divided into two basic types of operations: Bounce diving and saturation diving procedures.

Bounce Diving Procedures

A bounce dive is one in which the diver's exposure to the bottom pressure is usually limited to about 30–60 minutes in order to minimize their subsequent decompression period. This is achieved with the help of a diving bell which is first lowered to the working depth while maintaining internal atmospheric pressure. When the divers are ready to go for work, the internal pressure is raised rapidly by the divers until it reaches the external pressure at which point the outer door falls open and the diver is able to venture out of the bell. As soon as the diver finishes his work and returns to the bell, the inner door is closed and the bell immediately risen. Thereafter, decompression is commenced.

Saturation Diving Procedures

For some tasks the need for longer dive durations and more working divers necessitates the use of saturation techniques. Saturation diving systems are much larger than bounce diving systems because up to some 16 divers will be maintained under pressure and for as long as 4 weeks. Such systems can operate 24 hours a day, and consequently, a larger surface support crew of 10–35 men working on a shift basis is also required.

Saturation Diving Gases

The gaseous mixture used in the saturation diving and maximum depth are given in **Table 17.1**.

Nitrogen-Oxygen (Nitrox) Saturation Dive

N_2-O_2 saturation dive basically involves shallow depth of up to 40 meters because of the narcotic property of nitrogen. The oxygen partial pressure in the mixture is kept at 0.2 to 0.43 kg for avoiding chronic O_2 toxicity.

Advantages

- Cheaper than helium.
- Suitable for shallow depths up to 40 m and excursions possible up to 60 m.
- No chance of pulmonary O_2 toxicity.
- Negligible risk of high pressure nervous syndrome (HPNS).

Disadvantages

- Long decompression time would be required.
- Greater chances of decompression sickness.

Helium-Oxygen Saturation Diving

Helium is commonly used with oxygen (Heliox), even though helium is expensive and has a high thermal conductivity, which potentiates heat loss and can make hypothermia a serious possibility on deep dives. Helium molecules are small so that the work of breathing is low even at great depths. It is relatively insoluble in lipids, minimizing bubble liberation on decompression. Its insolubility means that it lacks narcotic effects, but this unmasks another problem of diving deep, the HPNS.

Table 17.1: Gaseous mixture used in saturation diving.

Mixture gas	*Maximum depth*
Nitrogen-oxygen	40 m
Helium-oxygen	350 m
Helium-oxygen-nitrogen	650 m
Hydrogen-oxygen	Unlimited

Advantages

- Colorless, odorless, tasteless, light weight, non-toxic, non-explosive inert gas.
- Suitable for deep diving up to 600 meters and more.
- Low density gas.
- Limited narcotic properties.

Disadvantages

- Good conductor of heat (especially below 300 meters) at least five times as rapidly as air.
- Voice distortion due to 'Donald duck' effect.
- HPNS.

During heliox dives, the partial pressure of oxygen is maintained at 0.35 to 0.43 kg for preventing chronic pulmonary oxygen toxicity. The habitat is to be pressurized gradually to avoid hyperbaric arthralgia and HPNS. Compression is kept slow from 9 to 18 meters/minute at shallow depth to 0.05 meters at deeper depths. The habitat temperature is regulated between 20–22°C. However, at depths greater than 300 meters, the temperature control gets more difficult in view of helium's high thermal conductivity and the temperature is to be maintained at 31–32°C. The relative humidity is maintained between 55 to 65%. Saturation excursion either deeper or shallower can be carried out from a particular storage depth of the habitat.

Trimix (Helium-Oxygen-Nitrogen) Saturation Diving

In order to prevent HPNS of heliox mixture, the narcotic properties of nitrogen is advantageously used in this mixture. In trimix, the partial pressure of N_2 is maintained below 1.5 kg. Trimix can be used up to a depth of 600 meters or more.

Hydrogen-Oxygen (Hydrox) Saturation Diving

The world's helium resources are gradually diminishing. Hence, there is a need to find gases to take man down to even greater depths than have been achieved with helium. Future deep diving operation will depend upon the substitute of helium in the breathing mixture. Hydrogen-oxygen saturation dive is still in experimental stage, but the diminishing supply of helium may make H_2–O_2 mixture an attractive alternative in the future.

Advantages of Hydrogen

- Colorless, odorless, tasteless gas and lighter than all gases.
- Being a low-density gas it offers lowest resistance to breathing.
- Diffuses faster than any other gas due to high diffusion coefficient. H_2 absorption and elimination from tissues is more rapid and thereby reduces decompression time.
- Minimal narcotic activity based on the solubility.
- No HPNS.
- Can be obtained from electrolysis of water and is thus potentially more abundant.
- Can be used for dives beyond 600 meters.

Disadvantages

- It is highly inflammable and explosive when the oxygen content in the mixture exceeds 4%.
- High thermal conductivity like helium.
- Voice communication is as bad as in a helium dive.

A young Swedish engineer, Arne Zetterstorm, made the first successful dive using H_2-O_2 mixture to depths of 110 meters and 160 meters in 1945. The French have conducted various experimental saturation dives using H_2-O_2 mixtures starting from the first Comex saturation dive - Hydrox I in 1972 at 60 meters to Hydrox IX in 1989 to a depth of 600 meters. In the future, the deepest dives can be achieved by using H_2-O_2 mixture.

Diving Problems

Diving injuries are increasing because of a tremendous increase in the popularity of SCUBA diving. Most diving emergencies are related to changes in the behavior of gases due to pressure changes. During descent, there is an increase in the partial pressure of gases in the blood and tissues. Barotrauma may result especially from compression of air present in the middle air, sinuses and lungs. Medical problems may occur during or even after 24 hours of diving. Immersion pulmonary edema (IPE) may result from an increase in the hydrostatic pressure. Decompression results on ascent after re-exposure to normal or lower ambient pressures when the gases dissolved in the body fluids may bubble out and cause decompression sickness which may present with varied clinical manifestations. High Pressure Nervous Syndrome (HPNS) appears during deep helium diving (150–180 m), with motor and sensory symptoms. Nitrogen narcosis while diving, occurs following a significant increase in partial pressure of nitrogen with change in level of consciousness and neuro-sensory state. Oxygen toxicity can result from the use of enriched air or closed-circuit rebreather during diving due to oxidative injury from oxygen free radicals affecting the brain, lungs and eyes. Central nervous system oxygen toxicity (CNS-OT) is one of the most harmful effects of Enriched Air Nitrox (EAN) diving and it is related to oxidative stress and inflammation causing convulsions with sudden loss of consciousness, nausea, vomiting, palpitations, visual field constriction, tinnitus and auditory hallucinations, which are probably preventable by administering anticonvulsant drugs.

An intensive medical fitness examination is important for deep sea and military divers. Routine during medical examination includes a pressure test in the hyperbaric chambers. Oxygen tolerance tests under hyperbaric conditions is important for divers who use oxygen rebreather devices.

SUGGESTED READING

1. Bennett PB, Elliot DH (Eds). The Physiology and Medicine of Diving, 4th edition. London: WB Saunders Company Ltd, 1993.
2. Bosco G, Rizzato A, Moon RE, Camporesi EM. Environmental physiology and diving medicine. Front Psychol. 2018;9:72. doi: 10.3389/fpsyg.2018.00072.
3. Bove AA, Davis JC. Diving Medicine, 2nd edition. Philadelphia: WB Saunders, 1990.
4. DeGorordo A, Vallejo-Manzur F, Chanin K, Varon J. Diving emergencies. Resuscitation. 2003;59:171–80.
5. Emerson GM. What you need to know about diving medicine but won't find in a textbook. Emerg Med. 2002;14:371–6.
6. Kot J, Sicko Z. Delayed treatment of bubble related illness in diving – review of standard protocol. Int Marit Health. 2004; 55:103–20.
7. Sport Diving. The British Sub-Aqua Club Diving Manual, 11th edition. London: Stanley Paul, 1993.
8. Strauss RH. Diving medicine. Am Rev Respir Dis. 1979;119: 1001–23.
9. Tetzlaff K, Shank ES, Muth CM. Evaluation and management of decompression illness: An intensivist's perspective. Intensive Care Med. 2003;29:2128–36.
10. Weiss M. Standards on medical fitness examinations for navy divers. Int Marit Health. 2003;54:135–43.
11. Wilmshurst P. ABC of oxygen, diving and oxygen. BMJ. 1998; 317: 996–99.

Chapter 18

Hyperbaric Oxygen Therapy

PS Tampi

INTRODUCTION

Hyperbaric oxygen therapy is the administration of oxygen at a pressure greater than that at sea level, which is one atmosphere. Hyperbaric medicine owes its origin to the problems encountered by deep-sea, divers exposed to high pressure diving sports, commercial or military expeditions at depths of 10 meters or more. In clinical medicine, this is simulated by exposing a patient to hyperbaric atmosphere in a closed monoplace or multiplace chamber. In either case, the partial pressure of oxygen (PaO_2) will approach 1500 mm Hg at a pressure equivalent of 33 feet of seawater. A century of research in oxygen administration has established that the effects are dose related, and the hyperbaric environment merely provides the opportunity to give higher doses than can be achieved at sea level.

HISTORY OF HYPERBARIC MEDICINE

Development of Hyperbaric Air Therapy

The British physician Henshaw used compressed air for medical purposes in 1662 in an airtight room called a "domicilium" in which variable climatic and pressure conditions could be produced, with pressure provided by a large pair of bellows. According to Henshaw, "In times of good health, this domicilium is proposed as a good expedient to help digestion, to promote insensible respiration, to facilitate breathing and expectoration, and consequently, of excellent use for the prevention of most afflictions of the lungs." There is however, no account of any application of Henshaw's proposed treatment, and there were no further developments in the field of hyperbaric therapy for nearly two centuries.

In the nineteenth century, there was a rebirth of interest in hyperbaric therapy in France. In 1834, Junod built a hyperbaric chamber to treat pulmonary afflictions using pressures of two to four absolute atmospheres (ATA). In 1837, Pravaz built the largest hyperbaric chamber of that time and treated patients with a variety of ailments. Fontaine, in 1877, developed the first mobile hyperbaric operating theater, and by this time hyperbaric chambers were available in all major European cities. Interestingly, there was no general rationale for hyperbaric treatments, and prescriptions therefore varied from one physician to another. During the second half of the nineteenth century, hyperbaric centers were advertised as being comparable to health spas. Junod referred to his treatment as "Le Bain d'air comprimd" (the compressed-air bath). In 1855 Bertin wrote a book on this topic and constructed his own hyperbaric chamber.

The first hyperbaric chamber on the North American continent was constructed in 1860 in Oshawa, Ontario, Canada, just east of Toronto. It was the first such chamber in the United States, and later shifted to New York, to treat nervous disorders. The chamber that was built by Dr Orville Cunningham, a professor of anesthesia, received the most publicity, and was the most actively used in Kansas City in the 1920s. Cunningham claimed to have achieved remarkable improvement in patients who were cyanotic and comatose. Cunningham reasoned that a barometric factor was therefore involved. However, one night a mechanical failure resulted in a complete loss of compression and all his patients died. This tragedy was a sobering lesson but ultimately did not deter Dr Orville Cunningham. His enthusiasm for hyperbaric air continued, and he started to treat diseases such as syphilis, hypertension, diabetes mellitus, and cancer. Its reasoning was based on the assumption that anaerobic infections played a role in the etiology of all such diseases. In 1928 Cunningham constructed the largest chamber ever built (five stories high and 64 feet in diameter), referred to as the "Steel Ball Hospital" in Cleveland. Each floor had one bedroom with all the amenities of a good hotel. At that time it was the only functioning hyperbaric chamber in the world. The Cunningham chamber was dismantled for scrap in 1937, which brought to a temporary end of the era of hyperbaric air therapy for medical disorders.

Development of Hyperbaric Oxygen Therapy

Oxygen was not "discovered" until 1775, when the English scientist Joseph Priestley isolated what he called "dephlogisticated air." Although hyperbaric air had been used as early as 1662, oxygen was not specifically added to early hyperbaric chambers. The toxic effects of concentrated oxygen reported by Lavoisier and Segiom in 1789 were reason enough for hesitation to use it under pressure. Paul Bert, the father of pressure physiology, discovered the scientific basis of oxygen toxicity in 1878. The potential benefits of using oxygen under pressure for the treatment of decompression sickness were first realized by Drager, who in 1917 devised a system for treating diving accidents. It was not until 1937—the very year that Cunningham's "air chamber" hotel was demolished, that Behnke and Shaw actually used hyperbaric oxygen (HBO) signifying the arrival of the era of HBO therapy.

It was in the year 1956 that the first clinical paper was published on HBOT by Ite Boerema, the Chief of Surgery at the University of Amsterdam, Netherlands. Till then HBOT was often marketed as a miracle cure for every conceivable illness known to mankind ranging from common influenza to even cancers. Boerema and his colleagues reported the use of hyperbaric oxygen during cardiac surgery, to prolong safe operating times and the beneficial effects in the management of ischemic non-healing leg wounds and necrotizing infections. It is not surprising that Ite Boerema has been recognized as the Father of hyperbaric medicine.

Rationale of Hyperbaric Oxygen

An increased atmospheric pressure increases the partial pressure of O_2 in the alveolar air and arterial blood provided the fractional concentrations of oxygen remains the same. This is easily derived from the alveolar air equation. Since the oxygen dissolved in the plasma depends upon PaO_2, the dissolved O_2 content of blood is also increased. This is independent of Hb levels of the blood. Therefore, under hyperbaric conditions the total oxygen carrying capacity of the blood is significantly more **(Table 18.1)**. At 1 atmosphere (sea level) with a person breathing 100% O_2, the PaO_2 is about 670 mm Hg and the total oxygen content of 18.7 mL/dL. Increasing the pressure to 3 atmospheres, the PaO_2 increases to about 1700–1800 mm Hg and the total O_2 content to 22 mL/dL. Of this, about 25% (i.e. 5.5 mL/dL) is dissolved in plasma. This in fact is equivalent to the total oxygen

Table 18.1: Different components of oxygen content of the blood at different atmospheric pressures at constant plasma hemoglobin of 14 g/dL, when breathing 100% O_2.

Pressure (atmospheres)	*PaO_2 (mm Hg)*	*Dissolved O_2 (%)*	*Total O_2 content (mL/dL)*
1	670	11	18.7
2	1200–1300	18	20
3	1700–1800	25	22

content of blood under normal conditions at much lower Hb level of 4 g%. Therefore under hyperbaric conditions, it is possible to maintain adequate oxygen content of blood as well as delivery to the tissues with a very low or no hemoglobin at all. However, it should be remembered that the whole of the tissue oxygen requirements can be met by dissolved oxygen only if PaO_2 is around 2025 mm Hg.

Other Physiological Effects of Hyperbaric Oxygenation

- **Effect on $PaCO_2$:** An increased hemoglobin saturation of venous blood reduces its ability to carry CO_2, and results in carbon dioxide accumulation (Haldane effect).
- **Vasoconstriction:** It occurs due to increase in PaO_2 and has a therapeutic value.
- **Angiogenesis:** The mechanism by which this occurs is not known but occurs only when oxygen is administered at more than 1 ATA, and does not occur with 100% oxygen at 1 ATA.

Beneficial Effects of HBO

Hyperbaric oxygen administration achieves two principal objectives:

1. It increases PaO_2 and tissue PO_2 to levels higher than those obtained at 1 ATA. This has got several potential therapeutic benefits. The oxygen delivery to the tissues is increased, which may promote healing; the phagocytosis and antibiotic action on the microorganism are augmented. Hyperoxia induces vasoconstriction, which reduces tissue edema. Finally, the oxygen dissolved in the plasma is available to the tissues without any increase required in the hemoglobin level. This is not associated with any increase by blood transfusions. Problems of increased blood viscosity are therefore, avoided.

2. There is an increase in the ambient pressure which increases interstitial tissue pressures as well. This is used to treat decompression sickness, which may occur in divers. Similarly, presence of air or gas in the blood either injected accidentally during some procedure or due to embolization can be absorbed with HBO therapy.

Mechanism of Action of HBO

- HBO increases dissolved oxygen in the plasma, which readily diffuses into the hypoxic tissues.
- Increased oxygenation results in vasoconstriction at the site resulting in induced transudation, reduction in capillary pressure and thereby decreasing the tissue edema and reducing inflammation by clamping down on the release of proinflammatory cytokines.
- The reduction in tissue edema reduces compression of the cells thereby enhancing the reabsorption of fluid.
- With edema being less, barriers of diffusion are reduced and oxygen diffusion to the tissue improves resulting in improvement in tissue functions.
- Improved vascularization due to neovascularization as a result of increase in vascular endothelial growth factor (VEGF), tumor growth factor-beta (TGF-β), angiopoietin 2, capillary tube formation and endothelial stem cells from bone marrow, aids in speedy recovery of the tissues and gives way to tissue regeneration. There is an increase in fibroblast growth factor (FGF), fibroblast migration and proliferation, collagen production and cross linking, leading to increase in extracellular matrix formation.
- Oxide, hydro-peroxide and superoxide radicals of oxygen are toxic, and interfere with cell metabolism of bacteria and thereby destroy the bacteria.
- HBO modulates the immune system and helps in the faster elimination of virus.
- Bacterial killing effect of leukocytes is impaired in the hypoxic state. Increased oxygenation will enhance the leukocyte bactericidal activity, increase the macrophage chemotaxis and decrease neutrophil beta 2 integrin adhesion.

Hyperbaric oxygen therapy (HBOT) overcomes the hypoxia, impaired angiogenesis and longstanding inflammation, so commonly associated with chronic non-healing wounds, through several mechanisms thereby promoting neovascularization, decreasing inflammation and improving wound healing.

Indications for Hyperbaric Oxygen Treatments

Enthusiasm with the use of HBO_2 now is almost similar to what was seen with use of normobaric oxygen in the 19th century when its therapeutic applications were first discovered. But this enthusiasm has helped to discover its beneficial role as an adjunct in the treatment of diverse clinical conditions. Indications may vary in different countries in different settings. Some of the more definite indications are the decompression sickness, air embolism, gas gangrene and carbon monoxide poisoning. In 1976, the Undersea and Hyperbaric Medical Society (UHMS), (at the time, Undersea Medical Society) drew up a list of clinical conditions for which HBOT could be used. This list is updated every 2 years based on emerging clinical evidence. The indications apprised by the Undersea and Hyperbaric Medical Society are rather limited and rely on the proof of efficacy of controlled studies. At present there are 14 UHMS approved indications for the use of HBOT as given in **Box 18.1**.

Decompression Sickness

Decompression sickness occurs when the ambient air pressure is allowed to lower rapidly after a prolonged exposure to a higher pressure. This is commonly seen in the deep sea divers after emerging

Box 18.1: Indications for hyperbaric oxygen therapy.

1. Air or gas embolism
2. Carbon monoxide poisoning
3. Clostridial myositis and myonecrosis (gas gangrene)
4. Crush injury, compartment syndrome, and other acute traumatic ischemias
5. Decompression sickness
6. Arterial insufficiencies
7. Severe anemia
8. Intracranial abscess
9. Necrotizing soft tissue infections
10. Osteomyelitis (refractory)
11. Delayed radiation injury (soft tissue and bony necrosis)
12. Compromised grafts and flaps
13. Acute thermal burn injury
14. Idiopathic sudden sensorineural hearing loss

from a diving juggernaut and occasionally in the aviators or astronauts on reaching the outer atmosphere or space. Due to a sudden lowering of pressure, the inert gases dissolved in body fluids bubble out in both intravascular and extravascular compartments resulting in multiple symptoms. The common clinical manifestations include musculo-skeletal pains, neurological symptoms such as paresthesias and sensori motor deficits, nausea, vomiting, nystagmus, tinnitus, sub-sternal pain, cough, dyspnea, hoarseness of voice and occasionally shock and death.

Hyperbaric oxygen and recompression to about 60 feet constitute the mainstay of therapy. Both steps help in the reduction and resolution of the bubbles and maintenance of tissue oxygenation. Increased occurrence of oxygen toxicity under higher pressure conditions limits the duration of use of hyperbaric oxygen. Relapse may occur after discontinuation of therapy. Short-term observation especially in patients with neurological symptoms for at least 6 hours is generally recommended. Some people advocate the provision of observation units for about 24 hours after hyperbaric therapy.

Air Embolism

Air bubbles may form in the venous circulation, due to sudden decompression (e.g. decompression sickness) or more commonly get introduced during central venous instrumentation, invasive medical and surgical procedures, hemodialysis, chest trauma or positive pressure ventilation, employing high levels of positive end expiratory pressures (PEEP). These air bubbles finally end up in the lungs causing obstruction of pulmonary circulation and presenting a picture of pulmonary air embolism. It may occasionally be fatal if a large pulmonary vessel gets blocked. Bubbles may also form in the arterial circulation but are rare because of the higher hydrostatic pressure in the larger vessels. Cerebral air embolism is uncommon but more serious in nature.

Treatment of air embolism employs resuscitative and restorative measures for pulmonary circulation through removal and/or absorption of air from the pulmonary vessels. Attempts to remove the air bubbles include the direct needle aspiration, Trendelenburg position or removal through a central venous catheter. Administration of 100% oxygen helps reabsorption of air. Hyperbaric oxygen administration rapidly reduces the bubble size. Generally 50% O_2

at a pressure of 165 feet is administered initially for a few minutes followed by intermittent periods of 100% oxygen at a lower pressure of 65 feet. A recent report on the use of USN TT6 suggests this use of oxygen filled monoplace hyperbaric chamber as better tolerated and safer from oxygen toxicity point of view than a multiplace chamber for the treatment of both decompression sickness and air embolism.

Gas Gangrene and Other Necrotizing Infections

There is an increased evidence to suggest a major role of HBO_2 on inflammatory cytokines and mediators. It is shown to cause cytokine down-regulation and growth factor up-regulation. HBO_2 therefore is likely to promote wound healing by suppressing inflammation and facilitating repair. It also augments the antibacterial actions of leukocytes which gets otherwise inhibited under hypoxic conditions and thereby improves the efficacy of antibiotics. These effects has been shown in a few trials and clinical experience as an adjunct treatment for gas gangrene, non-healing wounds (e.g. diabetic foot), osteomyelitis and necrotizing fasciitis. It is also shown to shorten the treatment with antibiotics for soft tissue infections.

Hyper-oxygenation in particular is valuable in gas gangrene since it inhibits the growth of the causative anaerobic micro-organisms i.e., clostridia and prevents formation of toxins responsible for necrotizing myositis and myonecrosis. Reports on the useful role of HBO_2 are available for treatment of all kinds of clostridial infections including necrotizing fasciitis of upper extremities, orbital gas gangrene, recurrent crepitant cellulites with extensive subcutaneous emphysema. It has been also used in patients with refractory mycoses and leprosy.

Carbon Monoxide Poisoning

Carbon monoxide (CO) a byproduct of incomplete combustion of coal is a poisonous gas. It is a common cause of death in miners and other personnel working with coal furnaces in foundaries and factories. CO poisoning in India occurs in people burning indoor coal for heating and cooking during winter months in ill ventilated houses. Deaths in this scenario are commonly reported in individuals sleeping in closed rooms. Malfunctioning air conditioning system in cabins have been occasionally blamed for CO poisoning.

CO poisoning is generally insidious. Neurological complications are most frequent. Some of the common symptoms include headache, confusion, dizziness, nausea and vomiting. In more serious forms, syncope, seizures and coma may precede death. Cardiac arrhythmias and pulmonary edema may also occur.

CO has an affinity for hemoglobin almost 300 times that of oxygen. Exposure to CO therefore quickly results in displacement of oxygen and formation of carboxy hemoglobin (HbCO).

Treatment of CO poisoning needs to be prompt and aggressive. A great degree of evidence supports that hypoxia occurs late in CO poisoning. But the treatment of both the actually poisoned persons as well as the environmental exposures are based on a hypoxic theory of toxicity. Oxygen therapy is the mainstay of therapy besides other supportive care. Oxygen accelerates the dissociation of CO from hemoglobin and other heme proteins. Oxygen with an FiO_2 100% is administered with a high flow and the response is quick provided the treatment is started in time before any organ damage has occurred.

Hyperbaric oxygen has been used in a few trials. It rapidly decreases blood COHb. It may also delay the occurrence of delayed brain injury. But there is no conclusive evidence to support its use. Firm guidelines regarding the use of hyperbaric oxygen cannot be established from the available literature.

Adjunct to Treatment of Cancers

HBO_2 may improve the treatment of malignant tumors by increasing the tumor sensitization to radiotherapy. A significant improvement is reported with HBO_2 followed by radiotherapy for local tumor control and mortality for cancers of the head and neck and local tumor recurrences in cancers of head and neck and uterine cavity. It also improves the response to photodynamic and chemotherapy possibly by raising intra-tumoral oxygen tension. It was also shown to improve survival in locally advanced breast cancer undergoing neo-adjuvant chemotherapy. It may also promote new vessel growth into areas with reduced oxygen tension thereby promoting healing of radiation-induced tissue injury.

HBOT AND COVID-19

The current pandemic caused by corona virus SARS-CoV-2 affects the respiratory system primarily and often leads to severe bronchopneumonia, acute respiratory distress syndrome and respiratory failure. HBOT has been tried as an off-label use to treat Covid- 19 pneumonia. The pathogenesis of Covid-19 pneumonitis involves a hyperinflammatory response, the "cytokine storm", against which, the use of HBOT has shown to mitigate this inflammatory response. A multicentre study on the use of HBOT in Covid-19 is in progress and the results are eagerly awaited.

CONTRAINDICATIONS

Contraindications for HBO therapy can be divided into the absolute contraindication which include untreated tension pneumothorax and relative contraindications which include upper respiratory infections, emphysema with CO_2 retention, symptomatic pulmonary lesions seen on chest X-ray, history of thoracic or ear surgery, uncontrolled high fever, pregnancy, claustrophobia, seizure disorders, hyperthyroidism, congestive heart failure and malignant diseases.

COMPLICATIONS

The complications in the use of HBO are related to pressure changes and the toxic effects of oxygen. They include barotrauma to ear sinuses, or lungs. Trauma to ears or sinuses may be averted with slow compression, the use of decongestants, patient education and rarely myringotomy. Pulmonary barotraumas is very rare, perhaps occurring 1 in 50,000 treatments. It can be prevented by careful pretreatment screening for pulmonary blebs, air trapping caused by bronchospasm or secretions, preexisting pneumothorax, central lines and ventilatory support. Oxygen toxicity with occurrence of grand-mal seizures are noticed beyond a depth of 3 ATA (66 feet or 20 meters of sea water). Damage of lung tissue, manifested by decrement in vital capacity and irritation to large airways may occur due to oxygen toxicity following HBO. Increased pressure causes increased gas density and airway resistance. This produces an altered voice called the "Donald Duck voice" and an increased awareness of breathing. Hypoventilation may result especially in a patient with the underlying obstructive lung disease. Increased partial pressure of nitrogen causes symptoms of mild euphoria at pressure of 2.5 atmospheres progressing to frank intoxication and decreased performance at over 4 atmospheres. Accumulation of O_2

may occur in the event of an exposure for several days. Hyperpnea and occasionally respiratory acidosis may result. Other toxic substances or pollutants, which may continue to accumulate in a closed chamber and reach toxic pressures, include alcohol (from disinfectant solution), sulfur dioxide, hydrocarbons, carbon monoxide, volatile substances and mercury vapors. A regular monitoring is required for their concentrations. The nursing and medical personnel looking after the patient in a hyperbaric chamber may suffer from decompression sickness due to tissue bubble formation. The risk is rather low because the chamber is kept warm; exposure is short and decompression rate slow. Risk of an accidental fire is greater in hyperbaric conditions. All inflammable material should therefore be kept away. Refractive changes (myopia), cataracts in the lens of the eye and retinal changes may occur as a complication of prolonged HBOT. Pulmonary edema and exacerbation of congestive heart failure can occur. Claustrophobia may be a problem in up to 10% of patients especially in the monoplace chamber.

HYPERBARIC CHAMBERS

The main facility required for hyperbaric medicine is of course the hyperbaric chamber itself. This is essentially a chamber constructed to withstand pressurization so that oxygen can be administrated inside at a pressure greater than at sea level. The size, shape and pressure capabilities of the design chambers vary considerably. The technical details of each model now available are provided by the manufacturers and a classification of various types of chambers is shown below:

Types of Hyperbaric Chambers

- Monoplace chamber **(Fig. 18.1)**.
- Multiplace or "walk-in" chambers **(Fig. 18.2)**.
- Mobile or portable:
  - **Monoplace:** Transportable by air, sea or land, e.g., a portable hyperbaric bag like the Gamov bag, in which the patient is placed, the bag is sealed and then inflated with a foot pump.
  - **Multiplace:** A chamber that can be driven from place to place.
- Chambers for testing and training divers.
- Small hyperbaric chambers.
- For neonates.
- For animal experiments.

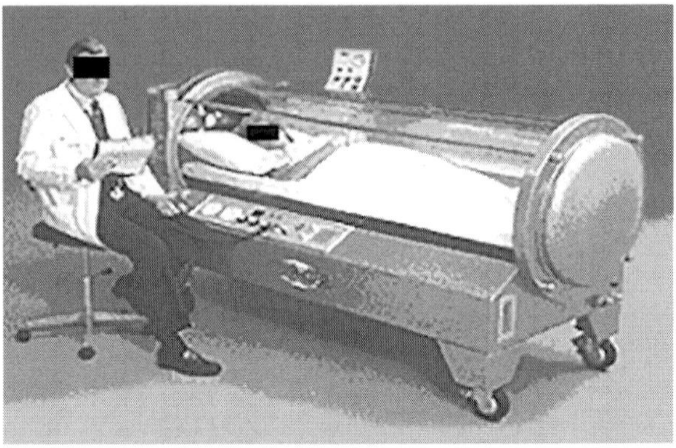

Fig .18.1: Monoplace hyperbaric chamber.

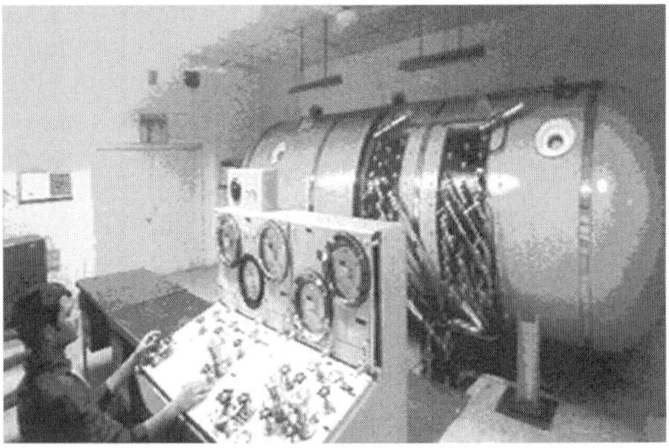

Fig. 18.2: Multiplace hyperbaric chamber.

Techniques of Hyperbaric Oxygenation

The hyperbaric technician follows the prescribed instructions for the hyperbaric physician about pressure, duration, and frequency of treatment. Most of the treatments are given at pressures between 1.5 and 2.5 ATA, and the usual duration of a hyperbaric session is 60 minutes. Of this 10 minutes are required for compression and 5 minutes for decompression if a pressure of 1.5 ATA is used. Thus, the maximal oxygen saturation is maintained for about 50 min. In the case of infections, the treatment duration is doubled. The treatment sessions for most chronic conditions are given daily, including on weekends.

World Distribution of Hyperbaric Chambers

Some idea of the quantity of hyperbaric medical facilities in the world can be obtained by a review of the statistics regarding the distribution of hyperbaric chambers in various countries. Accurate information on this subject is difficult to obtain. The largest number of chambers is located in Russia (over 1200). The USA has 361 hyperbaric centers of which only 43 are equipped to treat the high acuity patients (2020). South Korea has the largest number per million inhabitants (4.9 compared with 3.6 in Russia). Within Europe, excluding Russia, Italy has the largest number of installations (34.1% of the European total) and also the largest number per million inhabitants (1.75). The number of hyperbaric chambers per million inhabitants has risen progressively since 1968 in all countries except Germany, where the number has actually declined. The fastest rise has been in China and Japan. The number of chambers does not necessarily correlate with the number or the number of treatments given. There is no separation of multiplace and monoplace chambers in the statistics.

Hyperbaric Chambers in India

As the medical professionals in India are not all aware of the benefits of hyperbaric treatment, the availability of such facilities is also considerably less in number in India. A few years ago, of the 16 hyperbaric chambers in India, nine chambers were available with defence services and seven chambers were with civil hospitals in metropolitan cities. However, there is a rapid increase in the commercial use of hyperbaric chambers with several corporate hospitals now offering hyperbaric oxygen therapy with monoplace chambers of course, the hyperbaric chambers available with the defence services are also being utilized by the civil population. But considering the magnitude of hyperbaric chamber requirements in India, for over 1.3 billion population, the availability of chambers is grossly inadequate.

CONCLUSION

Hyperbaric oxygen therapy has been in medical use for several decades now. There are few specific indications for the use of HBOT as the primary modality of treatment like decompression sickness, air embolism, carbon monoxide poisoning, etc. However, the vast majority of indications use HBOT as an adjunct to standard therapy. HBOT acts by increasing neovascularization and decreasing inflammation and thereby aids healing in especially chronic non-healing wounds in diabetics, post radiation and even chronic osteomyelitis. It is currently used for the treatment of 14 clinical conditions as listed by UHMS where its efficacy is based on evidence from appropriate clinical studies. The full beneficial effects of HBOT will require more data from larger randomized clinical trials.

SUGGESTED READING

1. Al-Waili NS, Butler GJ, Beale J, Hamilton RW, Lee BY, Lucas P. Hyperbaric oxygen and malignancies: A potential role in radiotherapy, chemotherapy, tumor surgery and phototherapy. Med Sci Monit. 2005; 11: RA279–89.
2. Al-Waili NS, Butler GJ. Effects of hyperbaric oxygen on inflammatory response to wound and trauma: Possible mechanism of action. Scientific World Journal. 2006; 3:425–41.
3. Bennett, PB, Elliot DH (Eds). The Physiology and Medicine of Diving, 4th edition. London, WB Saunders Company Ltd., 1993.
4. Bennett M, Feldmeier J, Smee R, Milross C. Hyperbaric oxygenation for tumour sensitization to radiotherapy. Cochrane Database Syst Rev. 2005; 19:CD005007.
5. Boerema I, et al. Life without blood: A study of the influence of high atmospheric pressure and hypothermia on dilution of the blood. J Cardiovascular Surg. 1960;1:133–46.
6. Dauwe PB, Pulikkottil BJ, Lavery L, Stuzin JM, Rohrich RJ. Does hyperbaric oxygen therapy work in facilitating acute wound healing: A systematic review. Plast Reconstr Surg. 2014;133:208e–15e.
7. Davies JC, Hunt TK (Eds). Hyperbaric Oxygen Therapy. Bethesda, MD: Undersea and Hyperbaric Medical Society, 1977.
8. Gretl L, Rocky F, Frank LR, Ernest SC. Hyperbaric oxygen therapy: Exploring the clinical evidence. Adv Skin Wound Care. 2017;30(4):181–90.
9. Latham E. https://emedicine.medscape.com/article/1464149-overview, updated Nov16, 2020.
10. Lumb AB. Hyperoxia and oxygen toxicity. Nunn's Applied Respiratory Physiology, 5th edition, Oxford, Butterworth-Heinemann 2000; 491–512.
11. Mayer R, Hamilton-Farrell MR, Van der Kleij AJ, Schmutz J, Granstrom G, Sicko Z, Melamed Y, Carl UM, Hartmann KA, Janset EC, Ditri L, Sminia P. Hyperbaric oxygen and radiotherapy. Strahlenther Onkol. 2005; 181:113–23.

12. Moon RE, Camporesi EM. Clinical care at altered environment pressure. In: Miller RD (Ed). Anaesthesia. Churchill Livingston, New York. 1994; 2277-2306.
13. Moon RE. Hyperbaric oxygen treatment for air or gas embolism. Undersea Hyperb Med. 2014;41:159-66.
14. Perry BN, Floyd WE 3rd. Gas gangrene and necrotizing fasciitis in the upper extremity. J Surg Orthop Adv. 2004;13:57-68.
15. Sahni TK, Hukku S, Jain M, Prasad A, et al. Recent advances in hyperbaric oxygen therapy: Medicine update. Assoc Physicians India. 2004;14:632-9.
16. Sahni TK, Singh P, John MJ. Hyperbaric oxygen therapy : Current trends and applications. JAPI. 2003; 51:95-99.
17. Strauss RH. Diving medicine. Am Rev Respir Dis. 1979;119:1001-23.
18. Sugihara A, Watanabe H, Oohashi M, Kato N, Murakami H, Tsukazaki S, Fujikawa K. The effect of hyperbaric oxygen therapy on the bout of treatment for soft tissue infections. J Infect. 2004;48:330-3.
19. Tetzlaff K, Shank ES, Muth CM. Evaluation and management of decompression illness—an intensivists perspective. Intensive Care Med. 2003; 29:2128-36.
20. Trivedi DR, Rout VV. Role of hyperbaric oxygen therapy in the rapid control of gas gangrene infection and its toxaemia. Postgrad Med J. 1990; 36:13-15.
21. Undersea and Hyperbaric Medical Society. COVID-19 Information. Available at https://www.uhms.org/covid-19-information.html. November 11, 2020; Accessed: November 16, 2020.
22. Undersea and Hyperbaric Medical Society. Indications for Hyperbaric Oxygen Therapy. https://www.uhms.org/resources/hbo-indications.html. Last accessed January 25, 2017
23. Wang C, Schwaitzberg S, Berliner E, Zarin DA, Lau J. Hyperbaric oxygen for treating wounds: A systematic review of the literature. Arch Surg. 2003;138:272-9
24. Weaver LK. Monoplace hyperbaric chamber use of US navy Table 6: A 20 year experience. Undersea Hyperb Med. 2006;33:85-8.

Chapter 19

Complications of Oxygen Therapy

Vijay Hadda, Rohit Vadala, Hariharan Iyyer

Oxygen has been used not only for the correction and prevention of hypoxemia but for the relief of dyspnea as well. Importance of optimal body oxygenation may be understood with the fact that oxygen saturation is included as a 'fifth vital sign' for all breathless and/or critically ill patients, as it is a good and readily available indicator of oxygen status. Although, oxygen supplementation is commonly used in critical care; however, overzealous use of oxygen may lead to the toxicity with adverse effects on almost all the organ systems. Oxygen toxicity is an iatrogenic condition arising from the use of high partial pressure of inspired oxygen during the course of oxygen therapy. The oxygen toxicity on lungs closely mimics acute respiratory distress syndrome. There is no specific therapy for treating oxygen toxicity; hence, its prevention remains the cornerstone of management. Therefore, it is important that everyone prescribing oxygen therapy should be cognizant and vigilant of risks and benefits of this therapy. This chapter provides a brief overview of the pathogenesis and effects of oxygen toxicity.

INTRODUCTION

Oxygen has been administered since ages for the correction of hypoxemia, prevention of hypoxemia or for the relief of dyspnea. Importance of optimal body oxygenation may be understood with the fact that oxygen saturation is included as a 'fifth vital sign' for all breathless and/or critically ill patients which is a good and readily available indicator of oxygen status. The achievable target saturation for most acutely ill patients is 94–98% and 88–92% for those at risk of hypercapnic respiratory failure. Monitoring oxygen therapy and maintenance of target saturation is an important part of management which warrants stringent vigilance to avoid unnecessary and excess oxygen supplementation. This is because although lifesaving, inappropriate and excess use of oxygen therapy results in hyperoxia leading to free radical mediated alveolar toxicity. The degree of oxygen toxicity is directly proportional to partial pressure of oxygen delivered and the duration of exposure. The current understanding of the toxic effect of oxygen is attributed to the seminal work of J Lorrain Smith on animal models in the early part of 19th century. A thorough understanding on various aspects of oxygen therapy is necessary to prevent avoidable complications with prudent use. The discussion in this chapter focuses on oxygen therapy mediated tissue damage to various organs.

HYPEROXIA AND HYPEROXEMIA

Hyperoxia refers to the administration of high inspired concentration of oxygen, whereas hyperoxemia refers to high levels of oxygen in the blood. A PaO_2 of more than 100 mm Hg is a reflection of hyperoxia.

The alveolar gas equation calculates the oxygen level in the alveolus using the following formula:

$$PaO_2 \approx PiO_2 - PaCO_2/RER$$

In this equation, PaO_2 represents partial pressure of oxygen at the alveolar level and $PaCO_2$ represents partial pressure of carbon dioxide at the alveolar level and RER is the respiratory exchange ratio or the ratio of carbon dioxide production to oxygen consumption. Inspired PO_2 (PiO_2) = FiO_2 × (barometric pressure (100 kPa, 750 mm Hg) - water vapor pressure (~6 kPa, 45 mm Hg)). Although hyperoxia can be caused by hyperoxemia and polycythemia, the term hyperoxia is used to describe situations only when the PaO_2 is raised. Hyperoxemia can only exist in the presence of high PiO_2 or low $PaCO_2$ (resulting from hyperventilation). Hyperoxia leads to adverse effects on the body. The pathophysiological effects of hyperoxia on various organ systems are given in **Table 19.1**.

PATHOPHYSIOLOGY OF HYPEROXIA AND OXYGEN TOXICITY

Oxygen toxicity is caused by a high partial pressure of oxygen during the course of oxygen supplementation, and occurs due to excessive amount of reactive oxygen species (ROS) that overwhelms the natural anti-oxidant defense capacity. Exposure time, atmospheric pressure,

Table 19.1: Pathological effects of hyperoxia.

Organ system	*Effects and risks*
Respiratory system	Decreased ventilation leading to ventilation/perfusion mismatch and absorption atelectasis, respiratory acidosis and failure
Cardiovascular system	Myocardial ischemia, reduced cardiac output, reduced coronary blood flow, increased blood pressure due to increased reactive oxygen species
Metabolism	Decreased 2, 3-DPG, decreased CO_2 carriage (Haldane effect) attributed to increased reactive oxygen species
Nervous system	Decreased cerebral blood flow due to vasoconstriction of carotid and downstream cerebral arteries
Renal system	Decreased renal blood flow

and fraction of inspired O_2 (FiO_2) determine the cumulative oxygen dose leading to toxicity. Oxygen is toxic to the lungs when high FiO_2 (>0.60) is administered over extended exposure time (≥24 hours) at normal barometric pressure. This type of exposure is referred to as low pressure O_2 poisoning, or the Lorraine Smith effect. There exists an inverse relation between the FiO_2 administered and the amount of time needed to produce pathological changes in the lung. At FiO_2 of 100%, these pathological changes can be seen within 24 hours.

The pathogenesis of oxygen toxicity involves complex interaction between ROS, the anti-oxidant defense system and the host response. One of the main mechanisms of oxygen toxicity on the lungs is mediated via production of free radicals. The free radical mediated lung damage has four phases—initiation, inflammation, proliferation and fibrosis **(Fig. 19.1)**. Extent of damage depends on degree of severity and reversibility of injury. The pathophysiological mechanism of pulmonary toxicity due to high exposure to oxygen is linked to the eventual formation of free radicals. Free radicals (ROS) are generated as a cascade during the process of conversion of elemental molecular O_2 to ionic O_2 thereby making O_2 usable for ATP generation within cells. ROS generation occurs by a three-step process reducing O_2 to water by addition of four electrons yielding three reactive oxygen species—superoxide anion (O_2^-), hydrogen peroxide (H_2O_2) and hydroxyl radical (HO^-). The generation of these free radicals results in oxidant/antioxidant imbalance leading to damage of alveolar

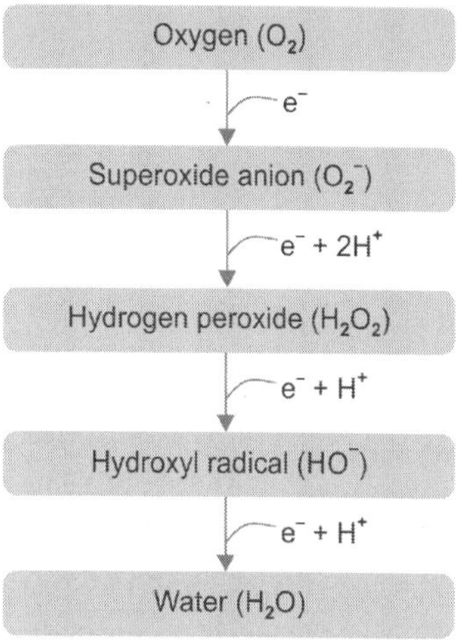

Fig. 19.1: Reactive oxygen species (ROS) generation cascade where oxygen is reduced to water yielding three reactive oxygen species.

epithelium and capillary endothelium. Injury to the alveoli leads to release of cytokines and other pro-inflammatory molecules which in turn activate macrophages to recruit neutrophils to the site of tissue injury. A cascade of response ensues with activation of molecules such as leukotrienes, oxidants, platelet activating factor and proteolytic enzymes. These molecules further damage capillary endothelium and alveolar epithelium, disrupting the barriers between the alveolar capillaries and air spaces.

The inflammatory or exudative phase results in edema fluid, proteins, and cellular debris to flood the air spaces and pulmonary interstitium, causing disruption of surfactant, airspace collapse, ventilation-perfusion mismatch, shunting, and stiffening of the lungs with decreased compliance and pulmonary hypertension. Dependent parts of the lungs are most frequently affected. Finally, the terminal fibrotic phase is irreversible with accumulation of collagen and pulmonary interstitial thickening leading to lung fibrosis.

The damaging effects of hyperoxia mediated initially by cytokine storm eventually leads to cell death and acute lung injury (ALI). The pathological changes associated with hyperoxia mediated ALI mimic the ALI triggered by other conditions such as hemorrhagic shock, reperfusion injury, pneumonia, sepsis, or inhalation of toxic chemicals **(Fig. 19.2)**.

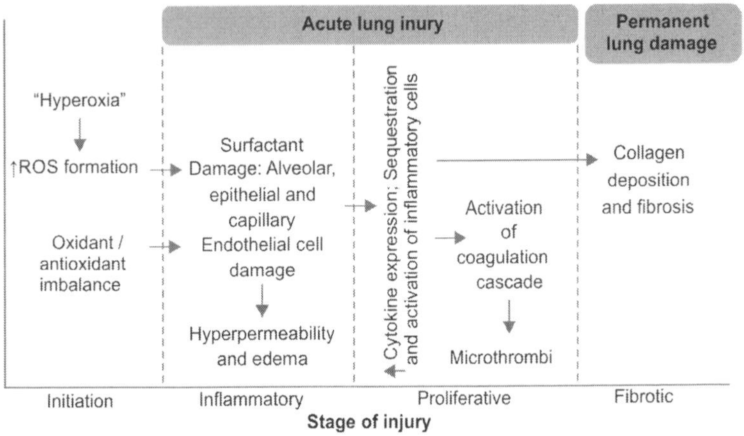

Fig. 19.2: Various phases of pathological changes occurring due to hyperoxia.

POTENTIATORS OF OXYGEN TOXICITY

The oxygen toxicity may be increased by simultaneous use of certain drugs such as bleomycin, paraquat, nitrofurantoin and disulfiram. These drugs are known to potentiate the effects of oxygen toxicity by disturbing the balance between oxidants and anti-oxidants. Similarly, deficiency of antioxidant vitamins such as vitamin A and E can also aggravate oxygen toxicity.

SYSTEMIC EFFECTS OF OXYGEN THERAPY

Toxic effects due to excess oxygen can be seen in various organs. These are mainly due to vasoconstriction in various organs, linked to the action of ROS released as a result of hyperoxia. These effects in various organ systems are discussed below.

Cardiac Emergencies

High-dose oxygen is associated with a variety of hemodynamic alterations that may increase myocardial ischemia and impair cardiac performance. In patients with acute myocardial infarction, studies have demonstrated utility of supplemental oxygen only when saturation is less than 90%. Detrimental effects such as sinus tachycardia and greater rise of myocardial enzymes have been reported due to excess oxygen delivery in such patients. This is possibly due to hyperoxia induced coronary vasoconstriction.Prolonged exposure of high oxygen is also known to cause decrease in stroke volume and cardiac output in healthy subjects,the effects are more in patients with congestive cardiac failure.Therefore, target peripheral oxygen saturation in such patients should be 90–94%, particularly if the clinical condition of the patient is stable.

Lungs

Approximately after 12 hours of oxygen exposure, fluid accumulation in the lungs occurs with airway congestion, absorption atelectasis (Lorraine Smith effect) and pulmonary edema. The pathophysiology of oxygen toxicity mediated lung damage has already been discussed above.

In COPD as such, hypoxic drive refers to the patient being dependent chronically on low levels of arterial blood oxygen (PaO_2) to stimulate breathing. If too much O_2 is given to such patients who rely on hypoxic drive to breathe, the blood O_2 levels as well as CO_2 levels rise, leading to CO_2 retention and respiratory acidosis and failure (Haldane effect). Studies have demonstrated significantly lower mortality rate in patients with COPD receiving titrated oxygen rather than high concentration of oxygen, thereby necessitating strict monitoring of oxygen saturation in such patients to maintain SpO_2 between 88–92%.

Central Nervous System (CNS)

Vasoconstrictive effects of oxygen therapy have been noted in carotid and cerebral arteries. Inhalation of oxygen at high atmospheric pressure leads to a constellation of symptoms which has been referred to as Paul Bert effect. CNS toxicity of hyperoxia manifests as seizures followed by coma in most people within 30 to 60 minutes. Seizures often occur without warning and are likely to be lethal.

Similarly, in various medical conditions such as stroke, the rationale of supplemental oxygen administration is questionable with no proven beneficial effects on mortality or functional disability. In fact, one of the trials was terminated due to deleterious effects of hyperoxia among this group of patients. As a result, the American Stroke Association does not support the use of supplemental oxygen for most patients with acute ischemic stroke.

Septic and Hemorrhagic Shock

Peripheral vasoconstriction induced by hyperoxia is known to be beneficial in patients with septic and hemorrhagic shock by reducing the need for vasopressors and volume resuscitation. Hyperoxia is hypothesized to have antimicrobial and anti-inflammatory effects. However, on the contrary there are no studies available to support benefits of supra-normal oxygen levels in sepsis wherein hyperoxia is known to impair oxygen consumption by tissues. The surviving sepsis campaign does not advocate hyperoxia in sepsis and ARDS patients but recommends peripheral oxygen saturation between 88 and 95%.

Cardiopulmonary Resuscitation

Clinically, hyperoxia during cardiopulmonary resuscitation is associated with poor neurological outcome post resuscitation. Various studies suggest the deterioration and relative risk of mortality to be high among patients who are resuscitated using high oxygen concentration (PaO_2 >300 mm Hg). This may be due to excessive oxidative stress mediated by hyperoxic reperfusion.

CLINICAL MANIFESTATIONS AND MANAGEMENT OF OXYGEN TOXICITY

Mortality related to acute lung injury and acute respiratory distress syndrome (ARDS) has improved over the past decade; however, it still ranges between 30 and 75%. Hyperoxia may also result in ARDS that usually presents within 24 to 48 hours after a direct or indirect trigger. The diagnosis of pulmonary oxygen toxicity depends on the correct association of non-specific symptoms and abnormal pulmonary functions in a proper clinical setting.

Common symptoms and signs include dyspnea, cough, chest pain, tachypnea, tachycardia, cyanosis, mottled skin, abnormal breath sounds. Visual changes, nausea, dizziness and confusion are initial signs of CNS toxicity. Seizure is the most dramatic sign of O_2 toxicity but reversible as the inspired PO_2 is reduced. Physical examination may reveal signs of pulmonary interstitial or alveolar edema.

Arterial blood gas analysis may reveal worsening hypoxia with widening of alveolar-arterial oxygen gradient. Chest radiograph reveals infiltrates consistent with signs of pulmonary edema and diffuse alveolar damage. Pulmonary function tests may show decrease in vital capacity, lung compliance and carbon monoxide diffusion capacity. Molecular assays may reveal presence of genes expressed as a result of oxidative stress, anti-proteolytic function and decreased surfactant function. Tissue examination reveals signs of microthrombi due to endothelial injury, red blood cells, and cellular fragments and eroded basement membrane epithelium.

There is no specific therapy for pulmonary oxygen toxicity. Prevention of oxygen toxicity remains the most important step in the management. The goal of oxygen therapy is to ensure the adequacy of tissue oxygenation with minimal oxygen toxicity. Therefore it is of utmost importance that the patient receiving oxygen therapy be monitored closely for adequate oxygenation through use of arterial blood gas analysis, pulse oximetry and looking for signs and symptoms of potential oxygen toxicity. A thorough knowledge of various oxygen therapy devices and proper patient selection along with patient tailored treatment target saturation goal is essential to prevent oxygen toxicity.

The first and foremost step after suspecting oxygen toxicity is to reduce the FiO_2 and thereby decrease the oxygen levels in the blood. Treatment includes lung protective mechanical ventilation strategies for ARDS, precise titration of oxygen guided by arterial blood gas analysis and treatment of the underlying cause. Ascorbic acid has also been shown to improve and reverse hyperoxia related effects in patients with cardiac emergencies due to its antioxidant properties.

HYPERBARIC OXYGEN THERAPY AND ITS CONSEQUENCES

Hyperbaric oxygen therapy (HBOT) has found its medical application as a useful primary or adjunctive therapy for a diverse range of medical conditions which includes decompression sickness, arterial gas embolism, carbon monoxide or cyanide poisoning and aggressive soft tissue infections like gas gangrene and necrotizing fasciitis. Typically, hyperbaric therapy is administered with pressurized oxygen or air in a closed chamber where the pressure is usually maintained between 2.5 and 3.0 atm and the treatment duration lasts from 45 to 300 minutes depending upon the indication. Exposure to high pressures exceeding 2.8 to 3.0 atm, particularly over prolonged periods especially beyond 90 to 120 minutes, exponentially increases the risk of both neurologic and pulmonary oxygen toxicity.

Potential complications of HBOT which are documented include middle ear barotraumas and seizures due to oxygen toxicity. Seizures should be managed by reducing the inspired oxygen concentration to that of air ($FiO_2 = 0.21$), administering anticonvulsant therapy, and if possible, terminating hyperbaric treatment. Oxygen toxicity may be prevented by alternating between short (five minute) intervals of air and longer intervals (30 minutes) of 100 percent oxygen, to limit oxygen free radical formation.

SUGGESTIONS TO AVOID OXYGEN TOXICITY

It is essential that oxygen therapy be considered as a medication and be prescribed with a clear mention of flow rate, appropriate device/interface and target oxygen saturation as per the underlying disease. It is also essential that the need for oxygen use be monitored regularly with discontinuation of the same when the target is achieved. This target is usually 94–98% (88–92% for patients like COPD who are at risk of hypercapnic respiratory failure). If these parameters are strictly adhered to, one can avoid unnecessary oxygen therapy and thereby its toxicity.

KEY POINTS

- Oxygen therapy is a double-edged sword with beneficial and harmful effects.
- Oxygen toxicity primarily affects the lung which is the maximum exposed tissue. Effects of O_2 toxicity appears as early as 24–48 hours in lungs.
- Oxygen should be considered as a drug that requires a dose titration based on the target oxygen saturation or PaO_2.
- Hyperoxia (which often simply accepted) should be avoided and efforts should be made to maintain normoxia.
- The ideal oxygenation target in a critically ill patient remains uncertain; however, the most recent data suggests that 'conventional' levels of 9–13 kPa or oxygen saturations of 94–98% are acceptable.
- With the widespread availability of the pulse oximetry, routine care should include the titration of oxygen therapy based on the target oxygen saturations.

- Overuse and toxicity of oxygen can be avoided with a proper prescription that includes the dose (flow), device, and oxygen target (oxygen saturation).
- There is no specific therapy for oxygen toxicity; hence, the prevention remains the cornerstone for the management.

LIST OF ABBREVIATIONS

BTS	British Thoracic Society
O_2	Oxygen
CO_2	Carbon dioxide
SaO_2	Arterial oxygen saturation
PAO_2	Alveolar oxygen tension
PaO_2	Arterial oxygen tension
$PACO_2$	Alveolar carbon dioxide tension
PIO_2	Inspired oxygen tension
RER	Respiratory exchange ratio
FiO_2	Fraction of inspired oxygen
2,3 DPG	2,3 diphosphoglycerate
ATP	Adenosine triphosphate
ATM	Atmospheric pressure
ROS	Reactive oxygen species
HALI	Hyperoxic acute lung injury
HBOT	Hyperbaric oxygen therapy

SUGGESTED READING

1. Brugniaux JV, Coombs GB, Barak OF, Dujic Z, Sekhon MS, Ainslie PN. Highs and lows of hyperoxia: Physiological, performance, and clinical aspects. Am J Physiol Regul Integr Comp Physiol. 2018;315:R1–R27.
2. Cabello JB, Burls A, Emparanza JI, Bayliss S, Quinn T. Oxygen therapy for acute myocardial infarction. Cochrane Database Syst Rev. 2010, (6):CD007160.
3. Camporesi EM. Side effects of hyperbaric oxygen therapy. Undersea Hyperb Med. 2014; 41(3):253–7. PMID: 24984321.
4. Cornet AD, Kooter AJ, Peters MJL, Smulders YM. The potential harm of oxygen therapy in medical emergencies. Critical Care. 2013;17:313.

5. Hafner S, Beloncle F, Koch A, Radermacher P, Asfar P. Hyperoxia in intensive care, emergency, and peri-operative medicine: Dr. Jekyll or Mr Hyde? A 2015 update. Ann Intensive Care. 2015;5(1):42. doi: 10.1186/s13613-015-0084-6. Epub 2015 Nov 19. PMID: 26585328; PMCID: PMC4653126.
6. Horncastle E, Lumb AB. Hyperoxia in anaesthesia and intensive care. BJA Education. 2019;19(6):176–82.
7. Kallet RH, Matthay MA. Hyperoxic acute lung injury. Respir Care. 2013; 58(1):123–41. doi:10.4187/respcare.01963.
8. Mach WJ, Thimmesch AR, Pierce JT, Pierce JD. Consequences of hyperoxia and the toxicity of oxygen in the lung. Nurs Res Pract. 2011; 2011:260482. doi: 10.1155/2011/260482. Epub 2011 Jun 5. PMID: 21994818; PMCID: PMC3169834.
9. McNulty PH, Robertson BJ, Tulli MA, Hess J, Harach LA, Scott S, Sinoway LI. Effect of hyperoxia and vitamin C on coronary blood flow in patients with ischaemic heart disease. J Appl Physiol. 2007;102:2040–45.
10. O'Driscoll BR, Howard LS, Davison AG. BTS guideline for emergency oxygen use in adult patients. British Thoracic Society. 2008;36(6), vi1–68, doi: 10.1136/thx.2008.102947.
11. O'Driscoll BR, Howard LS, Earis J, et al. on behalf of the British Thoracic Society Emergency Oxygen Guideline Group. British Thoracic Society guideline for oxygen use in adults in healthcare and emergency settings. Thorax. 2017; 72:i1–i90.

Part D

Special Issues

Chapter Outline

Chapter 20

Alternate Oxygen Carriers

Priya N, Balamugesh T

Allogenic blood transfusion has some problems like availability of donor, storage, shelf life, also some complications like immunogenicity due to allo-immunisation and acute lung injury. Hence a wide variety of compounds has been tried as oxygen carriers. An ideal blood substitute should have good efficacy, low cost, no side effects, easy clearance from blood and low allergenicity. So far none of these compounds have proven to be ideal. The two broad categories of blood substitutes are hemoglobin based oxygen (HBOC) and perfluorocarbons (PFCs). The HBOC are further classified into acellular and cellular varieties. These compounds are either human or bovine Hb molecules which are genetically modified and are made to offload oxygen delivery to the tissues in need. PFCs are emulsion particles which absorb oxygen within and then deliver even into the small capillaries due to the very small size of the particles. Each of these compounds has own side effects. There have been other modalities like extracorporeal membrane oxygenation (ECMO) which have been found useful in severe respiratory failure and ARDS. Heliox therapy is one another modality which has been tried in diseases with acute airway obstructions.

INTRODUCTION

"The life of every living thing is in the blood" (The Bible). Even with many advancements in biotechnology, there has been so far no ideal substitute for blood. One of the main function of the blood is transport of oxygen and carbon dioxide. Artificial blood came to importance after the emergence of HIV transmission in 1980. Thereafter research efforts have been directed towards constituting products that perform oxygen carrying and other transport functions of blood.

BLOOD SUBSTITUTES

Allogenic blood transfusion which is commonly used to improve oxygen delivery to tissues, has numerous drawbacks as follows:

- The red blood cells (RBC), if stored more than 15 days have a decreased ability to deliver oxygen efficiently, and these aged RBCs can undergo increased adhesion to the endothelial cells. In a critically ill patient, this imposes an increased risk of causing organ dysfunction by impairing the microcirculation.
- Allogenic blood transfusion also can cause immune activation leading on to transfusion-related acute lung injury (TRALI), transfusion related graft-versus-host disease and the risk of allo-immunization.
- The non-availability of allogenic blood in cases of emergencies, trauma because of the lack of universal donor-type blood, limited blood bank stock.

Hence there is a need for artificial oxygen carrier to replace our dependance of blood. This is important in cases of hemorrhagic shock due to acute blood loss in which massive volumes of blood needs to be replaced. Also blood substitutes are of value in situations in which blood is not an option (due to religious convictions) or blood is unavailable due to incompatibility. An ideal blood substitute should have the following qualities to function effectively in the circulation:

- Ability to transport oxygen
- Low cost
- No need for any Rh typing
- No risk of any contamination and transmission of infections
- Storage and extended half-life period
- Non immunogenicity and non-antigenicity
- Able to be excreted fully without toxicity.

The blood substitutes that have been developed are of two categories:

1. Hemoglobin-based oxygen carriers (HBOCs)
2. Perfluorocarbons (PFCs).

Hemoglobin-based Oxygen Carriers

In hemoglobin based oxygen carriers (HBOCs), the hemoglobin (Hb) is either of mammalian origin (human or of bovine) or genetically engineered by recombinant technology, with the ability to off-load and deliver oxygen to tissues by reducing its oxygen affinity. HBOCs may be either in aqueous solution of hemoglobin or micro-encapsulated hemoglobin particles (neo red cells). Large molecules (hemoglobin polymers) are preferred as it reduces the penetration of these polymers into the vessel wall.

Some problems associated with HBOCs were:

- Significant nephrotoxicity, when the natural tetramer Hb molecule degrades into dimer and monomer Hb species.
- Outside the RBCs, the hemoglobin and 2,3 DPG molecules are separated resulting in increased oxygen affinity, thereby releasing oxygen only at very low oxygen tension only.
- The Hb dimers scavenges the NO molecules, thereby causing hypertension due to vaso-constrictive effect. This vasoconstriction can be detrimental especially in those patients who are already suffering from blood loss and hemodilution.

To overcome these problems, the Hb molecules are chemically modified and are classified into two groups:

1. Acellular HBOC
2. Cellular HBOC.

Acellular HBOC

Acellular HBOCs are now in various phases of clinical trials and are classified into three categories:

1. **Cross-linked variety:** In cross-linked variety, an intramolecular covalent bond was formed between the globin chains to prevent detachment. However, it was not beneficial considering the increase in mortality in phase 3 clinical trials, due to the renal toxicity and due to the lack of the ability to out regulate the oxidative state of iron in their heme group, which in turn leads to increase in Met Hb levels and further toxicity.
2. **Polymerised variety:** Polymerized HBOCs (PolyHb) are another variety of acellular HBOC, wherein the Hb molecules are cross-linked intermolecularly to increase the molecular size. Each PolyHb molecule is composed of 4–5 Hb molecules, and various kinds of PolyHb molecules have been produced so far in various names. Hemopure is polymerized bovine Hb which is in its phase 3 clinical trial. Poly heme is another pyridoxylated Hb but has been rejected by US FDA due to its vasoactivity and hypertension. One another is Poly Hb with fibrinogen, which has both the capacity of oxygen delivery and coagulation properties. They help in situations of massive bleeds.

3. **Conjugated variety:** Conjugated HBOC are those acellular HBOCs where inert molecule is attached to the surface of Hb molecule, which does not have immunogenicity or antigenicity and also has a longer half life period. PEG, hydroxyethyl starch and albumin are used as conjugates.

Of these three, nano technology based polymerised Hb and conjugated HBOC varieties are found to be effective, however due to low half life in blood and many side effects, these products did not achieve the criteria for routine use.

- **Recombinant HBOC:** The Hb molecules are best functional when they are within the RBCs. So recombinant technology has been used to produce various modifications to increase the half life of these molecules and to reduce immunogenicity. These are genetically modified polymers to overcome the side effects like increased oxygen affinity and to improve Hb vasoactivity. But these have not been very popularly used. They have not been licensed for therapeutic use by the US FDA due to vasoactivity and shorter half-life.

Cellular HBOC

In this cellular HBOC, the Hb molecules are encapsulated in a phospholipid layer to liposome like molecules or nanosomes where the Hb molecules are linked to another molecule. These liposomes and nanosomes ensure better stability and resistance to heat, and mechanical activity. They serve as carriers of oxygen molecules, providing a long half-life in the blood. After delivery of oxygen to tissues, these molecules are biodegradable as well, causing less immunogenicity. However the production of these molecules is time consuming and very costly as well.

Perfluorocarbon-based Oxygen Carriers

These are molecules which are totally inert and where the fluorine atoms replace the hydrogen ions. They are hydrophobic and hence have to be emulsified for intravenous usage. Unlike HBOCs, they do not bind to oxygen gases. They are efficient solvents and dissolve significant amounts of oxygen and hence when used, the patients should be on high oxygen concentration supplementation. They have a half life of approximately 48 hours. These were the first tried molecules even before HBOCs and they were tried in traumatic brain injury patients, sickle cell crisis and wound care with compromised oxygenation. Once administered into circulation, they are finally taken up by the reticuloendothelial system, which determines the half life. They are also well tolerated with minimal side effects like flu like reaction, mild thrombocytopenia and delayed febrile reactions. PFCs are very useful to perfuse even in microcirculation due to the very small size of the emulsion particles and it is in this area they augment oxygen delivery to tissues in conditions like spinal cord ischemia, acute limb ischemia, emergency surgery when blood is not available and decompression sickness. They are also being tried for organ preservation in transplantation.

But considering that there was increased risk of stroke, the recent perflubron (the latest perfluorocarbon) has been terminated after phase III clinical trial.

None of the HBOCs are currently licensed by the FDA for routine use in the United States.

EXTRACORPOREAL MEMBRANE OXYGENATION

Extracorporeal membrane oxygenation (ECMO) is a technique for providing rest to the natural lungs in cases of severe acute respiratory distress syndrome with either hypoxemic or hypercapnic respiratory failure. It is a kind of cardio-pulmonary bypass machine, which involves connecting the patient's circulation to an external pump, then to a membrane oxygenator, wherein the gas exchanges take place. Then the blood flows back via cannulas into the patient's arterial or venous circulation. During circulation in the machine, anticoagulation is also being done to prevent blood clotting in the circuit.

Based on the vascular access techniques, ECMO is classified as veno-venous (VV ECMO), and veno-arterial (**Figs. 20.1A and B**).

For only respiratory failure without severe circulation defect, the VV ECMO configuration provides adequate ventilator support. In conditions where there is ARDS with severe sepsis in shock or severe left ventricular dysfunction veno-arterial ECMO is used.

ECMO is useful in patients with severe hypoxemia or severe hypercapnia, resulting in low pH (usually < 7.20) in spite of adequate lung-protective mechanical ventilation. ECMO support is often tried after failed attempts at multiple rescue therapies such as prone positioning, alveolar recruitment maneuvers, and the use of nitric oxide, alone or in combination. The use of ECMO also has both

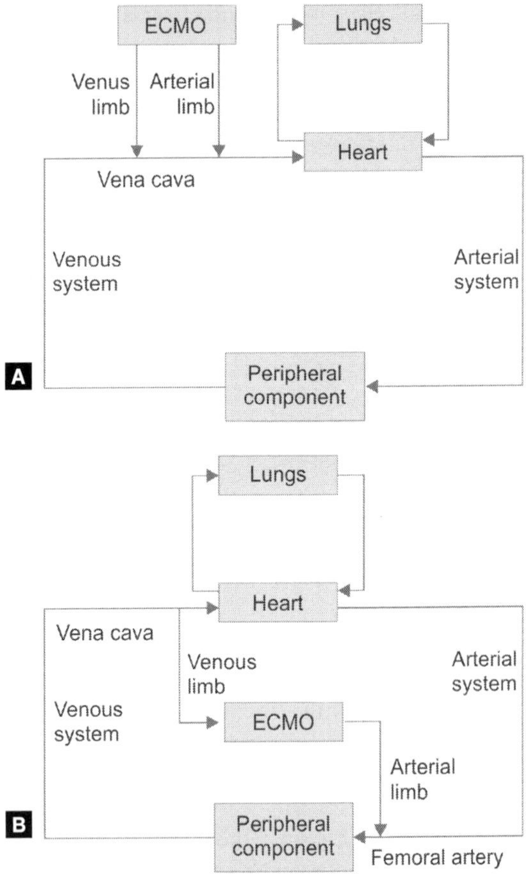

Figs. 20.1A and B: A. Veno-venous ECMO—the ECMO is in series with the lungs and provides respiratory support to the lungs; B. Veno-arterial ECMO—the ECMO is parallel to both heart and lungs and provides both respiratory and circulatory support.

mechanical and patient related complications. Mechanical problems like pump failure, cannula displacement, tubing disruption, pump malfunction can occur. Patient related problems like coagulopathy, other organ failure, infections can occur.

Age more than 75 years is a relative contraindication and being in mechanical ventilation more than 7 days prior to ECMO also carries poor prognosis and high mortality. The expenses of ECMO are very high and require analgesia, sedation and ICU care.

HELIOX THERAPY

Heliox therapy is a low-density mixture of helium and oxygen, commonly used in deep diving at > 6 ATM, therapeutically for decompression sickness. The first recorded use of Heliox in medicine was by Barach during the mid-1930s when Heliox mixtures were administered to patients in an effort to reduce dyspnea associated with asthma and other obstructive airway diseases. Heliox therapy reduces the airflow resistance within the bronchial tree and it reduces the work of breathing and hence improves pulmonary efficiency.

Heliox therapy is a mixture of 79% helium and 21% oxygen and hence it is at least 6 times at a lower density and viscosity than the atmospheric air and is available in portable cylinders. It causes significantly lower turbulence in the distal airways by causing laminar flow and hence reduces the peripheral airway resistance. It is non-toxic, non-carcinogenic and usually the benefits are seen within one hour of usage. They do not have long lasting side-effects.

USE OF HELIOX IN COPD

Heliox therapy in COPD patients has been studied in various small trials. The main aim of management of stable COPD patients is to reduce dyspnea and improve the quality of life. Due to its lower density, inhalation of heliox results in significantly lower turbulence, particularly in the more distal portions of the lung. This decrease in turbulence translates to a greater proportion of laminar flow and, as a direct result, lower overall airway resistance. In stable COPD, heliox has been found to result in modest improvement of lung physiology and exercise tolerance. However, the substantial cost of heliox as compared to supplemental oxygen therapy makes less useful in clinical practice. Further studies are also needed to verify the utility of heliox as a synergistic aid to training in pulmonary rehabilitation.

Heliox therapy is also being studied among patients with COPD exacerbations. It reduces work of breathing, improves respiratory acidosis, however it does not prevent noninvasive ventilation (NIV) failure or mortality. Giving heliox therapy in COPD patients post extubation along with NIV has been also found to reduce the inspiratory effort in these patients without significant changes in gas exchange parameters. Still larger controlled studies are required to prove its benefits. Because of the elevated cost of helium, it will be also interesting to see if helium sparing devices will be developed in the near future.

USE OF HELIOX THERAPY IN ASTHMA

Heliox therapy in acute asthma has been studied in various trials and no studies in adults have demonstrated an advantage of heliox over standard oxygen therapy. The reason is the heliox administration causes the increased expiratory airflow. At that point, the inspiratory airflow will also be theoretically increased to some parts of lung parenchyma, leading on to the increased risk of barotraumas and dynamic hyperinflation.

Heliox has also been studied as a driving gas for bronchodilator nebulization in acute asthma. A meta-analysis demonstrated significant improvement in peak expiratory flow especially in those with severe disease. The recent Global Initiative for Asthma (GINA) guidelines suggest that there is no clear role for heliox therapy in routine standard care of asthma patients. There may be role in patients not responding to the usual therapy, but due it its high cost and technical requirements it is not widely used.

HELIOX THERAPY IN CRITICALLY ILL PATIENTS

Heliox therapy has been studied in mechanically ventilated patients with respiratory failure. In few patients, reduction of carbon dioxide levels was noted. However, there is no definitive evidence to support it use.

In pediatric patients, heliox therapy has been tried for upper airway obstruction and has been found to be beneficial in certain clinical conditions like post extubation stridor, croup, laryngomalacia, laryngeal stenosis, bronchiolitis. But there is no definite evidence available so far of clinically important benefits justifying its routine use.

SUGGESTED READING

1. Barbosa, Fabiano Timbó et al. Artificial oxygen carriers as a possible alternative to red cells in clinical practice. Sao Paulo Med. J. [online]. 2009, vol. 127, n.2.

2. Davies A, Jones D, Bailey M, Beca J, Bellomo R, Blackwell N, Forrest P, Gattas D, Granger E, Herkes R, Jackson A. Extracorporeal membrane oxygenation for influenza A (H1N1) acute respiratory distress syndrome. JAMA. 2009;302(17):1888–95.
3. Jolliet P, Ouanes-Besbes L, Abroug F, Ben Khelil J, Besbes M, Garnero A, Arnal JM, et al. ECHO ICU trial investigators: A multicenter randomized trial assessing the efficacy of helium/oxygen in severe exacerbations of chronic obstructive pulmonary disease. Am J Respir Crit Care Med. 2017; 1;195(7):871–80.
4. Moradi S, Jahanian-Najafabadi A, Roudkenar MH. Artificial blood substitutes: First steps on the long route to clinical utility. Clin Med Insights Blood Disord. 2016;9:33–41. Published 2016 Oct 27. doi:10.4137/CMBD.S38461.
5. Neil D Eves, Stewart R Petersen, Mark J Haykowsky, Eric Y Wong, Richard L Jones. Helium-hyperoxia, exercise, and respiratory mechanics in chronic obstructive pulmonary disease. American Journal of Respiratory and Critical Care Medicine. 2006;174:7, 763–71.
6. Palange P. Lighter than air: Heliox breathing improves exercise tolerance in COPD. Eur Respir Rev. 2010;19(115):1-3.
7. Rodrigo G, Pollack C, Rodrigo C, Rowe BH. Heliox for nonintubated acute asthma patients. Cochrane Database Syst Rev. 2003;(4):CD002884. doi: 10.1002/14651858.CD002884. Update in: Cochrane Database Syst Rev. 2006;(4):CD002884. PMID: 14583955.
8. Rodrigo GJ, Rodrigo C, Pollack CV, Rowe B. Use of helium-oxygen mixtures in the treatment of acute asthma: A systematic review. Chest. 2003;123(3):891–6. doi: 10.1378/chest.123.3.891. PMID: 12628893.
9. Romano TG, Mendes PV, Park M, Costa EL. Extracorporeal respiratory support in adult patients. J Bras Pneumol. 2017;43(1):60–70. doi:10.1590/S1806-37562016000000299.
10. Valli G, Paoletti P, Savi D, Martolini D, Palange P. Clinical use of heliox in asthma and COPD. Monaldi Arch Chest Dis. 2007;67(3):159–64. doi: 10.4081/monaldi.2007.488. PMID: 18018756.

Chapter 21

Oxygen Delivery Devices

Venkata Nagarjuna Maturu, Virender Pratibh Prasad

OXYGEN DELIVERY DEVICES

Oxygen therapy is defined as the administration of oxygen to a patient at a concentration greater than the oxygen concentration in the ambient air. Several types of oxygen delivery devices (ODD) are available and it is important for the treating physician to have an understanding of these devices.

Oxygen delivery devices can be broadly categorized as being a low flow device or a high flow device **(Table 21.1)**.

Low Flow Oxygen Delivery Devices

These devices are also called as "variable performance oxygen delivery devices". These provide oxygen at a flow which is lesser than the patients inspiratory flow. As a result, when the patient breathes in, oxygen which is delivered by the device gets diluted with room air, and the degree of dilution depends on the patient's inspiratory flow.

Table 21.1: Low flow and high flow oxygen delivery devices.

	Low flow oxygen delivery device	*High flow oxygen delivery device*
Also called as	Variable performance oxygen delivery device	Fixed performance oxygen delivery device
Flow rate of delivered oxygen	Less than the person's inspiratory flow	More than the person's inspiratory flow
FiO_2 delivered	Variable	Fixed
Device types	Nasal cannula, simple oxygen masks, partial rebreather mask, non-rebreather mask	Venturi mask, high flow nasal cannula, mechanical ventilator

As a result, the inspiratory oxygen fraction (FiO_2) is not fixed and varies with changing ventilatory demand of the patient. Some of the low flow oxygen delivery devices include:

- Nasal cannula (low flow)
- Nasal catheter
- Simple oxygen mask
- Oxymask
- Partial rebreather mask
- Non-rebreather mask.

Nasal Cannula (Low Flow)

Nasal cannula is the most widely used oxygen delivery device, used for patients with mild hypoxemia. It consists of an oxygen supply tubing with two soft prongs that are inserted into the patient's anterior nares. **(Fig. 21.1)**. Oxygen flows from the oxygen source via a humidifier through the cannula into the nasopharynx where it mixes with room air.

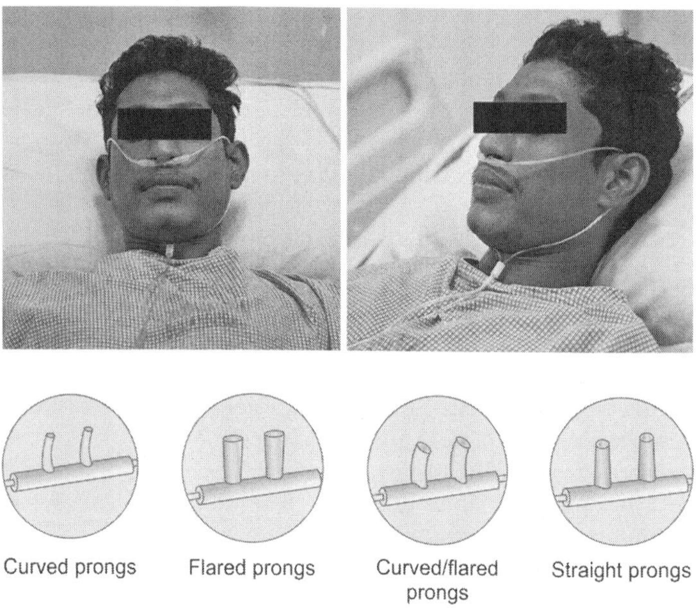

Fig. 21.1: Oxygen delivery by low flow nasal cannula. Different types of nasal prongs are shown in the image.

The oxygen flow is usually set between 1 and 6 liters per minute (Lpm). Flow rates of oxygen > 6 Lpm should be avoided as it can dry the nasal mucosa, leading to crusting and epistaxis. In newborns and infants, flow rates greater than 2 Lpm are not recommended. The FiO_2 delivered depends on several factors which include flow rate of oxygen, patients respiratory rate, tidal volume and extent of mouth breathing. The FiO_2 increases by approximately 4% with increase of every liter of oxygen per minute. A low flow nasal cannula can deliver FiO_2 upto 40–45%. Increase in flow rate beyond 6 Lpm makes the flow turbulent and does not lead to higher FiO_2 being delivered.

FiO_2 delivered by nasal cannula = 21% + (oxygen flow rate × 4%)

Advantages

- It is the most convenient oxygen delivery device as the person can talk and eat while receiving oxygen.
- It is light in weight.
- It can be tolerated well even by claustrophobic individuals.
- It is the cheapest oxygen delivery device.

Disadvantages

- The main disadvantage of nasal cannula is that it cannot deliver higher FiO_2 (>45%) of oxygen and hence may not be ideal in patients with severe hypoxemia.
- They can be easily dislodged if not worn properly (especially during sleep).
- The delivered FiO_2 cannot be accurately controlled.

Nasal cannulae are available in different sizes—adult, pediatric and infant. It is important to choose the correct size to improve the patient comfort. There are also several types of the nasal cannula available. The commonly available types include **(Fig. 21.1)**:

- **Curved prongs:** The prongs have a gentle curve and lead to improved anatomical fit and a greater comfort.
- **Flared prongs:** The prongs have a wider circumference at the distal end. This slows down the flow of oxygen and is more comfortable for the patient.
- **Curved/flared prongs:** These combine the benefits of both the above designs.
- **Straight prongs:** These are less comfortable and have a longer prong length to deliver oxygen deeper into the nares.

Nasal Oxygen Catheter

It is a 40 cm long single lumen flexible rubber or a plastic tube with several holes at the distal end. The catheter is inserted via one nostril and advanced such that the distal end lies in the nasopharynx. The other end of the catheter is connected to the oxygen source. Oxygen at low flows of 2 to 3 Lpm can provide FiO_2 upto 35–40%.

It has been earlier hypothesized that the oxygenation would be better when the oxygen delivered via catheter. However, studies comparing nasal catheter and nasal cannula have shown that the oxygenation is not much different.

Disadvantages

- Nasal catheters are more uncomfortable for the patient when compared to cannula.
- Placement of these catheters is uncomfortable and can cause trauma to the nares in people with nasal obstruction.
- These have to be changed every 8 hours to prevent breakdown, and are hence not ideal for long term use.
- If placed too deep in the pharynx, they can lead to aerophagia and gastric distension.
- As the natural humidifying mechanisms of the upper airway are bypassed with the catheter, the oxygen delivered to the airways is less humidified.

Because of the above reasons, the nasal cannula has replaced nasal catheters as the preferred oxygen delivery device in patients needing low FiO_2.

Simple Oxygen Face Mask

A simple face mask is a transparent mask which fits loosely over the patient's nose and mouth and can be set to deliver oxygen between 6 and 10 lpm. Oxygen concentration (FiO_2) of 35–50% can be administered, depending on the mask fit, flow rate of oxygen and the patient's ventilatory demand.

The mask itself acts as a reservoir for oxygen that is delivered through the tube attached to it. The side of the mask has two exhalation ports/holes. Exhaled air can exit through these ports. During inspiration, room air enters through these ports and dilutes the oxygen entering the mask **(Fig. 21.2)**. An oxygen flow rate greater than

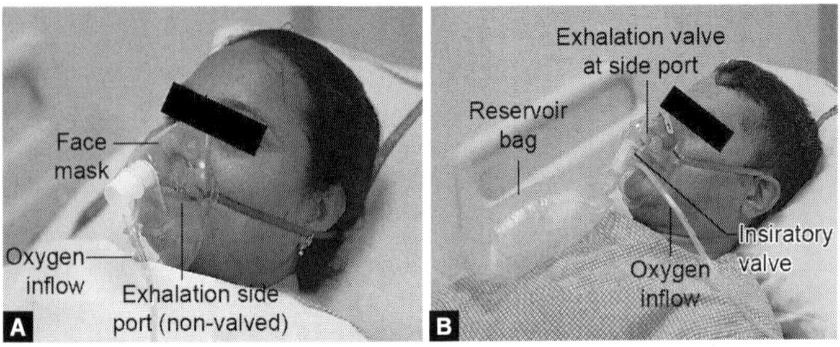

Figs. 21.2A and B: A. Oxygen delivery by simple oxygen mask; B. Non-rebreather oxygen mask

5 Lpm is required while using this mask to prevent rebreathing of the exhaled carbon-dioxide from the mask.

Advantages

- Face mask can deliver FiO_2 of upto 50%, which is higher than that can be delivered by a nasal cannula.
- It is easily available and not expensive.

Disadvantages

- Patient cannot eat or drink with the mask on.
- Some people may feel claustrophobic using the face mask.
- It may increase the risk of aspiration in patients who vomit.
- FiO_2 delivered is variable and cannot be accurately controlled.
- FiO_2 higher than 50% cannot be achieved using a simple oxygen mask.

Oxymask

In contrast to a simple face mask, the oxymask is a mask which uses a diffuser system that directs the oxygen towards the mouth and nose. The oxymask can provide higher FiO_2 at a lower oxygen flow rates. Studies have shown that the oxymask can deliver FiO_2 from 25–80%, by adjusting the oxygen flow rates from 1.5 to 30 Lpm. However, the clinical evidence for use of this type of mask is limited. Further, these oxymasks are not widely available in developing countries.

Partial Rebreather Mask

A partial rebreather mask consists of a simple oxygen mask with an attached reservoir bag of one liter capacity.

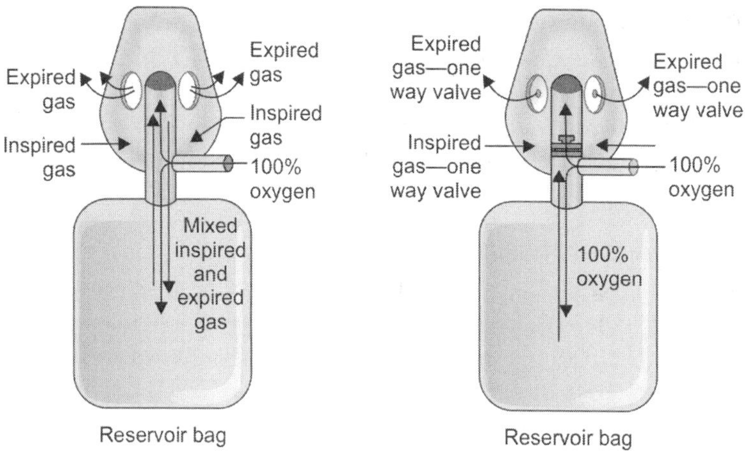

Fig. 21.3: Schematic diagram depicting the flow of gases during inhalation and exhalation in a partial rebreather mask (A) and a non-rebreather mask (B).

The reservoir bag gets filled with oxygen which flows into it during the exhalation phase. As there is no valve between the face mask and the reservoir, some of the exhaled air also enters the reservoir bag **(Fig. 21.3)**. Despite some exhaled air entering the reservoir bag, the gas in the reservoir is considered to be oxygen rich, as the early exhaled air which enters the reservoir bag is from the respiratory dead space (which has higher oxygen and lesser carbon dioxide). In order to maintain high percentage of oxygen in the reservoir bag and to prevent rebreathing, the oxygen flow rate must be adjusted such that the reservoir is always fully inflated.

During inspiration, air is drawn from the fresh oxygen flowing in as well as from the oxygen rich gas in reservoir bag. This is diluted by the air which enters in from the exhalation side ports. Since this not a tightly sealed mask, some amount of air can enter from the gap between the mask and the face. As a result, the FiO_2 delivered is between 60% and 80% with flow rates of 10–12 Lpm.

Advantages

- Higher oxygen concentrations can be achieved as compared to a simple face mask.
- It is more comfortable for the patient than a non-invasive ventilation mask.

Disadvantages

- Patient cannot eat or drink with the mask on.
- It is not widely available.
- FiO_2 delivered is variable and cannot be monitored.
- FiO_2 delivered is lesser than which can be delivered via a non-rebreather mask.

Non-rebreather Mask

A non-rebreather mask (NRBM) is the device which can provide a high FiO_2 (60–100%), similar to a high flow nasal cannula (HFNC) in patients breathing spontaneously. However, unlike in HFNC, the FiO_2 cannot be controlled while using NRBM. An NRBM can improve oxygenation but cannot improve ventilation. Non-invasive ventilators (NIV) and invasive mechanical ventilators can deliver high FiO_2 in addition to providing ventilatory support.

A non-rebreather mask is similar to a partial rebreather mask, and has a reservoir bag attached to the face mask. In addition, it has two types of one way valves—inspiratory valve and expiratory valve **(Figs. 21.2 and 21.3)**. A comparison of partial and non-rebreather masks is given in **Table 21.2**.

One Way Valves

- An inspiratory one-way valve is present between the reservoir bag and the mask. This allows unidirectional flow from the reservoir to the mask during inspiration and prevents the exhaled air from entering the reservoir bag. As a result, the reservoir bag is filled only by oxygen from the inflow (100% oxygen).
- Exhalation one way valves are present at the side holes on the face mask. These valves allow the exhaled air to exit the mask but prevent room air from entering the mask during inspiration.

Because of these one-way valves, the gas which the patient inhales (mixture of gas from inflow and reservoir bag) is rich in oxygen and can deliver FiO_2 as high as 80–95%. When both exhalation ports have valves and a tight mask seal is achieved, a non-rebreather mask (NRBM) can deliver FiO_2 of 95% with flow rates of 10–15 Lpm.

However, there is a remote risk of suffocation if both exhalation ports have one-way valves, and the oxygen supply is inadvertently interrupted. To avoid this, most commercially available NRBMs have a single one-way exhalation valve. The other exhalation port is left open.

Table 21.2: Comparison of partial rebreather and a non-rebreather mask.

	Partial rebreather mask	*Non-rebreather mask*
FiO_2 delivered	50–80%	60–95% Single valve: 60–80% Double valve: 80–95%
Type of device	Low flow device	Low flow or a high flow device
Valves in the device	None	Two types of valves: 1. Inspiratory valve between the reservoir bag and the mask 2. Expiratory valve(s) at the exhalation side ports
Gas in the reservoir bag	Mixture of pure oxygen and exhaled air	Pure oxygen (100%) as there is an inspiratory valve which prevents exhaled air from entering the reservoir
Inhaled air	Mixture of: • Pure oxygen from inflow • Oxygen rich gas from reservoir • Room air entering from the side ports • Room air entering from the gap between the mask and the face	Mixture of: • Pure oxygen from inflow • Pure oxygen from reservoir • Room air entering from the gap between the mask and the face
Exhaled air	Exits through the exhalation side ports and some amount also enters the reservoir bag	Exits through the exhalation side ports
Risk of suffocation	Not present	If oxygen delivery gets interrupted, there is a risk of suffocation

This allows for room air to enter the mask during inadvertent oxygen interruptions. During inspiration, the non-valved exhalation port allows room air to enter the mask and as a result, the FiO_2 delivered is usually around 80% with an NRBM which has a single exhalation valve.

Advantages

- It provides the highest possible FiO_2 without intubation/NIV.
- It is suitable for spontaneously breathing patients with severe hypoxemia.

Disadvantages

- Patient cannot eat or drink with the mask on.
- Not suitable for long term use as high FiO_2 can lead to oxygen toxicity.
- Inadvertent oxygen interruption may lead to CO_2 build up and suffocation in an NRBM with two exhalation valves.

High Flow Oxygen Delivery Devices

These devices are also called as "fixed performance oxygen delivery devices". These devices provide oxygen at flows higher than the patient's inspiratory demand. As a result, the delivered oxygen is not diluted by ambient air, and the FiO_2 delivered remains constant. High flow devices are important when the FiO_2 delivered has to be accurately controlled (e.g. COPD exacerbation). Examples of high flow devices include:

- Venturi mask
- High flow nasal cannula
- Non-invasive or invasive mechanical ventilators.

All the above devices (high flow as well as low flow) deliver oxygen continuously during inspiration as well as expiration, and are called "continuous oxygen delivery systems". Since the oxygen is delivered even during the expiratory phase, there is some wastage of oxygen. However, to decrease such wastage of oxygen, there are certain devices available known as "oxygen conserving devices" (see section below).

Venturi Mask

A venturi mask is a high flow device that allows precise measurement of the delivered FiO_2. The proximal end of the mask has a venturi device which allows for controlled entrainment of room air. Venturi device has a constriction aperture at the centre which increases the velocity of oxygen gas as it enters the device. The device also has side ports to allow entrainment of ambient air. This mixture of oxygen and ambient air then enters the face mask **(Fig. 21.4)**.

A venturi mask works on the venturi modification of the Bernouli principle **(Fig. 21.5)**. When a gas flows through a constriction, the velocity of the gas increases. This increased velocity leads to a fall in the pressure adjacent to the flow. This fall in pressure leads to entrainment of room air from the side holes of the venturi device. The smaller the orifice, the greater is the velocity of gas across the orifice

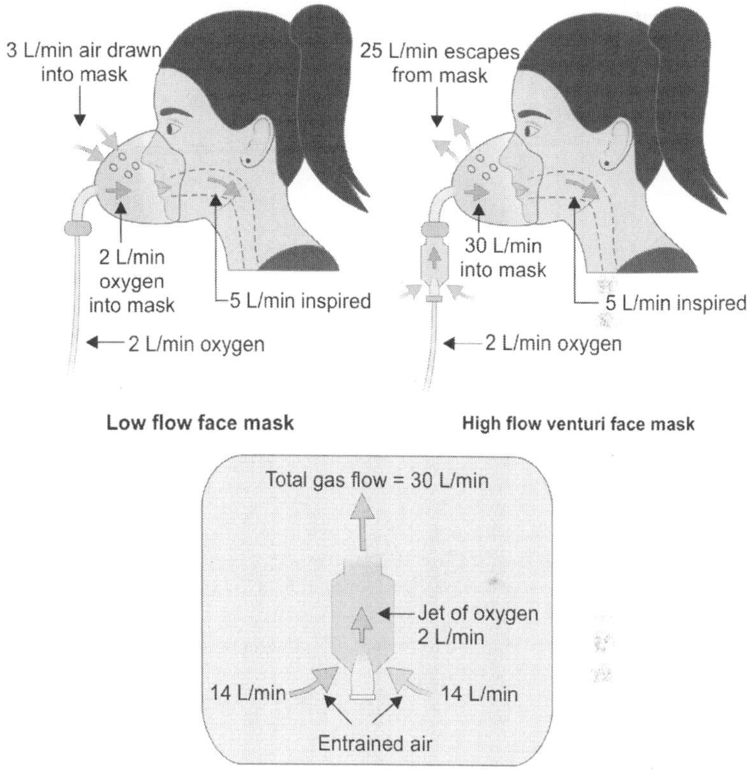

Fig. 21.4: Oxygen and air inflow with a simple oxygen mask and a venturi mask.

and therefore, greater is the negative pressure generated and more is the amount of ambient air entrained. Hence, smaller the orifice of the aperture, lesser is the delivered FiO_2.

The venturi devices are color coded **(Fig. 21.5)**, and are marked with the recommended flow rate of oxygen to be used so as to achieve the desired oxygen concentration. There are calibrated adjustable venturi devices also available, where we can adjust the FiO_2 by adjusting the a knob. Venturi masks can deliver FiO_2 from 24- 60% at flow rates varying from 3 to 15 Lpm.

Advantages

- Delivery of controlled FiO_2 (especially useful in patients with COPD where controlled oxygen needs to be delivered).

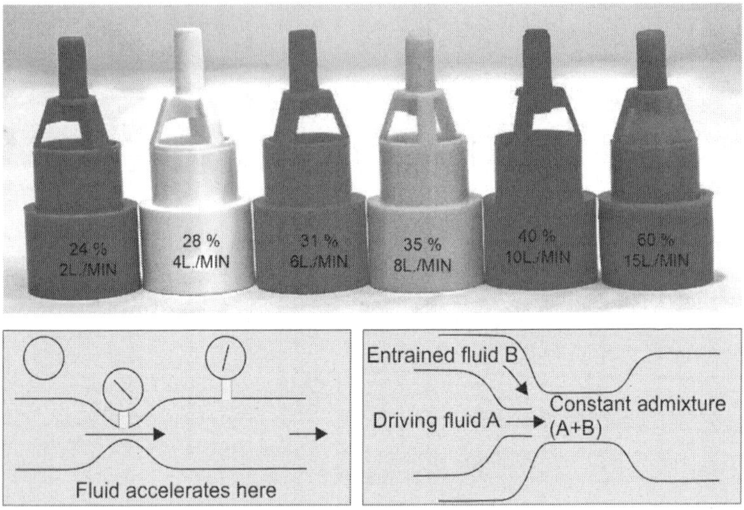

Figs. 21.5A to C: A. Schematic representation of Bernoulli principle; B. Schematic representation of Venturi principle; C. Venturi devices (colour coded) showing the FiO_2 delivered and the oxygen flow needed to achieve the same

- Accurate monitoring of the trend of of oxygen requirement as there is a control over the FiO_2 delivered.
- Can be used to deliver both lower FiO_2 (24%) and higher FiO_2 (50–60%).

Disadvantages

- Patient cannot eat or drink with the mask on.
- It is more expensive than a simple face mask.
- It cannot deliver FiO_2 higher than 60%.

OXYGEN CONSERVING DEVICES

Oxygen conserving devices are designed to improve the efficiency of oxygen therapy by reducing the wastage of oxygen which is delivered during the expiratory phase of patient's respiration. There are three ways by which oxygen is conserved:

1. By using a reservoir which gets filled with oxygen during expiration. The oxygen in the reservoir bag along with the oxygen from fresh inflow is inhaled during the next inhalation.
2. By delivery of oxygen only during the inspiratory part of the respiratory cycle which is called "pulsed oxygen delivery". This is

made possible by specially designed nasal cannula which has a sensor to detect the inspiratory flow.

3. By bypassing the anatomical dead space and directly delivering oxygen to the lower airway oxygenation can be maintained by using lower flows of oxygen. This is the principle of "trans tracheal oxygen delivery".

Reservoir Nasal Cannula

These were the first oxygen conserving devices to be used. They store oxygen during exhalation, making available a bolus of concentrated oxygen for delivery during the early portion of the subsequent inhalation. They enable a reduction in oxygen flow setting by appropriately 25 to 50% while maintaining the same oxygen saturation. There are two types of reservoir cannula **(Fig. 21.6)** available:

1. **Moustache cannula:** Also called as oxymizer, this utilizes a storage chamber under the nose. This is more noticeable on the face and may not be acceptable to some.
2. **Pendant cannula:** Also called as oxymizer pendant, this has a reservoir bag attached to the cannula that rests on the anterior chest wall of the patient. This is less noticeable than a moustache cannula, but less comfortable to wear.

Pulsed Oxygen Delivery

Also called as "demand oxygen pulse devices". These devices deliver oxygen only during the initial phase of inspiration. There is no flow of oxygen during the terminal inspiration and the expiration, thus reducing the wastage of oxygen. The reason for delivering oxygen only during the initial phase of inspiration is because the second half of the inspiration (around 150 mL) is used to fill the anatomic dead space, and does not contribute to oxygenation.

The nasal cannula has a specially designed sensor that detects the inspiratory flow as a pressure swing. When this is detected, the machine delivers a bolus of oxygen, the magnitude of which can be adjusted on the device. These have become the most widely available oxygen conserving devices currently being used. Portable oxygen concentrators utilize this principle to deliver oxygen for longer duration.

It is important to ensure that the delivered bolus of oxygen is sufficient to maintain oxygenation for the patient. The numerical setting on the device does not indicate the flow of oxygen but indicates

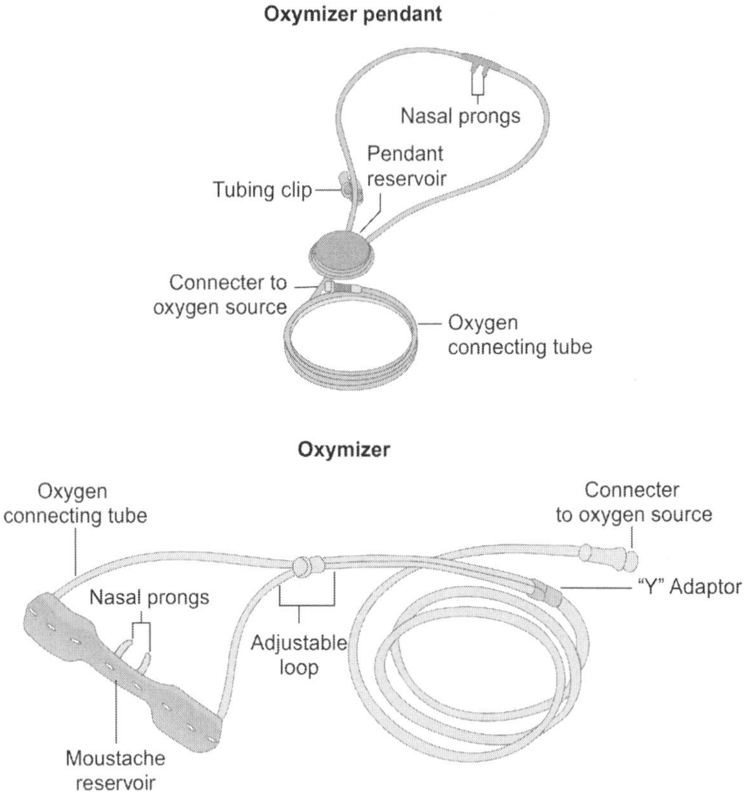

Fig. 21.6: Schematic diagram of reservoir nasal cannula—oxymizer and oxymizer pendant.

the relative size of the bolus of oxygen delivered. There is a wide variation in the performance of these devices and hence each device has to be titrated to each individuals' requirement.

Transtracheal Oxygen Delivery

Oxygen is delivered **(Fig. 21.7)** by a catheter which is introduced into the trachea. The catheter is inserted by either the modified seldinger technique or by creating a trachea-cutaneous fistula (Lipkins procedure). This delivery has been shown to reduce the oxygen usage, increase patient comfort (as there is no device on the face) and reduce the work of breathing. However, as it is invasive and has the potential to get infected, it is not widely utilized.

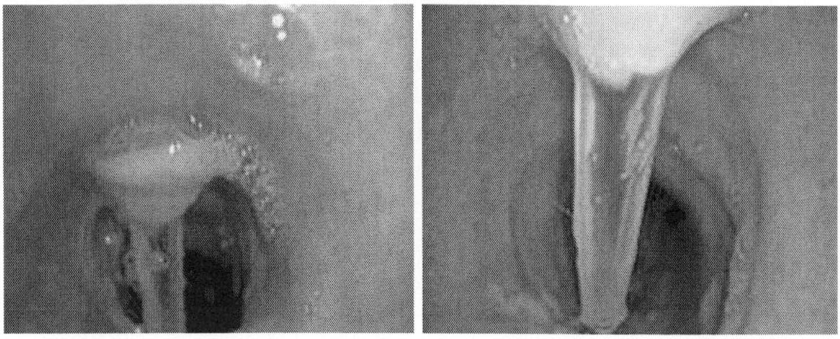

Fig. 21.7: Bronchoscopic image of a transtracheal oxygen catheter.

Table 21.3: Oxygen flow rates, FiO_2 delivered and aerosol generating potential of the various oxygen delivery devices.

	Oxygen flow rate (Lpm)	*FiO_2 delivered*	*Aerosol generating potential*
Low flow nasal cannula	1–6 Lpm	24–45%	++
Simple oxygen mask	6–10 Lpm	30–50%	+
Venturi mask	3–15 Lpm	24–60%	+++
Oxymask	3–30 Lpm	40–80%	+++
Partial rebreather mask	8–12 Lpm	50–70%	++
Non-rebreather mask	10–15 Lpm	60–95%	+/–

OXYGEN DELIVERY DEVICES IN PATIENTS WITH COVID-19

All oxygen delivery devices generate different amount of aerosols, which pose the threat of nosocomial infection to health care workers and other patients. When choosing an oxygen delivery device for a patient with COVID-19, it is important to consider the aerosol generating ability of the device in addition to its clinical efficacy. Aerosol generating ability of various oxygen delivery devices is given in **Table 21.3**.

Practical Points to Consider in Patients with Covid-19

- Placing a N95 mask or a surgical facemask over nasal cannula (low or high flow) decreases the aerosol spread.
- Ensuring the cannula are properly placed within the nasal cavity.

- When using a face mask, it is important to ensure a tight seal with the face to decrease the aerosol spread.
- Increasing the oxygen flow rates proportionately increase the aerosol dispersion and hence it is recommended to use the least oxygen flow rate that is required to maintain adequate oxygen saturation.
- Of the various masks, a NRBM has the least potential for aerosol spread while delivering the highest FiO_2.
- Avoid nebulizers whenever possible as they increase the aerosol generation. Switch over to inhaler with spacers.

SUGGESTED READING

1. Beecroft JM, Hanly PJ. Comparison of the oxymask and venturi mask in the delivery of supplemental oxygen: Pilot study in oxygen-dependent patients. Canadian Respiratory Journal. 2006;13:247–52.
2. Coudroy R, Frat JP, Girault C, Thille AW. Reliability of methods to estimate the fraction of inspired oxygen in patients with acute respiratory failure breathing through non-rebreather reservoir bag oxygen mask. Thorax. 2020;75:805–7.
3. Eckmann DM. Transtracheal oxygen delivery. Critical Care Clinics. 2000;16:463–72, vii.
4. Ergul AB, Calıskan E, Samsa H, et al. Using a high-flow nasal cannula provides superior results to oxymask delivery in moderate to severe bronchiolitis: A randomized controlled study. European Journal of Pediatrics. 2018;177:1299–307.
5. Hardavella G, Karampinis I, Frille A, Sreter K, Rousalova I. Oxygen devices and delivery systems. Breathe (Sheffield, England). 2019;15:e108–e16.
6. Jensen AG, Johnson A, Sandstedt S. Rebreathing during oxygen treatment with face mask. The effect of oxygen flow rates on ventilation. Acta Anaesthesiologica Scandinavica. 1991;35:289–92.
7. Lamb K, Piper D. Southmedic OxyMask (TM) Compared with the Hudson RCI ® Non-Rebreather Mask (Tm): Safety and performance comparison. Canadian Journal of Respiratory Therapy : CJRT = Revue Canadienne de la Therapie Respiratoire: RCTR. 2016;52:13–5.
8. Marriott HL. Oxygen administration by nasal catheter. British Medical Journal. 1936;1:154–7.
9. Martí S, Pajares V, Morante F, et al. Are oxygen-conserving devices effective for correcting exercise hypoxemia? Respiratory Care. 2013;58:1606–13.
10. McCoy R. Oxygen-conserving techniques and devices. Respiratory Care. 2000;45:95-103; Discussion 4.

11. Milross J, Young IH, Donnelly P. The oxygen delivery characteristics of the hudson oxy-one face mask. Anaesthesia and Intensive Care. 1989;17:180–4.
12. Muhe L, Degefu H, Worku B, Oljira B, Mulholland EK. Comparison of nasal prongs with nasal catheters in the delivery of oxygen to children with hypoxia. Journal of Tropical Pediatrics. 1998;44:365–8.
13. Palwai A, Skowronski M, Coreno A, Drummond C, McFadden ER, Jr. Critical comparisons of the clinical performance of oxygen-conserving devices. American Journal of Respiratory and Critical Care Medicine. 2010;181:1061–71.
14. Paul JE, Hangan H, Hajgato J. The OxyMask (TM) Development and performance in healthy volunteers. Medical Devices (Auckland, NZ). 2009;2:9–17.
15. Roy A, Singh A, Khanna P. Oxygen delivery devices in Covid-19 patients: Review and recommendation. Bali Journal of Anesthesiology. 2020;4:3–7.
16. Siddiqui FM, Campbell S, Ie S, Biscardi F, Rubio E. Three decades of transtracheal oxygen therapy: A review of the associated complications with an illustrative case presentation. Lung India: Official Organ of Indian Chest Society. 2017;34:448–51.
17. Tantum KR. Comparison of nasal catheter and nasal cannula inpatients recovering from general anesthesia. Anesthesiology. 1969;31:376–7.
18. Tiep B, Carter R. Oxygen conserving devices and methodologies. Chronic respiratory disease. 2008;5:109–14.
19. Weber MW, Palmer A, Oparaugo A, Mulholland EK. Comparison of nasal prongs and nasopharyngeal catheter for the delivery of oxygen in children with hypoxemia because of a lower respiratory tract infection. The Journal of Pediatrics. 1995;127:378–83.

Chapter 22

High-flow Oxygen through Nasal Cannula

Inderpaul Singh Sehgal, Valliappan Muthu

INTRODUCTION

Supplemental oxygen is the first-line therapy for hypoxemic patients, and is provided via nasal cannula, face masks, venturi mask, and rebreathing mask. Further, the oxygen is humidified through bubble humidifiers. At high flow rates, there is insufficient humidification of oxygen with bubble humidifiers that leads to poor tolerance. Also, the conventional oxygen delivery devices can deliver oxygen at a maximum flow rate of 15 liters per minute. During acute respiratory failure (ARF), the inspiratory flow demands of the patients vary from 30 liters/minute to as high as 80 liters/minute. The high inspiratory flow demand results in a large difference between the required (patient's flow rate) and the delivered flow rates causing a lower delivery of fraction of oxygen in inspired air (FiO_2) than expected.

High-flow nasal cannula (HFNC) delivers humidified oxygen at high flow using a nasal cannula. HFNC has an air-oxygen blender, an active humidifier, a single heated circuit, and a nasal cannula. HFNC has been primarily used for ARF in pediatric population and has also gained popularity in adults. Herein, we discuss the physiological basis, indications, and current evidence on the use of HFNC in managing ARF in adults.

PHYSIOLOGICAL EFFECTS OF HFNC

At high flow, heated and humidified oxygen has the following physiological effects:

- **High flow washes out carbon dioxide in the anatomical dead space:** HFNC is an open system and thus does not increase the tidal volume. However, the use of HFNC improves thoracoabdominal synchrony due to reduced work of breathing and a lesser anatomical dead space. As the flow rate of HFNC is increased, there is a reduction in respiratory rate and minute ventilation without an increase in the $PaCO_2$.

- **Meets the high flow requirements of patients with ARF and assures constant FiO_2:** During ARF, the inspiratory flow and the tidal volume vary breath-by-breath. Thus, the delivered FiO_2 is not stable with low-flow oxygen delivery devices. With HFNC, the delivered FiO_2 is closer to the depicted FiO_2, especially at high flow. Most patients with ARF breathe through the open mouth. With HFNC, the delivered FiO_2 is higher with open mouth than with closed mouth. The high flow creates an anatomic reservoir in the nasopharynx and thus providing high FiO_2despite mouth breathing.
- **Provides a positive end-expiratory pressure (PEEP):** In vitro models have shown that at high gas flow, the airway pressures are increased. In a previous study of healthy volunteers, the airway pressures increased on increasing flow rates. In another study, HFNC could provide a PEEP of up to 3 cm H_2O with the closed mouth but not with the mouth open. As most patients with ARF breathe through the open mouth, it is unlikely that HFNC provides clinically significant PEEP. At a higher flow rate, HFNC improves end-expiratory lung volumes, dynamic lung compliance, oxygenation, homogenizes the ventilation distribution, and reduces the respiratory rate.
- **Provides heated humidified oxygen facilitating the mucociliary function of the airways:** The gas delivered through HFNC is actively humidified similar to critical care ventilators. The absolute humidity of the expelled air is greater at higher flow rates than at lower flow rates. Also, the absolute humidity is higher for a newer generation of HFNC machines than previous versions at similar flow rates.

INDICATIONS FOR HFNC IN RESPIRATORY FAILURE

The HFNC has been primarily evaluated in acute hypoxemic respiratory failure (AHRF), after extubation, in postoperative patients, in pre-oxygenation before airway intubation, and during bronchoscopy.

Acute Hypoxemic Respiratory Failure

Most evidence for HFNC in adults is in AHRF. Several studies (five in ICU setting and four in emergency department) have prospectively compared HFNC to conventional oxygen therapy in AHRF. The use of HFNC significantly reduced [relative risk (95% confidence interval), 0.85 (0.74-0.99)] the need for intubation compared to conventional oxygen therapy. However, the use of HFNC did not reduce the mortality, the ICU, or the hospital length of stay. Most studies on HFNC have included a heterogeneous population (community-acquired pneumonia, cardiogenic pulmonary edema, immunocompromised patients, and others). Thus, it is not clear which subgroup of patients would benefit the most with the use of HFNC. In the Florali study, 80% of subjects had PaO_2:FiO_2 ratio of <200 and had bilateral infiltrates on chest radiograph (fulfilling all the criteria for ARDS except PEEP). The use of HFNC avoided intubation in 50% subjects. Messika et al. found the success rate of HFNC in subjects with ARDS to be 60%. Thus, in patients with ARDS not requiring immediate intubation, a trial of HFNC may be given. However, close monitoring will be needed with a timely escalation of therapy. The hazard of HFNC is delayed intubation, which can increase mortality. Other reasons for increased mortality with HFNC include self-inflicted lung injury that occurs due to prolonged spontaneous breathing. Also, oxygen supplementation through HFNC rapidly improves oxygen saturation but the underlying disturbances (ventilation-perfusion mismatch, alveolar hypoventilation that require inspiratory pressure support and extrinsic PEEP) are insufficiently corrected. Patients may gradually worsen to the point of respiratory muscle fatigue, cardiac dysfunction, and organ failure leading to a worse prognosis. Therefore, close monitoring of patients on HFNC is mandatory and a delay in airway intubation must be avoided.

Hypercapnic Respiratory Failure

The HFNC has been used in the management of hypercapnic respiratory failure. Most of these are physiological studies and only a few have used HFNC in critically ill patients. Lee at al. compared HFNC with non-invasive ventilation (NIV) in acute exacerbation of COPD found no difference in the intubation rates and 30-day mortality between the groups. There was also no difference in PaO_2,

$PaCO_2$, and pH at 6 and 24 hours of admission. In a study by Kim et al. HFNC significantly reduced $PaCO_2$ compared to conventional oxygen therapy. HFNC complements the management of patients during NIV off periods, where its use results in better unloading of diaphragmatic muscles than conventional oxygen therapy. Ricard et al demonstrated that the use of HFNC during NIV off period resulted in better patient comfort, respiratory rate, and control of dyspnea than standard oxygen. More evidence is needed before HFNC can be routinely used in managing hypercapnic respiratory failure.

Post-extubation Respiratory Failure

Five trials have compared HFNC to conventional oxygen therapy and four studies have compared HFNC to NIV in subjects at high-risk for reintubation. The high-risk features included age >65 years, heart failure, moderate to severe COPD, APACHE II score >12, BMI >30 kg/m^2, difficult weaning, presence of two or more co-morbid illnesses, or mechanical ventilation for >7 days. The HFNC reduced reintubation [RR (95% CI), 0.32 (0.12–0.88)], and post-extubation respiratory failure [RR (95% CI), 0.54 (0.3–0.94)] compared to conventional oxygen therapy. However, HFNC was not different than NIV in preventing reintubation or the development of post-extubation respiratory failure. Most studies have examined the prophylactic use of HFNC after extubation. There is a scarcity of evidence to support the routine use of HFNC in those with post-extubation respiratory failure.

Pre-intubation Oxygenation

A few studies have compared HFNC to conventional oxygen therapy or NIV in pre-oxygenating patients before intubation. Most trials have been done in patients undergoing surgery under general anesthesia and a few in critically ill patients requiring elective airway intubation. Pre-oxygenation with HFNC did not reduce [RR (95% CI), 0.98 (0.68-1.42)] the incidence of hypoxemia or apneic time compared to conventional oxygen therapy or NIV. The study population of trials included in the meta-analysis was heterogeneous making it difficult to identify a subgroup that will benefit from HFNC for pre-oxygenation. There is a lack of evidence for the utility of HFNC during intubation in high-risk group, including obese patients, those with PaO_2:FiO_2 ratio <150 mm Hg, and difficult to intubate patients.

Postoperative Period

Few studies have compared HFNC to conventional oxygen therapy and one trial compared HFNC to NIV as prophylactic therapy in the immediate postoperative period. Most studies included patients undergoing cardiac or thoracic surgeries. The HFNC significantly reduced [RR (95% CI), 0.32 (0.12–0.88)] the reintubation rate and escalation of respiratory support [RR (95% CI), 0.54 (0.31–0.94)] compared to oxygen supplementation with face mask. However, HFNC did not reduce mortality, the incidence of postoperative hypoxia, the ICU, and the hospital length of stay.

As Palliative Therapy

The NIV is the most used respiratory support as a palliative measure in terminally ill patients with do-not-intubate (DNI) status. However, NIV is associated with patient discomfort, the risk for pressure ulcers, claustrophobia, and the inability of patients to communicate or eat. The HFNC is theoretically an attractive alternative in DNI patients but the evidence supporting its use is limited in these circumstances.

A few studies have described HFNC use in palliative patients. HFNC improved oxygenation and breathing patterns in patients with DNI orders who presented with hypoxemic respiratory failure. HFNC was well-tolerated, improved oral intake, communication, and reduced the respiratory rate. Hui et al. randomized 30 patients with advanced cancer to NIV or HFNC and demonstrated comparable improvement in physiologic parameters and alleviation of dyspnea. In another study Hui et al. demonstrated that the use of HFNC led to a rapid and clinically significant reduction of dyspnea at rest in hospitalized non-hypoxemic patients with cancer.

HFNC during Bronchoscopy

Respiratory drive and mechanics are altered during bronchoscopy owing to procedural sedation and partial occlusion of the airway by the bronchoscope. As a result, oxygen saturation may fall below 90% despite oxygen supplementation. The NIV can prevent hypoxemia during bronchoscopy, but mask intolerance and difficulty in manipulating the scope through the mask limits its routine use. The HFNC permits oral passage of the bronchoscope and may improve oxygenation during the procedure. Lucangelo et al. randomized patients undergoing bronchoscopy (under midazolam sedation) to

HFNC set at 40 liters/minute with 50% FiO_2, HFNC set at 60 liters/minute with 50% FiO_2, or Venturi mask with 50% FiO_2. The HFNC at a flow rate of 60 liters/minute produced higher oxygen saturation at the end of the procedure than HFNC at 40 liters/minute or Venturi mask (98% vs. 94% and 92%, respectively). In another study, Simon and colleagues randomized patients with respiratory failure (PaO_2:FiO_2 < 300) undergoing bronchoscopy to 50 liters/minute of HFNC or NIV. The HFNC and NIV produced similar nadirs in oxygenation during the procedure (92±7% and 95±5%, respectively). One patient in the HFNC group and three patients in the NIV group required intubation within 24 hours of the procedure. La Combe et al. reported similar results in 30 patients undergoing bronchoscopy with hypoxemia. Five patients required escalation of respiratory support within 24 hours of the procedure (two intubations, three NIV). These studies suggest that HFNC can provide support for hypoxemic patients undergoing bronchoscopy and should be considered when evaluating procedural risks and benefits in high-risk populations.

Setting up of HFNC and Monitoring

An HFNC unit comprises of a flow meter that can deliver flow between 15-60 liters/minute, an air-oxygen blender, active humidifier, heated inspiratory circuit, and a nasal cannula with contoured ends for a better fit **(Table 22.1)**. The nasal cannula is attached to the patient with a head strap that has cheek pads to reduce pressure on the face. The nasal cannula comes in three sizes (small, medium, and large). For an average built adult, a medium size is most commonly used. In addition, there is also an interface for the tracheostomy tube and mask. Before each use, we disinfect the HFNC unit by using the disinfection kit and using the disinfection mode inbuilt in some HFNC machines. The disinfection process takes about an hour to complete.

Initiation, titration, and weaning: In patients with acute hypoxemic respiratory failure, we start the HFNC at a flow rate of 40 liters/minute and we then titrate the flows according to the respiratory rate and patient comfort. The FiO_2 is set at 100% at initiation, and we then adjust the FiO_2 to achieve a target SPO_2 between 92 and 94%. During titration, we also monitor the respiratory rate, use of accessory muscles of respiration, sensorium, and hemodynamics. We escalate the respiratory support (NIV or invasive mechanical ventilation) if there is, tachypnea (respiratory rate is >35 breaths/minute), intolerance

Table 22.1: Specifications for high flow nasal cannula.

Flow rate range	2–60 Lpm
FiO_2 range	21–100%
Assured FiO_2	At least 90% at a flow rate of 60 Lpm
Humidifier	Inbuilt active humidifier with auto-fill function
Temperature range for heating air	32–37°C
Tubings	Inbuilt spiral heater wire to prevent condensation
Disinfection	Inbuilt thermal disinfection for disinfection of internal blower (preferable) using a dedicated disinfection kit
Patient interface • Nasal cannula size • Tracheostomy interface • Mask interface	Small, medium, and large

to HFNC, use of accessory muscles of respiration or paradoxical breathing, hemodynamic compromise (arrhythmias, shock), or worsening of sensorium. We also measure the ROX index, which is the ratio of oxygen saturation as measured by pulse oximetry/FiO_2 to respiratory rate [(SPO_2/FiO_2)/RR]. A ROX index of >4.88 at 12 hours after initiation of HFNC predicts success while a ROX index of <3.85 at 12 hours predicts failure. At our center, we use a ROX index cut-off of 5 at 1-2 hours of initiation of HFNC and clinical features as a guide to escalate respiratory support **(Fig. 22.1)**. Once there is resolution of respiratory failure, we wean the patient from HFNC by reducing the flow in decrements of 10 liters/minute every 2-4 hours, till the patient is comfortable at a flow rate of 20 liters/minute and an FiO_2 of ≤50%. If the respiratory rate is <25 breaths/minute, SPO_2 is ≥92%, and there is no use of accessory muscles or patient discomfort at these settings, we shift the patient to a Venturi mask. If any time during weaning, the patient's respiratory rate increases to >30 breaths/minute or if there is use of accessory muscles of respiration or patient discomfort we switch back to HFNC at settings that the patient was comfortable before weaning.

In conclusion, HFNC is a high-flow oxygen delivery device that improves patient comfort and clinical outcomes. HFNC has been found useful in acute hypoxemic respiratory failure, peri-

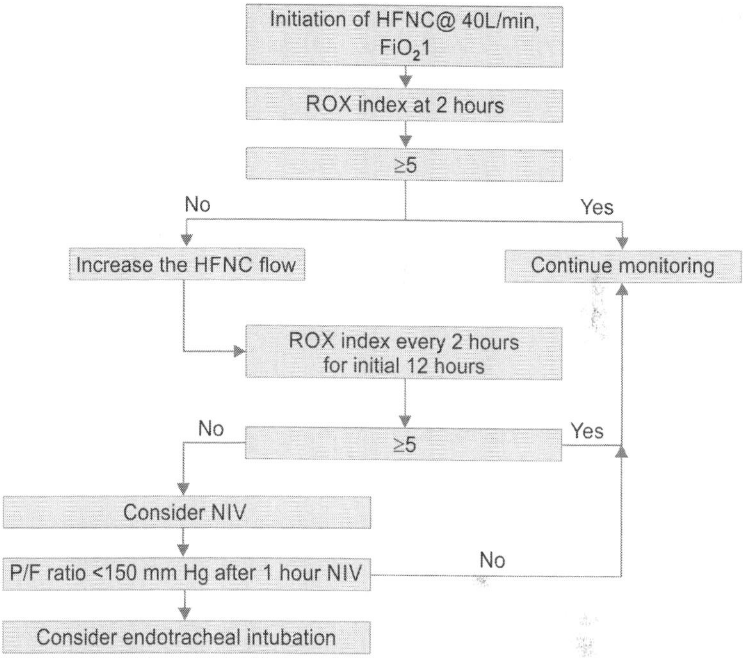

Fig. 22.1: A suggested algorithm describing the use of high-flow nasal cannula (HFNC) for management of patients with acute respiratory failure. ROX index is the ratio of oxygen saturation as measured by pulse oximetry/FiO_2 to respiratory rate [(SPO_2/FiO_2)/RR].

NIV: non-invasive ventilation

operative setting, and post-extubation. It can also be used during bronchoscopy, especially in those with hypoxemia requiring diagnostic bronchoscopic procedures.

SUGGESTED READING

1. Bräunlich J, Beyer D, Mai D, et al. Effects of nasal high flow on ventilation in volunteers, COPD and idiopathic pulmonary fibrosis patients. Respiration. 2013; 5(4): 319–25.
2. Bräunlich J, Dellweg D, Bastian A, et al. Nasal high-flow versus noninvasive ventilation in patients with chronic hypercapnic COPD. Int J Chron Obstruct Pulmon Dis. 2019;14: 1411–21.
3. Bräunlich J, Köhler M, Wirtz H. Nasal highflow improves ventilation in patients with COPD. Int J Chron Obstruct Pulmon Dis. 2016; 1: 1077–85.

4. Bräunlich J, Mauersberger F, Wirtz H. Effectiveness of nasal highflow in hypercapnic COPD patients is flow and leakage dependent. BMC Pulm Med. 2018;18(1):14.
5. Bräunlich J, Seyfarth HJ, Wirtz H. Nasal high-flow versus non-invasive ventilation in stable hypercapnic COPD: A preliminary report. Multidiscip Respir Med. 2015;10(1): 27.
6. Chanques G, Constantin JM, Sauter M, et al. Discomfort associated with underhumidified high-flow oxygen therapy in critically ill patients. Intensive Care Med. 2009; 35(6): 996–1003.
7. Chanques G, Riboulet F, Molinari N, et al. Comparison of three high flow oxygen therapy delivery devices: A clinical physiological cross-over study. Minerva Anestesiol. 2013;79(12): 1344–55.
8. Chaudhuri D, Granton D, Wang DX, et al. High-flow nasal cannula in the immediate postoperative period: A systematic review and meta-analysis. Chest. 2020;158(5): 1934–46.
9. Chaudhuri D, Granton D, Wang DX, et al. Moderate certainty evidence suggests the use of high-flow nasal cannula does not decrease hypoxia when compared with conventional oxygen therapy in the peri-intubation period: Results of a systematic review and meta-analysis. Crit Care Med. 2020;48(4): 571–78.
10. Chikata Y, Izawa M, Okuda N, et al. Humidification performance of two high-flow nasal cannula devices: A bench study. Respir Care. 2014;59(8): 1186–90.
11. Epstein AS, Hartridge-Lambert SK, Ramaker JS, Voigt LP, Portlock CS. Humidified high-flow nasal oxygen utilization in patients with cancer at memorial sloan-kettering cancer center. J Palliat Med. 2011;14(7): 835–9.
12. Fraser JF, Spooner AJ, Dunster KR, Anstey CM, Corley A. Nasal high flow oxygen therapy in patients with copd reduces respiratory rate and tissue carbon dioxide while increasing tidal and end-expiratory lung volumes: A randomised crossover trial. Thorax. 2016; 71(8): 759–61.
13. Frat JP, Thille AW, Mercat A, et al. High-flow oxygen through nasal cannula in acute hypoxemic respiratory failure. N Engl J Med. 2015; 372(23): 2185–96.
14. Hernández G, Vaquero C, González P, et al. Effect of postextubation high-flow nasal cannula vs conventional oxygen therapy on reintubation in low-risk patients: A randomized clinical trial. JAMA. 2016;315(13): 1354–61.
15. Hui D, Hernandez F, Urbauer D, et al. High-flow oxygen and high-flow air for dyspnea in hospitalized patients with cancer: A pilot crossover randomized clinical trial. Oncologist. 2021;26(5): e883–e892.
16. Hui D, Mahler DA, Larsson L, et al. High flow nasal cannula therapy for exertional dyspnea in cancer patients: A pilot randomized clinical trial. Oncologist. 2020.

17. Kim ES, Lee H, Kim SJ, et al. Effectiveness of high-flow nasal cannula oxygen therapy for acute respiratory failure with hypercapnia. J Thorac Dis. 2018; 10(2): 882–88.
18. Koyauchi T, Hasegawa H, Kanata K, et al. Efficacy and tolerability of high-flow nasal cannula oxygen therapy for hypoxemic respiratory failure in patients with interstitial lung disease with do-not-intubate orders: A retrospective single-center study. Respiration. 2018;96(4): 323–29.
19. La Combe B, Messika J, Labbé V, et al. High-flow nasal oxygen for bronchoalveolar lavage in acute respiratory failure patients. Eur Respir J 2016;47(4): 1283–6.
20. Lee MK, Choi J, Park B, et al. High flow nasal cannulae oxygen therapy in acute-moderate hypercapnic respiratory failure. Clin Respir J. 2018; 12(6): 2046–56.
21. Lucangelo U, Vassallo FG, Marras E, et al. High-flow nasal interface improves oxygenation in patients undergoing bronchoscopy. Crit Care Res Pract. 2012; 2012: 506382.
22. Mauri T, Alban L, Turrini C, et al. Optimum support by high-flow nasal cannula in acute hypoxemic respiratory failure: effects of increasing flow rates. Intensive Care Med. 2017; 43(10): 1453–63.
23. Messika J, Ben Ahmed K, Gaudry S, et al. Use of high-flow nasal cannula oxygen therapy in subjects with ARDS: A 1-year observational study. Respir Care. 2015;60(2): 162–9.
24. Nagata K, Kikuchi T, Horie T, et al. Domiciliary high-flow nasal cannula oxygen therapy for patients with stable hypercapnic chronic obstructive pulmonary disease: A multicenter randomized crossover trial. Ann Am Thorac Soc. 2018; 15(4): 432–39.
25. Peters SG, Holets SR, Gay PC. High-flow nasal cannula therapy in do-not-intubate patients with hypoxemic respiratory distress. Respir Care. 2013;58(4): 597–600.
26. Pilcher J, Richards M, Eastlake L, et al. High flow or titrated oxygen for obese medical inpatients: A randomised crossover trial. Med J. 2017; 207(10): 430–34.
27. Pisani L, Betti S, Biglia C, et al. Effects of high-flow nasal cannula in patients with persistent hypercapnia after an acute COPD exacerbation: A prospective pilot study. BMC Pulm Med. 2020; 20(1):12.
28. Pisani L, Fasano L, Corcione N, et al. Change in pulmonary mechanics and the effect on breathing pattern of high flow oxygen therapy in stable hypercapnic COPD. Thorax. 2017; 72(4): 373–75.
29. Ricard JD, Dib F, Esposito-Farese M, Messika J, Girault C. Comparison of high flow nasal cannula oxygen and conventional oxygen therapy on ventilatory support duration during acute-on-chronic respiratory failure: Study protocol of a multicentre, randomised, controlled trial. The 'high-flow ACRF' study. BMJ Open. 2018; 8(9): e022983.

30. Ritchie JE, Williams AB, Gerard C, Hockey H. Evaluation of a humidified nasal high-flow oxygen system, using oxygraphy, capnography and measurement of upper airway pressures. Anaesth Intensive Care. 2011; 39(6): 1103–10.
31. Rochwerg B, Einav S, Chaudhuri D, et al. The role for high flow nasal cannula as a respiratory support strategy in adults: A clinical practice guideline. Intensive Care Med. 2020;46(12): 2226–37.
32. Rochwerg B, Granton D, Wang DX, et al. High flow nasal cannula compared with conventional oxygen therapy for acute hypoxemic respiratory failure: A systematic review and meta-analysis. Intensive Care Med. 2019; 45(5): 563–72.
33. Sehgal IS, Dhooria S, Agarwal R. High-flow nasal cannula oxygen in respiratory failure. N Engl J Med. 2015;373(14): 1374.
34. Simon M, Braune S, Frings D, et al. High-flow nasal cannula oxygen versus non-invasive ventilation in patients with acute hypoxaemic respiratory failure undergoing flexible bronchoscopy—a prospective randomised trial. Crit Care. 2014;18(6): 712.
35. Sztrymf B, Messika J, Bertrand F, et al. Beneficial effects of humidified high flow nasal oxygen in critical care patients: A prospective pilot study. Intensive Care Med. 2011;37(11): 1780–6.
36. Wettstein RB, Shelledy DC, Peters JI. Delivered oxygen concentrations using low-flow and high-flow nasal cannulas. Respir Care. 2005; 50(5): 604–9.

Chapter 23

Oxygen Therapy in Children and Neonates

Manvi Singh, S Venkatseshan, Anil Narang, Meenu Singh

INTRODUCTION

Oxygen is by far, the most frequently used intervention in the management of the critically ill child; whether there is respiratory disease or not. There is often, a casual attitude towards the administration of oxygen. We, often, forget that oxygen has well characterized and potentially toxic effects on the lungs and retina. Hypoxemia means low levels of oxygen in the blood (low blood oxygen saturation or content). Hypoxia is inadequate oxygen in tissues for normal cell and organ function, and hypoxia results from hypoxemia. While a number of diseases in children and neonates cause hypoxemia and hypoxia, therapy with oxygen remains the mainstay of treatment.

Soon after its discovery over two hundred years back, Priestly himself conjectured that oxygen is a double edged sword, both beneficial and hazardous to humans, a fact borne out by further experience with its (mis) use. Oxygen was given to babies more than any other medicinal product in the last 60 years. The free use of oxygen for abolishing periodic breathing in the 1940's led to a high incidence of retrolental fibroplasias. The first, largest landmark trial on oxygen use in neonatal medicine confirmed that although oxygen was a good thing, it was quite possible to have too much of a good thing. As a result, the environmental concentration of oxygen for premature babies was generally restricted to 40% from that time. However, it soon became clear that 40% oxygen was insufficient in many cases of the respiratory distress syndrome and led to a higher mortality rate. McDonald in a retrospective study of preterm babies born in the 1940s showed an inverse relationship between the incidence of retrolental fibroplasia and that of cerebral diplegia. Thus the obvious benefits and the less obvious risks of oxygen therapy are matters of great concern for neonatologists the world over. Significant advance has been made in the recognition of reactive oxygen species (ROS) mediated injury and the role of hypoxia—reperfusion in the pathogenesis of lot of neonatal illnesses. Recent advances in monitoring patient oxygenation together with a better understanding of the physiology of oxygen transport in health and disease have considerably advanced our knowledge in this area.

PHYSIOLOGY OF OXYGEN TRANSPORT

Partial Pressure of Oxygen (PO_2)

Oxygen enters the blood by diffusion across the pulmonary epithelium-vascular endothelium membranes according to oxygen pressure differences between the alveolus (PAO_2) and the plasma (PaO_2). The PO_2 incidentally is the expression of the 'activity' of oxygen molecules and quantitates the tendency of oxygen molecules to escape the gas or fluid in which it is present and is expressed as mm Hg. Physiologically, one can think of partial pressure as a 'driving force' that determines the degree to which oxygen will move from one compartment to another (e.g. plasma to tissue). The alveolar PO_2 is less than the atmospheric PO_2 due to dilution by CO_2 and water vapor.

Oxygen Capacity

Oxygen dissolves in the plasma and binds to hemoglobin. The amount of oxygen dissolved in the plasma is proportional to the PO_2. However with hemoglobin, the relationship is sigmoid. At any PO_2, more oxygen can be contained by hemoglobin than plasma. The maximal quantity of oxygen that can be carried by the hemoglobin is called the 'oxygen carrying capacity.' Each gram of adult or fetal hemoglobin can combine maximally with 1.34 mL of oxygen.

Oxygen Content

Oxygen content (CaO_2) is the total amount of oxygen present in a given, volume of blood and is expressed in volumes percent. It includes the oxygen that is combined with hemoglobin as well as that dissolved in plasma .

The largest portion (98%) of blood oxygen content is the oxygen bound to hemoglobin. For a normal newborn with 20 g hemoglobin per 100 mL blood, hemoglobin would carry 268 mL oxygen/L compared to only 4.5 mL/L of oxygen dissolved in the plasma water.

Oxygen Saturation

The oxygen saturation of blood expresses the relationship between the actual amount of oxygen bound to hemoglobin at a given PO_2 and the oxygen carrying capacity of the same blood, i.e., it is the percentage of the amount of oxygen bound to hemoglobin compared to the maximally possible amount. Oxygen content (CaO_2) can be calculated if oxygen saturation (SaO_2) and hemoglobin content (Hb) are known.

Oxygen saturation (SaO_2) of Hb and the amount of dissolved O_2 in plasma are directly related to the plasma oxygen partial pressure (PaO_2). Under this pressure, O_2 diffuses into the red blood cells where it reacts with the Hb to form a chemical compound $4O_2 + Hb = Hb(O_2)$. This relation is reflected by the oxygen-hemoglobin dissociation curve. Binding of oxygen with Hb activates further binding until it gets completely saturated. This is due to the "heme-heme interaction" (cooperative binding). In other words, the oxyhemoglobin dissociation curve relates the PO_2 to the oxygen saturation or to the amount of oxygen bound to hemoglobin.

The position of the dissociation curve is an expression of the affinity of hemoglobin for oxygen. In adult blood, complete saturation occurs at a PaO_2 of 90–100 mm Hg, whereas the dissociation curve of fetal blood is shifted to the left and at any given PaO_2 below 100 mm Hg, fetal blood binds more oxygen than does adult blood. The shift is the result of a lower content of 2, 3 diphosphoglycerate (DPG) in fetal Hb as well as a reduced sensitivity of HbF for 2, 3 DPG. The position of the curve (Hb-O_2 affinity) is primarily modified by four factors: Hydrogen ion concentration (H+), PCO_2, temperature and 2, 3 DPG concentrations. An increase in these factors, decrease the affinity and vice versa.

Chronic hypoxic conditions are handled with increased Hb-O_2 affinity in large variety of biologic situations. In these conditions, the Hb structure is altered such that Hb affinity for O_2 is increased, resulting in higher O_2 saturation and blood O_2 content at relatively lower PO_2 values. Though the ability of fetal hemoglobin to carry more oxygen at a given PO_2 may be advantageous to extract more oxygen from maternal blood, it reduces the ability of the hemoglobin to unload the oxygen to the tissues as well. This is clinically significant because the sick neonate's blood will take up more oxygen at an alveolar PO_2 of 40 mm Hg, but the tissue PO_2 will have to drop to a very low level in order to unload adequate amounts of oxygen.

Cyanosis is first observed at saturations of 75–85% which relate to oxygen tensions of 32–42 mm Hg in the fetal hemoglobin dissociation curve, a level well below the value of adult blood and approaching levels at which patho-physiological effects of hypoxia occur. In contrast, the flattening of the upper portion of the S-shaped dissociation curve makes it almost impossible to estimate oxygen tensions accurately above 60–80 mm Hg from arterial oxygen saturation.

Improved survival of low birth weight infants with severe respiratory distress syndrome following exchange transfusion has been known for some time. This is because infants given exchange with fresh blood, show an increase in P50 (shift to right) and 2, 3-DPG, especially if citrate phosphate dextrose blood is used which helps preserve the 2, 3 DPG for longer period. Thus replacement by blood with higher 2, 3 DPG content and therefore a more favorable ability to unload oxygen to the tissues would appear to be of benefit, provided the risks of the procedure itself can be tolerated by the infant.

In the thermoneutral zone, the oxygen consumption by the baby is minimal yet sufficient to maintain the body temperature. Placing the baby in an environmental temperature below the thermoneutral zone, results in large obligatory increases in oxygen consumption. However, if the baby is also hypoxic this response is abolished, i.e., oxygen consumption does not increase and the infant's body temperature drops. This paradoxical hypoxic response to a lowering of environmental temperature has been used as a means to physiologically determine the presence of hypoxia. Though a complicated test, its simple clinical counterpart would dictate that a falling rectal temperature associated with a constant thermal environment only slightly below the thermoneutral environment should suggest the possibility of hypoxia. In addition, it has also been shown that lowering the environment temperature also lowers the PaO_2 in healthy newborn infants.

The newborn has certain temperature stimulation zones especially in the trigeminal area of the face. Thus the use of cold, non-humidified oxygen via a face mask will result in large increases in oxygen consumption even if the baby is in the thermoneutral zone.

CLINICAL SIGNS OF HYPOXIA

Hypoxia occurs due to a ventilation/perfusion mismatch, due to pathology in the respiratory tract, the heart or the peripheral or central nervous system. The clinical signs depend on the cause of hypoxia. Respiratory system pathology is signaled by:

- Increased respiratory rate
- Nasal flaring
- Grunting
- Head nodding
- Intercostal and subcostal retractions
- Cyanosis.

Cardiac causes of respiratory compromise should be suspected when there are features of congestive cardiac failure prompted by:

- Elevated JVP
- Hepatomegaly
- Presence of murmur.

Nervous system pathology (peripheral or central) causes hypoventilation and can be identified clinically by:

- Depressed sensorium
- Decreased respiratory rate
- Irregular respiration
- Decreased chest expansion.

A pulse oximeter is a valuable bedside tool that can diagnose hypoxemia early. Investigators have defined hypoxemia from <96.6% to <90% oxygen saturation at sea level and <85% to <88% at higher altitudes. For simplicity, a couple of on-going international multicentre clinical trials for pneumonia therapy are using cut-offs of <90% at sea level and <88% at higher altitude to define hypoxemia.

HYPOXIA IN THE NEONATE

Cyanosis

This is a late sign of hypoxia and in the newborn it appears at PaO_2 of less than 40 mm Hg, well below the level at which pulmonary vasoconstriction occurs. However, in an ill premature baby, the peripheral circulation is slowed which may lead to a cyanotic appearance when in actuality, the PaO_2 is normal or high. On the other hand, in very immature infants with little subcutaneous fat nursed in a high oxygen concentration, one may observe a pink skin probably due to direct diffusion from the atmosphere, while the baby is actually hypoxemic. Guidelines to hypoxemia other than skin color are also less reliable in the newborn.

Heart Rate

The newborn may react to hypoxemia by a deceleration rather than acceleration in the pulse rate. A fixed heart rate of about 120/min is seen in hypoxic babies.

Pulmonary Changes

Respiratory response to hypoxia varies between a fetus, a preterm and a term neonate. Fetuses respond to hypoxia with a suppression of ventilation, and this is more marked in growth retarded fetuses. Very immature infants respond to hypoxia in a similar fashion to fetuses. Otherwise neonates have a biphasic response with an initial increase in ventilation followed by suppression. This response disappears by 12–14 days of age and then the adult pattern is established. However, hypoxic babies are tachypneic either due to underlying cardiopulmonary disorder or due to the metabolic academia secondary to the anaerobic metabolism induced by hypoxia. Hypoxia induces acute pulmonary vasoconstrictive response due to pulmonary artery smooth muscle spasm. This further aggravates the cyanosis both by decreasing pulmonary blood flow and by intracardiac right to left shunting. The synthesis surfactant is also seriously disturbed along with injury to the type II pneumocytes (surfactant producing cells).

Thermoregulatory Disturbances

A fall in the deep body temperature (core) may prove an indication of a fall in PaO_2 to a level of approximately 50 mm Hg. Fat thermogenesis is also affected by hypoxemia. In fact, skin temperature over sites of brown fat is the first to drop in this situation.

Metabolic Acidosis

Living organisms like humans are dependent on oxygen for energy. In the key reaction in the aerobic metabolism of glucose (oxidative phosphorylation), 38 moles of ATP are produced from each mole of carbohydrate in the presence of adequate amounts of oxygen.

Anaerobic conditions are far less efficient yielding only two moles of ATP in addition to causing metabolic acidosis. Hypoxemia induced pulmonary vasoconstriction is further augmented by acidosis. Together, this will compromise pulmonary blood flow inducing further hypoxemia which in turn will compromise the synthesis of lung surfactant.

Although the clinical guides to hypoxemia are poor, there are no signs whatsoever of hyperoxemia and given the dangers of hypoxemia and hyperoxemia, there is no substitute for proper monitoring of oxygenation in the newborn.

OXYGEN TOXICITY

Oxygen may prove toxic either directly via oxidation of tissue or indirectly through auto regulatory effects on blood flow. It also causes injury by production of reactive oxygen species (ROS) that interact with lung cell lipids. Oxygen induces both pulmonary functional and lung parenchymal changes. It acutely reduces ventilation and diffusing capacity as also induces pulmonary vasodilatation. Absorption atelectasis may result in reduction in vital capacity and increased intrapulmonary shunting. Surfactant production is initially reduced, with reduction in both dipalmitoylphosphatidylcholine (DPPC) and phosphatidylglycerol (PG) and so are mucociliary clearance, pulmonary alveolar macrophage viability and function.

Continuous exposure to high concentrations of oxygen cause endothelial and alveolar type I cell damage, leukocytic infiltration with resultant lymphatic distension, alveolar hemorrhage and edema eventually leading onto fibrosis.

O_2 toxicity has been considered to be one of the factors leading to the development of bronchopulmonary dysplasia (BPD). Although human neonate has some antioxidant defenses like glutathione peroxidase, which may even be greater than that of an adult, other defenses, such as catalase are lower in the neonate and even lower in the fetus. Oxidative stress affects a complex array of genes involved in inflammation, coagulation, fibrinolysis, extracellular matrix turnover, cell cycle, signal transduction and alveolar enlargement. Hyperoxia also augments the transdifferentiation of pulmonary lipofibroblasts to myofibroblasts (leads to fibrosis) and increases apoptosis. Neonates, however, seem to more resistant to pulmonary oxygen toxicity than adults.

The other disease related to oxygen toxicity is retrolental fibroplasia or its more modern synonym, retinopathy of prematurity (ROP). Though hypoxemia, hyper or hypocarbia and prostaglandins have been implicated in its pathogenesis, there is abundant clinical and epidemiological evidence incriminating oxygen (hyperoxemia) as a major causative factor. It is evident that careful control of oxygen administration reduces the incidence of ROP but it has proved impossible to define a safe level of oxygen. Current neonatal research is exploring the safe and upper limits of arterial oxygen saturation.

Hyperoxemic reduction in local blood flow in multiple areas of the central nervous system secondary to the vasoconstrictive action of oxygen on the cerebral blood vessels have been demonstrated and a number of brain lesions are attributed to this cause. Recently, in autopsies of human infants exposed to hyperoxemia, a specific lesion, pontosubicular necrosis has been demonstrated.

It is also known that hyperoxemia suppresses erythropoiesis and predisposes to hemolysis. Anatomical changes in the renal tubule and stimulation of the sympathoadrenal medullary system are other purported toxic effects of oxygen.

It has been suggested that oxygen is toxic due to the production of oxygen free radicals. Reactive oxygen species (ROS) are unstable chemical compounds with only one unpaired electron in the outer electron orbit. In the energy economy of the body, oxygen is the ultimate electron acceptor. It is reduced by a series of four single electron transfers to water, in which process superoxide radical, hydrogen peroxide and hydroxyl radical are generated. In addition, singlet oxygen is formed directly from the oxygen molecule. They are thus highly reactive and can injure cell membranes by peroxidation of the polyunsaturated free fatty acids, inactivation of sulfhydryl enzymes and damage to the nucleic acids.

One important oxygen radical generating system is the hypoxanthine-xanthine oxidase system. Hypoxic neonates have elevated concentrations of hypoxanthine in the tissues and when simultaneously treated with oxygen, may produce oxygen radicals far in excess of the body's defense systems against free radicals.

A series of conditions in neonates may be caused by free radicals, e.g., bronchopulmonary dysplasia, retinopathy of prematurity, necrotizing enterocolitis, intraventricular hemorrhage and patent ductus arteriosus. These conditions may constitute part of the so called neonatal oxygen radical disease.

Protection against oxygen free radicals is accomplished by protecting agents classified as scavengers (e.g. mannitol, superoxide dismutase), antioxidants (e.g. vitamin E, C and bilirubin), repair agents (e.g. reduced glutathione) and antioxidant enzymes (e.g. catalase, glutathione peroxidase). Therapeutic strategies to reduce oxygen toxicity would include aggressive treatment of infection, aspiration and pulmonary embolization which contribute to oxidant stress, to correct anemia, optimize cardiac output, treat fever and provide good nutrition. If oxygen concentration cannot be reduced to a $FiO_2 < 0.6$, it may be advantageous to add continuous positive airway pressure (CPAP) or to ventilate.

Pharmacologic approaches to prevent oxygen free radical diseases are mostly experimental and consist of strategies to reduce free radical generation like xanthine oxidate inhibition, calcium channel blockers or to increase free radical elimination, like use of allopurinol, N-acetyl cysteine and mannitol and perhaps the most promising would be the use of cimetidine or intravenous polyethylene glycol conjugated superoxide dismutase.

Vitamin A and its metabolites are important in lung development and maturation. Vitamin A supplementation attenuates hyperoxia induced lung injury in newborn rats. Randomized controlled trials have shown that vitamin A supplementation reduces BPD in infants. Inositol is required for maturation of surfactant components and supplementation has shown to reduce the incidence of BPD, ROP and intraventricular hemorrhage (IVH). Intratracheal administration of Cu-Zn-SOD for ventilated animals has been tried based on the observation that ventilated pre-term infants have reduced levels of Cu-Zn-SOD. Chang et al performed a novel study by continuous infusion of a catalytic antioxidant during 100% O_2 exposure and found that the histological changes due to ROS were partially reversed.

OXYGEN AND RESUSCITATION

Standard guidelines for resuscitation of asphyxiated newborn recommend use of 100% oxygen for assisted ventilation. Recent evidence suggests that resuscitation with high concentration of oxygen lead to excessive release of free oxygen radicals during the post-hypoxic reoxygenation phase. This has the potential to cause cellular and organ damage. These observations initiated several experimental studies to investigate the efficacy of room air in neonatal resuscitation. Experimental studies in piglets have indicated that outcome of resuscitation with room air is comparable to the outcome of resuscitation with 100% oxygen. Preliminary studies comparing room air with 100% oxygen for resuscitation of the asphyxiated newborn have indicated that room air is as effective as 100% oxygen. A recent multicentric quasirandomized trial comparing the short-term efficacy of room air versus 100% oxygen for resuscitation of asphyxiated neonates has shown that room air was as good as 100% oxygen for resuscitation of asphyxiated neonates. This trial has stimulated the need for studies assessing the long-term effects of room air resuscitation. As per the latest neonatal resuscitation programme (NRP) guidelines, positive pressure ventilation (PPV) may be initiated with room air in term and late preterm babies, and upto 30% oxygen in preterm babies. Pulse oximetry should be used to target the natural range of oxygenation in term babies.

INDICATIONS FOR OXYGEN THERAPY

Diagnostic

Oxygen has been used to differentiate the cause of cyanosis in infants. Breathing of 100% oxygen for 10 minutes—the hyperoxia test, would help differentiate a defect of diffusion in the lungs, from right to left shunting of blood, usually seen in congenital heart diseases. The rise in PO_2 above 100 mm Hg, usually to the tune of 150 mm Hg, rules out a right to left shunt. The hyperoxia-hyperventilation test is used to differentiate cyanosis due to a congenital heart disease from that due to persistent pulmonary hypertension of the neonate (PPHN). In this test, hyperventilation with 100% oxygen, to achieve a critical $PaCO_2$ level of 20–25 mm Hg, would lead to a rise in PaO_2 above 100 mm in PPHN, but not in congenital heart disease.

Therapeutic

Cardiac and respiratory causes of hypoxemia warrant oxygen therapy in both neonates and children.

Periodic breathing is abolished by oxygen enrichment but this being physiological, such therapy is not warranted. Though oxygen is needed in the treatment of a severe apneic episode and for a few minutes thereafter, its continued use is contraindicated if there is no ongoing hypoxia. If there is persistent hypoxemia between apneic episodes, the number of apneic periods can be reduced markedly if the oxygen concentration is increased slightly, but careful monitoring is required to prevent hyperoxia.

Though hyperbaric oxygen therapy has not been successful in the treatment of respiratory distress syndrome, it has been used with success in promoting wound healing in neonates. Hyper-oxygenation of the mother has been shown to have a beneficial effect on fetuses with intrauterine growth retardation and oxygen has also been used successfully for "in utero resuscitation" of the hypoxemic fetus. Further it has also been shown that significant amounts of oxygen are absorbed through the newborn skin and it has been suggested that transepidermal oxygen therapy can usefully supplement oxygen delivery to very premature infants with poor pulmonary gas exchange.

Oxygen administration has also been shown to improve right ventricular performance in neonates with chronic lung diseases and may help in the early detection of patients who can benefit from long-term oxygen therapy. Such carefully supervised oxygen therapy has been accomplished at home and so, at least in the West, home oxygen therapy has permitted the safe, early discharge of selected extremely low birth weight infants with chronic lung disease.

CONTRAINDICATIONS FOR OXYGEN THERAPY

While there are no absolute contraindications of oxygen therapy, caution has to be exercised in preterm babies due to the retino-toxic effects as well as the risk of bronchopulmonary dysplasia (BPD). Also, babies with ductus dependent cardiac lesions, relative hypoxia, using less oxygen has to be maintained as closure of the ductus and vasodilatation in the pulmonary vasculature due to administration of high concentrations of oxygen can precipitate cardiac failure in these children. Oxygen is an effective pulmonary vasodilator but if the inspired oxygen concentration is reduced rapidly, the vasoconstriction returns (flip-flop phenomenon) and then may not reverse. Closure of a patent ductus arteriosus with high oxygen breathing is generally temporary and the ductus tends to relax when the stimulus is withdrawn.

OXYGEN SOURCES AND TRANSPORTATION SYSTEMS

These include oxygen cylinders and oxygen concentrators.

Oxygen Cylinders

In most situations in developing countries, oxygen cylinders are the main source of oxygen. They are expensive, bulky and difficult to transport. A high pressure gauge is needed with individual cylinders. Full cylinders contain oxygen at a pressure of 132 atmospheres or bars (2000 psi or 13,400 kPa). When the pressure falls below 8 atmospheres or bars (120 psi or 800 kPa) the cylinder is nearly empty. A flow meter must be attached to the regulator to allow the precise flow of oxygen to the patient. One limitation of individual cylinder is assessing the remaining quantity of oxygen in order to prevent the risk of supply running out. Size and pressure of the cylinder and oxygen flow per minute can be used to calculate the remaining oxygen in the cylinder. Cylinders come in variable sizes. For example size 'D' contains 340 liters, size 'E' contains 680 liters, size 'F' contains 1360 liters and size 'G' contains 3400 liters. One can calculate how many hours the contents will last by using the formula V/F/60, where 'V' is numbers of liters remaining in the cylinder, 'F' flow of oxygen per minute (60 being minutes in an hour).

Oxygen for cylinders is produced by cooling air until it liquifies, and then distilling the liquid to separate pure oxygen from it. Because of the very low temperatures required, below –180°C, this process has a high-energy consumption and can only be done in large manufacturing plants. It is an expensive process. Oxygen cylinders are heavy and difficult to transport. The cylinders have to be transported back to the bulk supply depot to the refilled, as well as from the depot out to the point of use. Transport is often unreliable in developing countries and expensive, so there are often long periods when small hospitals in developing countries have no supplies of oxygen.

Medical oxygen is very expensive in some developing countries and may have to be imported, therefore consuming scarce foreign currency. Industrial oxygen is often much cheaper than medical oxygen may be easier to obtain as the principle of manufacture is identical to that of medical oxygen. Chemical impurities are unlikely in either form. Industrial oxygen is therefore usually safe for medical use and can be used instead of medical oxygen. If oxygen is obtained from an industrial source however, hospital administrators or persons incharge of oxygen supplies must make certain with the manufacturer that the cylinders do indeed contain oxygen and have not previously been used for other gases. The means of cylinder identification must be agreed with the supplier before cylinders are purchased.

Oxygen Concentrators

These were developed in 1960s are widely used in the industrialized world to provide oxygen at home to patients with chronic lung disorders. Their success is attributed to provision of oxygen at a low cost. WHO has identified some models that fulfill the requirements for use in high temperature, humidity and altitude. In resource poor settings, there is a need to look for more cost-effective ways of oxygen management. The use of oxygen concentrators and provision of oxygen by nasal prongs or catheter can reduce the cost of oxygen therapy tremendously. The use of pulse oximeter can improve the care of critically ill children and provide cost savings, especially if the oxygen source is cylinders.

An oxygen concentrator separates the nitrogen from the oxygen in air. Most machines use an electrically powered compressor to force compressed air through synthetic aluminium silicate (Zeolite), which reversibly binds nitrogen. They deliver approximately 2–4 L/min of gas containing over 90% oxygen: The concentration of oxygen is less at higher flow rates.

There have been recent improvements in the design and manufacture of oxygen concentrators, making them more reliable/ smaller, lighter and cheaper. A working group established WHO and the World Federation of Societies of Anaesthesiologists (WFSA) has drawn up requirements for concentrators to be used in adverse conditions, which are based on the International standard for oxygen concentrators. In order to meet the WHO specifications, concentrators are required to operate at temperatures of upto 43°C, a relative humidity of 90–95% and altitudes of upto 4000 m. A vibration test, to simulate hazards of transport over rough terrain, and a corrosion test are also specified. Machines meeting these specifications are now being field-tested to assure their suitability for use in developing countries. Their performance should be closely monitored since to date there is relatively little experience with their use in such settings. Existing concentrators require a regular AC power supply of about 300 watts from mains or a back-up generator. It is recommended that an oxygen cylinder be kept in addition as a back up in case of breakdown or power failure. Oxygen concentrators are much more reliable now than they used to be. Typically, all that is required for their regular maintenance is that the users wash a filter each day and replace two other filters every 3 to 6 months. Skilled mechanical maintenance is needed at intervals of about one year. Concentrators do malfunction occasionally, and their repair can require considerable expertise; worn parts on the compressor and valves may need replacement, so that adequate stocks of filters and spare parts must be included in the initial purchase.

Some malfunctions cause oxygen concentrators to pump out air rather than oxygen, so it is important to be able to test the oxygen concentrations delivered, and not just check for a gas flow. The models meeting the WHO specifications have a built-in device, called an oxygen concentration status indicator (OCSI), which measures the oxygen concentration just before the outlet. A warning is given when the concentration is low, and the machines switch off if the concentration of oxygen falls below 70%. In models, which are not fitted with such a device, the concentration of oxygen needs to be checked at regular intervals using a separate oxygen analyzer. It is advisable to check the concentration of oxygen in the models fitted with an OCSI as well, though less frequently (twice a year, for example). The measurement must be carried out about 10 minutes after switching the concentrator on, since this is the average time taken by the machine to build up the desired (90–95%) concentration of oxygen. Oxygen concentrators cost about US$ 1500-2000 each; because cylinders of oxygen are so expensive, concentrators can result in large savings in cost, but they should only be used where there is a reliable electricity supply and adequate maintenance and repair facilities. WHO recommends that only models meeting the technical specifications mentioned above be used in small hospitals in developing countries.

OXYGEN DELIVERY DEVICES

The administration of oxygen requires the selection of an oxygen delivery system that suits the weight, age and the need of the patient. A low flow system provides FiO_2 that varies with the patient's inspiratory flow rates, and includes nasal catheters, nasopharyngeal catheters, nasal cannula, simple mask, partial rebreathing mask and non rebreathing mask. A high flow system provides fixed FiO_2 at flows that meet or exceed the patient's own inspiratory flow requirements, which includes Venturi systems and the oxyhood.

The patient's own flow requirement depend on the minute ventilation (MV) and inspiratory/expiratory ratio (I:E ratio). Normal flow requirements are 3–4 times the MV and MV = Tidal volume (Vt) × Respiratory rate (RR). Average Vt is about 6 mL/kg. Therefore a 5 kg child breathing at 60/min needs about 6–7 L/min of the air oxygen mixture.

Low Flow Systems

Nasopharyngeal Catheter

This is a thin flexible tube, which is passed through the nose until its tip lies in the patient's throat, just beyond the soft palate. A catheter passed for a distance equal to that from the side of the nostril to the front of the ear usually reaches that point in the oropharynx. The tip of the catheter should be visible just below the uvula when the mouth of the child is open. The nasopharyngeal catheter is also known, in some places, as oropharyngeal catheter, because its tip lies in the patient's oropharynx.

The advantages of this method are that the lowest flow rate of oxygen is required to achieve a given concentration in the airways, the concentration is not reduced if the patient's nostrils are blocked, the catheter can easily be secured in place so that it is unlikely to be dislodged, and there is no danger of hypercarbia (carbon dioxide accumulation) if the oxygen is turned off or the tubing disconnects. With a nasopharyngeal catheter, an oxygen flow of 1 L/min delivers between 45% and 60% of oxygen to a 5 kg child. When oxygen is supplied from a cylinder with a flowmeter, the use of a nasopharyngeal catheter can result in considerable savings over other methods of administration.

However, the gas should be humidified (to avoid drying of the pharyngeal mucosa and reduce the likelihood of inspissated secretions which can block the catheter and cause airway obstruction), the catheter must not be pushed in too far (because gastric distension may result), the flow rate must not be greater that 2 L/min (because of the risk of gastric distension), and the catheter must be taken out and cleaned at least twice a day (so that mucus does not block the holes of the catheter). Some children will cough and gag, or even vomit, when a nasopharyngeal catheter is first put in. Some will deep on coughing and gagging, and the catheter should then be withdrawn slightly. Occasionally, a nasopharyngeal catheter will cause obstruction of the airways or even apnea; continuous and skilled nursing care is needed to prevent or treat these rare but potentially fatal complications. If a nasogastric tube and a nasopharyngeal catheter are used at the same time, they should be placed in the same nostril.

Nasal Catheter

This is a thin flexible tube which is passed through the nose and ends with its tip in the nasal cavity, or just within the nasopharynx. A catheter passed for a distance that is equal to the distance from the side of the nostril to the inner margin of the eyebrow usually reaches that point in the nasal cavity. The tip of the catheter should not be visible when the mouth of the child is open.

Nasal catheter are not as economical as nasopharyngeal catheters, when oxygen is supplied from a cylinder: They require a higher flow to achieve a given concentration of oxygen in the airways. They are usually well tolerated and unlikely to be dislodged. Humidification of oxygen is not necessary. Like nasopharyngeal catheters, they can become blocked with mucus; accumulation of mucus can also cause airway obstruction. The risk of displacement into the esophagus, and as a consequence the potential risk of gastric distension, is smaller. If a nasogastric tube and a nasal catheter are used at the same time, they should be placed in the same nostril.

Nasal Prongs

This is a device for oxygen therapy ending in two short tapered tubes (i.e., a fork or prong) designed to lie just with in the nostrils. It is also called nasal cannula in some places and by some manufacturers. Two soft prongs in the nostrils attached to the oxygen source are attached to the face. The flow is directed to the nasopharynx, which continues to do the work of humidification and heat exchange. The maximum accepted flow is 2–4 L/min. Irritation and nasal obstruction may occur but these are generally well tolerated. In small premature babies, some inadvertent positive end-expiratory pressure (PEEP) may be generated and this device has been used after extubation to provide some pressure, as when a very small size 2 or 2.5 mm endotracheal tube (ETT) is in place, the resistance with CPAP may be too high.

Nasal prongs are not as efficient as nasopharyngeal catheters for giving oxygen—the inspired oxygen concentration is limited to about 30–35%. The concentration delivered falls substantially if the child breathes through the mouth (for example, when the nose is blocked by mucus). Nasal prongs can be easily dislodged if they are not fixed to the upper lip with a piece of tape. On the other hand, nasal prongs are comfortable for the patient and there is no danger of gastric distension. Also, humidification is not required with nasal prongs. When used in combination with an oxygen concentrator and a flow splitter, nasal prongs are the cheapest method of oxygen administration.

Nasal cannulae are capable of delivering low-flow oxygen and provide FiO_2 in the range of 0.23 to 0.35. In general, 1 L/min of nasal cannula oxygen flow is approximately equivalent to an FiO_2 of 24% with each additional liter of flow, increasing the FiO_2 by approximately 3%. Flow rates exceeding 4 L/min, however, are not tolerated well because of drying of the nasal mucosa. An advantage of a nasal cannula is that the patient can eat and drink while receiving oxygen. Actual FiO_2 for a given oxygen flow, however, may fluctuate depending on whether the patient breathes by mouth or by nose. Although nasal cannulae usually are considered safe, complications, such as mucosal perforation leading to submucosal emphysema with airway obstruction, have been reported.

Administration of oxygen through nasal prongs/cannulas in sick neonates is not recommended. Newborns are obligate nose breathers. The cannulae occlude the nostrils and increase the airway resistance. However, it may be better to position the catheter across the infant's upper lip, with the distal end under the infant's nose and secure it by adhesive tape. Maximum flow should be limited to 2 L/mt. The exact concentration of oxygen delivered by cannula cannot be measured and flow rates are titrated by monitoring the PaO_2, $tcPO_2$ or pulse oximetry levels and by evaluating the clinical course. Excessive mucus drainage and mucosal edema are common side effects. Even though FiO_2 at the alveolar level is practically not possible to measure, attempts had been made to measure the FiO_2 level at the hypopharyngeal level and nomograms have been created to identify the flow requirements of air and oxygen to provide the desired FiO_2.

Masks

- **Simple masks:** A mask has perforations, which are exhalation ports. It fits the person's face without much discomfort. As children vary in size, the most comfortable size must be sought and care must be taken that there are not pressure points or eye damage. Precise FiO_2 is not the aim when using these masks and by their nature, they are used in conditions that are not severe.
- **Partial rebreathing masks:** These are simple masks with an additional reservoir that allows the accumulation of oxygen-enriched gas for rebreathing. A portion of the exhaled volume from the anatomical dead space is rich in oxygen. This is what enters the reservoir. Up to 60 percent can be delivered but the pitfalls are similar to those of the simple mask.
- **Non-rebreathing masks:** These are like the above masks, but have a valve at the exhalation port that allows only exhaled gases to enter the reservoir. It prevents room air from being entrained. A well-fitting mask can provide up to 100 percent oxygen. The oxygen percentages obtained with different systems are summarized in **Table 23.1**.

High Flow Systems

Air-entrainment or Venturi masks: These are dilutional masks that work on the Bernoulli principle. Oxygen is delivered through a narrow orifice at a high flow. Negative lateral wall pressure is created in the tubing system. There are openings (entrainment ports) near the nozzle that allow room air to be sucked in, diluting the oxygen. Changing the size of the nozzle, the flow rates, as well as ports, allows control of the amount of oxygen.

Table 23.1: Oxygen percentages with different masks.

Liters/min	*Simple*	*Partial rebreathing*	*Non-rebreathing masks*
5	40%		
6	45–50%	35%	55–60%
8		45–50%	60–80%
10		60%	80–90%
12		60%	90%
15		60%	90–100%

The advantages of a venturi system include: (i) A high flow device guarantees the delivery of a fixed FiO_2; (ii) The high flow comes from the air therefore saving on oxygen costs; (iii) Can be used for low FiO_2 also; (iv) Helps in deciding whether the oxygen requirement is really increasing or decreasing; (v) Humidification not needed; and (vi) Fairly cheap and reliable. Each device will have a table on the package insert as a guide to flow rates required by that particular device.

In children, the problem of fit and comfort is a daily issue. Infants too large for oxyhoods and too small for masks are the usual users. The average infant or even toddler is usually intolerant of a mask and will keep pulling it off. In fact, the infant that remains quiet when the mask is first fitted, is one that may be obtunded from hypoxia or too tired too fight.

Oxyhood

Oxygen hoods are enclosure systems designed to surround the head of the neonate and small infant to deliver a constant concentration of oxygen. It is the simplest and most effective way to deliver oxygen to a spontaneously breathing infant. However, the oxygen supplied has to be prewarmed and humidified and the FiO_2 inside the hood should be monitored periodically. The hood should be of appropriate size and flows >7 L/min is required to prevent carbon dioxide accumulation.

Incubator Enclosure System

Closed incubators provide a warm environment. Supplemental oxygen may be added to the incubators but oxygen concentration may dangerously rise if left unmonitored.

Ventilatory Therapy

Mechanical ventilation is an important therapeutic modality for managing respiratory failure. Though indications would vary depending on the facilities, generally a pH<7.25, PaO_2<50 mm Hg and $PaCO_2$>60 mm Hg on a FiO_2 of 0.6 would indicate the need for respiratory assistance. Types of ventilatory support available are: application of continuous positive airway pressure (CPAP), intermittent mandatory ventilation (IMV), High- frequency ventilation (HFV) and others.

Continuous positive airway pressure (CPAP) commonly is delivered by a tight-fitting mask with a continuous gas-flow rate (usually 15–30 L/min at a specified FiO_2) a reservoir bag, a one-way valve, a humidifier, and an expiratory pressure valve. Many patients, however, cannot tolerate a CPAP mask because of claustrophobia, aerophagia, or hemodynamic instability. In these patients, endotracheal intubation should be considered.

OXYGEN MONITORING

The mainstay of monitoring oxygen therapy in children is by arterial blood gas analysis and by pulse oximetry. The goal is to maintain the PO_2 level above 80 mm Hg or SpO_2 above 94%. In neonates undergoing oxygen therapy, there is only a fine line dividing the therapeutic benefits of oxygen and its manifold toxic effects. Therefore, the quality of respiratory care depends on the tools available to measure the effects of such therapy. Recent advances in electronic and computer technology have made available an array of sophisticated and reliable instruments for monitoring patient oxygenation.

FiO_2 Monitoring

The FiO_2 monitor/O_2 analyzer is recommended for use in any area where a continuous, accurate oxygen concentration is required for neonatal oxygen therapy, e.g., intensive care, during anesthesia etc. It consists of an oxygen sensor—a thermal conductivity analyzer type, a galvanic cell or a Clark electrode, which produces a voltage that is proportional to the oxygen concentration at its detecting surface. This data are fed into a microprocessor incorporating a monitor. The monitor assembly contains sophisticated circuitry that converts the sensor signal into a corresponding percent oxygen display. FiO_2 monitors should be employed to monitor inspired oxygen concentration every hour/continuously in all infants receiving supplemental oxygen.

Blood Oxygen Monitoring

Monitoring the partial pressure of oxygen in arterial blood is mandatory in all infants undergoing oxygen therapy in order to assess the adequacy of therapeutic interventions as well as to adjust the respiratory support acutely, thus minimizing oxygen toxicity.

Intermittent Monitoring

In its most basic form this involves intermittent sampling of arterial catheter, and in acute cases must be done at least four hourly. These samples however yield discontinuous information about patient's oxygenation. The pain, crying and breath holding, which accompany intermittent punctures, could affect the results. Moreover, the frequent sampling and the associated blood loss may be harmful especially for a preterm neonate. The delay in blood sampling, plus the delay in obtaining the results, means that this sort of analysis may be misleading. Despite these major impediments to serial measurements, arterial blood gas values are the most frequently ordered laboratory examinations in the intensive care unit (ICU).

Continuous Monitoring

Continuous blood gas monitoring initially used electro-chemical principles where blood gas electrodes (Clark type) were placed inline. An indwelling intra-arterial polarographic electrode built into the umbilical artery catheter has been used to continuously monitor PaO_2 so also an indwelling saturation monitor (co-oximeter). However there are many technical difficulties with their usage and the list of catheter related complications is formidable. More recently, electro-chemical principle has been replaced by a more accurate and user friendly technique—optode technology (using optical sensors).

Optode Technology

A further refinement in invasive blood gas monitoring has been the development of the PO_2 optode which works on the principle of photoluminescence quenching. An optode is a sensor that optically measures a specific substance. A chemical film is glued to the tip of the optical cable and the fluorescent property of this film varies with the varying concentration of the measured analyte. The fluorescence in an oxygen optode is maximum when there is no oxygen. When an oxygen molecule comes and collides with the film, it reduces the fluorescence in proportion to the number of colliding O_2 molecules. Several recent studies have examined its accuracy and it has been shown to function most precisely at low PO_2, a desirable feature. Thanks to its small diameter, the optode sensor can be placed either extra- arterial (EABG) or intra-arterial (IABG). Studies have shown that

EABG is slightly better than the IABG systems regarding the precision of PaO_2 analysis.

Non-invasive Monitoring of Oxygenation

Transcutaneous PO_2 Monitoring

The serious complications of invasive blood gas monitoring and the realization of the inadequacy and fallacy of intermittent blood gas monitoring led to the development of transcutaneous, non-invasive, continuous monitoring of blood gases in the newborn. The $tcPO_2$ electrode is a miniaturized heated, redesigned Clark electrode consisting of a platinum cathode and a silver reference anode encased in an electrolyte solution and separated from the skin by a membrane permeable to oxygen. The heating of the skin arterializes the capillary blood and oxygen diffuses through the membrane in to the electrode. There it is reduced by the cathode thereby generating an electric current which is converted into partial pressure measurements and displayed by the monitor. The $tcPO_2$ monitoring has received wide acceptance the world over. Data show good correlation with PO_2 values in healthy as well as sick neonates. Improper probe placement and poor peripheral perfusion are the two common conditions where the PO_2 measurement goes wrong. The $tcPO_2$ monitor has been widely used in ventilatory care facilitating maintenance of adequate oxygenation as well as faster weaning; it provides an excellent opportunity to have a continuous trend of oxygenation over the previous hours/days, which significantly helps in clinical and research activities. The $tcPO_2$ monitor has also been used in the diagnosis of right to left shunting by monitoring the preductal and postductal oxygenation. The $tcPO_2$ electrodes have been used in monitoring maternal and fetal oxygen during labour. Side effects are few and minor like local erythema, skin craters and blister formation.

Pulse Oximetry

Pulse oximeter provides a safe and simple method of assessing patient oxygenation. It has the advantages of being continuous, non-invasive, and reliable with a rapid response time, self-calibration and no risk of burns. It has the physiologic advantage of indicating adequacy of oxygen supply to the tissues, and hence the method is increasingly being used in neonatal intensive care units. Pulse oximetry is used to measure hemoglobin oxygen saturation and is based on the principles of plethysmography and spectrophotometry. The monitor displays percentage saturation of hemoglobin along with the pulse rate and pulse wave form.

In spite of these many benefits, pulse oximeter may not work well in the presence of hypotension and shock. Recent advances in pulse oximeter monitoring technologies (Masimo technology) which uses the signal extraction technology (SET) to reduce the false alarms following artifacts, has attempted to overcome these difficulties but this still remains to be proven in clinical trials. Vidyasagar et al claim that if the heart rate displayed by the ECG monitor correlates with the displayed pulse rate on the saturation monitor within a five beat range, it ensures adequacy of SpO_2 readings in low perfusion states. Errors in pulse oximeter recordings may occur due to the presence of abnormal hemoglobins like methemoglobin and carboxyhemoglobin, dyes like methylene blue and indigo carmine, artifacts like ambient light, low perfusion and motion, venous pulsation, technological problems like optical shunt, optical cross talk and electrical interference.

Even after accounting for so many sources of error, the accuracy of pulse oximeters is impressive. It has been suggested that the SpO_2 be kept at 92 ± 3% in sick neonates so that the corresponding PaO_2 values are between 45 and 100 mm Hg. A sensitivity-specificity analysis showed that the SpO_2 range of 92 ± 3% indicated a PaO_2 range of 45–100 mm Hg with 100% sensitivity and specificity. Hay et al recommended that the SpO_2 range of >98% should be considered as a goal for achieving and maintaining 'normal' blood oxygenation in newborn infants .

But till now the safe limits of saturation is controversial. A recent national survey of pulse oximetry before and after 2 weeks of life has shown that a saturation range ≤98% before 2 weeks and ≤92% after first 2 weeks of life led to a less number of severe ROP cases requiring ablative surgery. However, some correlation should be made between oxygen saturation and PO_2 at lower (85–90%) and higher (96–99%) saturation values before relying entirely on pulse oxygen saturation determinations for oxygen and respiratory management. Currently, randomized trials have been planned to look for early infancy outcomes (ROP and neurodevelopment) after a low (85–89%) vs. high (91–95%) target saturations and the results of these studies may through some light on this issue. Some hints on pulse oximetry can be found in **Table 23.2**.

Table 23.2: Hints on SpO_2 monitoring.

	Acute illness	*Chronic illness*
Acceptable limits	87–95%	90–95%
O_2 management parameters	Wean from O_2 when baby stable and SpO_2 consistently > 95%	Wean from O_2 when baby stable and SpO_2 consistently >95% 12–24 hours
Blood gas requirements	SpO_2 <85/>97% consistently over 15–30 min • Monitor whether ECG heart rate is correlating • Watch for poor peripheral perfusion	SpO_2 <87/>95% consistently over an hour

Other Methods of Assessing Oxygenation

Conjunctival PO_2

A miniaturized Clark electrode has been made to fit inside a polymethylmethacrylate ocular confirmer ring, and is directly applied to the palpebral conjunctiva. This is thus a true tissue oxygen monitor, does not need heating, has rapid equilibration time and helps detect changes in carotid blood flow. However, practical limitations are same as for any transcutaneous monitoring. Potential for ocular damage had to be kept in mind.

Invasive Hemoglobin Saturation Monitoring

Mixed venous PO_2 (PvO_2) and hemoglobin and saturation (SvO_2) reflect global tissue oxygenation and the ability of the cardiopulmonary system to transport sufficient oxygen to meet body oxygen needs. Based on this physiologic argument, continuous mixed venous oxygen monitoring using a fibreoptic system with the catheter tip in the pulmonary artery has been accomplished, although, it has not found wide acceptance in neonatology.

Cytochrome aa3 Saturation Monitoring

Cytochrome aa3 is a distal enzyme in the oxidative phosphorylation taking place in the mitochondria. Evaluating the redox state of this enzyme, by illuminating with a near-infrared optical scanner (NIROS)—scope that emits near infrared light, has been used to follow trends in mitochondrial oxygenation. The device, however, is not currently suitable for clinical use owing to its size, expense and limited data as to its accuracy. Nevertheless, it promises an exciting future for monitoring oxygen continuously and non-invasively at its ultimate destination, in living tissue.

GUIDELINES TO OXYGEN THERAPY

Oxygen is a drug and so should be given only for medical indications as detailed earlier. Regardless of the mode of administration, safe oxygen therapy should follow certain guidelines. The following recommendations have been made in accordance with the guidelines of the American Academy of Pediatrics and the American College of Obstetricians and Gynaecologists:

- No concentration of oxygen is safe. What is therapeutic for one infant may be toxic to another. Therefore, mere FiO_2 monitoring is not adequate.
- Give sufficient oxygen to maintain an arterial PO_2 of 50–80 mm Hg. If this is not possible, give just enough oxygen to alleviate cyanosis.
- Oxygen administration without some form of continuous monitoring of infant's oxygenation is not safe and so is not recommended.
- Administered oxygen should always be humidified (30–40%) and prewarmed to 31–34°C.
- Inspired oxygen concentration should be measured near the infant's nose continuously or at least hourly and recorded. FiO_2 monitors need 8-hourly calibration.
- Always try to maintain a constant FiO_2 so as to stabilize the PaO_2. All changes in FiO_2 must be gradual to minimize the risk of 'flip-flop' phenomenon.
- Close monitoring and recording of clinical parameters like color, respiratory effort, activity and circulatory response as also of FiO_2 concentrations and time of adjustments should be carried out. This helps determine the need for oxygen therapy.

FUTURE PERSPECTIVES

With the current state of our knowledge regarding oxygen's uses, hazards and dangers it must be administered with extreme caution. The administration must be done only when indicated and it should be rigorously monitored to prevent life threatening complications. In this regard, there has been development of devices that allow the automated delivery of oxygen, such that the auto-adjustment of the FiO_2 takes place based on the patients blood oxygenation status. These devices have shown to be effective in adults as well as neonates, in maintaining oxygenation within the target range, and reducing the need for manual titration. Large scale implementation and trials are subject to future research. Another exciting concept is the evolution of intravenous oxygen. A foam based microparticle self assembling lipid suspension with a core of oxygen has been developed, which has been shown to improve oxygenation in hypoxemic rodents. While much needs to be done to translate this research from bench to bedside, it is promising and may offer a solution to replace bulky oxygen cylinders and concentrators, especially in remote areas, and decrease the barotrauma and volutrauma associated with invasive ventilation.

SUGGESTED READING

1. Aziz K, Henry CL, Marilyn B. Part 5: Neonatal Resuscitation: 2020 American Heart Association Guidelines for Cardiopulmonary Resuscitation and Emergency Cardiovascular Care. Circulation 2020;142: S524-S550.
2. Black KJ, Lock AT, Thomson LM, Cole AR, Tang X, Polizzotti BD, et al. Hemodynamic effects of lipid-based oxygen microbubbles via rapid intravenous injection in rodents. Pharm Res. 2017;34(10):2156-62.
3. Cole CH, Wright KW, Tarnow-Mordi W, Phelps DL. Resolving our uncertainty about oxygen therapy. Pediatrics. 2003; 112:1415-19.
4. Darlow BA, Graham PJ. Vitamin a supplementation for preventing morbidity and mortality in very low birth weight infants. Cochrane Database Syst Rev. 2002; (4):CD000501
5. Hallenberger A, Poets CF, Horn W, Seyfang A, Urschitz MS, CLAC Study Group. Closed-loop Automatic Oxygen Control (CLAC) in Preterm Infants: A Randomized controlled trial. Pediatrics. 2014;133(2):e379-85.
6. Hay WW, Thilo E and Curlander JB: Pulse oximetry in neonatal medicine. Clin Perinatol. 1991;18: 441.
7. Hudak BB, Allen MC, Hudak ML and Loughlin GM: Home oxygen therapy for chronic lung disease in extremely low birth weight infants. Am J Dis Child. 1989;143:357
8. Kheir JN, Polizzotti BD, Thomson LM, O'Connell DW, Black KJ, Lee RW, et al. Bulk manufacture of concentrated oxygen gas-filled microparticles for intravenous oxygen delivery. Adv Healthc Mater. 2013;2(8):1131-41.

9. Martin DS, Grocott MPW. Oxygen therapy in critical illness: Precise control of arterial oxygenation and permissive hypoxemia. Crit Care Med. 2013;41(2):423–32.
10. Myers TR. AARC clinical practice guideline: Selection of an oxygen delivery device for neonatal and pediatric patients-2002 revision and update. Respir Care. 2002;47:707–16
11. Priestly J: The discovery of oxygen (1775). Alembic Club Reprints. No 7, University of Chicago Press, 1906.
12. Roberton NRC, Dahlenberg GW and Tizard JPM: Oxygen therapy in the newborn. Lancet. 1968;2:1323.
13. Veness-Meehan KA, Pierce RA, Moats-Staats BM, Stiles AD. Retinoic acid attenuates o2-induced inhibition of lung septation. Am J Physiol Lung Cell Mol Physiol. 2002;283:L971–80.
14. Walsh BK, Smallwood CD. Pediatric oxygen therapy: A review and update. Respir Care. 2017;62(6):645–61.
15. Weinberger B, Laskin DL, Heck DE, Laskin JD. Oxygen toxicity in premature infants. Toxicol Appl Pharmacol. 2002; 181:60–67.
16. Zapata J, Gómez JJ, Araque Campo R, Matiz Rubio A, Sola A. A randomised controlled trial of an automated oxygen delivery algorithm for preterm neonates receiving supplemental oxygen without mechanical ventilation. Acta Paediatr Oslo Nor. 1992. 2014;103(9):928–33.

Chapter 24

Oxygen Storage and Supply in Hospitals

Pankaj Arora, Navneet Dhaliwal

Medical oxygen is an essential part of patient treatment in hospitals. Several oxygen delivery methods, including oxygen cylinders, liquid oxygen from cryogenic vessels through manifold gas pipeline distribution systems, oxygen concentrators, and oxygen generators. Various accessories like pressure regulators, flow meters, control panels, and outlet point fixtures are required for providing oxygen to a patient. Installation of alarm systems and control panels are required for monitoring in the manifold room and at various points of the distribution network. Since oxygen is a highly inflammable gas, we must follow all necessary guidelines and standard operating procedures during operation. The manufacture, supply, and distribution, and storage of medical oxygen are governed by the Ministry of Commerce and Industry (Government of India), which has laid down certain rules and regulations. Herein, we provide an overview of oxygen storage and supply in hospitals.

INTRODUCTION

Oxygen, an essential element for life, is also the third most abundant element after hydrogen and helium. The importance of oxygen in health care establishments cannot be overemphasized. The events of the Gorakhpur tragedy in 2017, where more than 50 children died apparently due to lack of oxygen supply, is a stark reminder of the medicinal value of a gas found abundantly in the atmosphere. The COVID pandemic has reinforced the role of oxygen as a mode of treatment, and the measurement of SpO_2 has entered the lexicon of the common people.

USES OF OXYGEN

Industrial Use

Oxygen gas is widely used in the steel industry and o for manufacturing chemicals, namely hydrogen peroxide, epoxyethane, and others. Oxygen is used for oxyacetylene welding and cutting of metals and is also increasingly being used to treat sewage and effluent.

Medicinal Use

Oxygen is a drug according to the formulation prescribed in Indian Pharmacopoeia (IP) and has been affirmed as such by the Supreme Court of India (The State of Andhra Pradesh V/s M/s Linde India Ltd. Civil Appeal No. 2230 of 2020). Oxygen is prescribed for various ailments in varying doses and pressure depending upon the disease, e.g., high-flow nasal oxygen in severe COVID, hyperbaric oxygen in decompression sickness, and others.

MECHANISM OF DELIVERY OF OXYGEN IN THE HEALTH CARE FACILITY

Oxygen at the bedside can be delivered through oxygen cylinders, oxygen concentrators, and piped oxygen supply. The piped oxygen supply can have the following sources at the central location, including oxygen cylinders, oxygen generators, and liquid oxygen storage vessels. An health care facility (HCF) may have one or more mechanisms to provide oxygen to the patients depending upon the scope of its operation, the kind of patients being treated, and the resources available. For example, establishing a piped oxygen supply with liquid oxygen as a source may not be viable for an HCF with less than 200 beds.

SOURCES OF OXYGEN

Oxygen Cylinders

The delivery of oxygen gas for medical treatment through cylinders is one of the earliest methods of providing oxygen to patients. Substantial research has improved the design and structural safety of oxygen cylinders over the last few decades. The earlier cylinders were made of steel. Currently, chrome-molybdenum steel, which is resistant to corrosion and is lightweight, is being used in hospital setups. Composite material cylinders made of lightweight steel or aluminum and encased in carbon fiber or Kevlar material are used for rescue and search operations and patient transportation. The preference for composite cylinders is because they are lightweight, sustain high pressure, and hold more gas. Aluminum cylinders compatible during magnetic resonance imaging studies are being used for this purpose.

Size and Capacity of Oxygen Cylinders Used in Hospitals

Oxygen cylinders are named alphabetically based on their capacity (**Table 24.1**). Size A cylinders are the smallest and are not used in hospitals. Size E cylinders are commonly used in anesthesia machines and during patient transportation.

Color Coding and Labeling of Oxygen Cylinders

According to the international guidelines, oxygen cylinders are white. The USA has adopted green color, Germany uses blue, while in India, the cylinder is identified by a white shoulder with a black body. As per the Indian norms, these cylinders must conform to IS 7285 (Part 2): 2004 and be approved by the Chief Controller of Explosives, Nagpur, India. Cylinders are built based on standard specifications and marked permanently with symbols and numbers on the shoulder or head. The engravings on the cylinders usually consist of:

- Tare weight
- Test pressure with the date of the last test performed
- The chemical formula of the content of the cylinder.

Sometimes this information is mentioned in the ring around the neck of the cylinder. The suppliers attach labels to the cylinders that show the UN Number for compressed oxygen, hazard warning in the shape of a diamond, the size of the cylinder, and the gas pressure.

Table 24.1: Common cylinder sizes used in health care facility.

Type	*Nominal oxygen capacity (L)*	*Water capacity (L)*	*Dimensions (height × diameter in cm)*	*Normal service pressure (psi)*	*Approximate weight (kg)*
D	340	2.3	53.5 × 10.2	1987	3.9
E	680	4.7	86.5 × 12	1987	6.5
F	1,360	9.4	93 × 14	1987	17
G	3,400	23.6	132 × 17.8	1987	39
J	6,800	47.2	152 × 23	1987	78

Cylinder Components

The cylinder has a body, neck, valve, port, stem, handwheel, and a pressure-relief device. The neck is the top part of the cylinder and ends in a tapered screw into which the valve is fitted. The valves fitted on the cylinders are mostly pin index, bullnose, or integral types. Other valves are pin index side spindle valve, hand wheel valve, hand wheel side outlet valve, and digital valve. The pin index valve safety system is used for cylinders of size E or less. Pinholes bored on the face of the valve align with pins projecting from the yoke assembly of the cylinder. Pinholes are safety mechanism as valves compliant to a particular type of gas cylinder will only fit the pins on the yoke assembly of that cylinder.

Working of an Oxygen Cylinder

Oxygen gas is stored under pressure in the cylinder. Hence, a regulator is required to reduce the output pressure of the compressed oxygen when it flows out of the cylinder to prevent an explosive outflow of the gas. The regulator has two attached gauges, the pressure gauge, which measures gas pressure in pounds per square inch (psi) in the cylinder, and a flow gauge required to indicate and control the gas flow (L/min) out of the cylinder. Regulators are used to reduce the pressure and control the flow. The regulators are classified as single-stage, dual stage, or three-stage regulators. Line regulators monitor the pressure of oxygen near the point of delivery when the cylinders are located at a distant location.

Flow meter is the device used to measure the rate of oxygen flow from a cylinder, pipeline, or concentrator to the patient in terms of liters per minute. Flow meters are either integrated with regulators or independent for oxygen outlets at the patient's bedside. These are mainly Thorpe tube, Bourdon gauge, and dial/click types. Thorpe-type regulators are used where the distribution is through a pipeline or for large-sized cylinders. Bourdon type regulator is used for small portable cylinders. The dial/click style is used for piped oxygen distribution systems.

Filling of Gas in Cylinders

The gases stored in the cylinders are compressed and under high pressure. A cylinder with a capacity of 23.6 liters of water can contain compressed gas under pressure which can expand up to 3400 liters of volume under normal atmospheric pressure. As a compressed gas, the filling limit in the cylinder is 2000-2015 psi at 70°C, depending on the type of cylinder, and is called the service pressure. Normally, the cylinders should be able to withstand 1.66 times the service pressure. An equation proposed by Arlas can give the approximate time of cylinder emptying.

Approximate time remaining in hours = O_2 cylinder pressure in psi/200 × O_2 flow rate per minute.

Testing of Cylinders

Testing of cylinders is an essential part of the filling process that must be followed by manufacturers and is mandated under the rules and regulations for the manufacture, supply, sale, and distribution of medical gases. Visual, endoscopic, and ultrasonic examination of cylinders is done to detect external and internal defects. Ultrasonic examination locates and quantifies flaw size. This testing is done every 10 years for steel cylinders and five years for composite cylinders. Hydraulic testing, tensile testing, flattening test, impact test, and bend test are also done to ensure the safety of the oxygen cylinders.

Handling Oxygen Cylinders

When a full cylinder is to be used, it must be inspected for the suitable contents from the label, engravings, and color-coding. There should be no trace of oil, grease, or other impurities on the cylinder. Avoid lifting the cylinder from the neck or valve part. Purging of the cylinder before use must be done to clear any debris. After purging, the regulator is connected to the cylinder valve outlet, and the valve is released slowly. The cylinder should not be entirely emptied as loss of positive pressure may contaminate the cylinder with environmental air leading to internal damage.

Advantages of Gas Cylinders

- It does not require any power source.
- Inexpensive method for short term use.
- Silent when functional.

Disadvantages of Gas Cylinders

- The weight and transportation of the cylinder.
- Need for frequent replacement or refilling and are not cost-effective if required for long-term use.
- Cylinders can be used only for a limited number of beds.

Oxygen Concentrators

Oxygen concentrator is equipment that concentrates the atmospheric oxygen to deliver oxygen at about 95% to the patients. It utilizes a process called "Pressure Swing Adsorption" or PSA to concentrate oxygen from ambient air. The air is taken from the atmosphere and processed through filters, heat exchangers, and zeolite sieve beds. The nitrogen of the atmospheric air is removed in the process, and the concentrated oxygen is delivered to a reservoir where it is accumulated and released for patient use. The oxygen can be supplied up to the rate of 10 liters per minute (LPM). The significant advantage of this technology is its portability, i.e., it can easily be taken to the bedside and provides an "inexhaustible" source of oxygen. The major disadvantage is its dependence on the electrical supply to run the equipment and hence a constant source of electricity if required.

A battery-operated concentrator is also available, but they deliver oxygen at lower rates, usually up to 3 LPM, but increase the patient's mobility, including outdoor activities. The concentrators require regular maintenance for their operation and efficient functioning. The oxygen concentrators can be an essential source of oxygen in a primary health care setting and domiciliary use. A cylinder backup is required in the event of a non-reliable supply of electricity or the non-availability of an alternative source of power.

Oxygen Generator Plant

Oxygen Generator Plant also works on the same principle as the oxygen concentrator and uses "Pressure Swing Adsorption" technology to generate oxygen from ambient air. However, here the scale of operation is massive, and depending upon the requirement of the HCF, an oxygen generator plant of suitable capacity may be established to fulfill the demand. The oxygen generated can be piped directly to the outlets at the bedside or used to fill the cylinders. These cylinders can be connected to manifold systems or can be taken to the bedside for delivery. The oxygen generator plant has the advantage of being a potential source of an inexhaustible supply of oxygen. However, the major drawback is the high cost of establishment and maintenance and specialized workforce to maintain the equipment. Like concentrators, it will require a constant supply of electricity to run its operation. However, unlike concentrators, oxygen generator plants are capable of supplying oxygen at high pressures.

Liquid Oxygen

Liquid oxygen is a cryogenic liquid or a liquefied gas with a boiling point of -297°F (-183°C). Oxygen, though a gas, is stored as a liquid in a unique insulated cryogenic storage vessel or a tank. The tank is constructed like a vacuum flask. It has an inner vessel surrounded by an outer vessel with an insulating material in between, which keeps the liquid stored in the vessel at the desired low temperature. The liquid form is converted to gaseous oxygen before supply through a system of coils knows as vaporizers. The gaseous oxygen is then supplied to the patient through the pipeline system, which is controlled through a central manifold. The liquid oxygen manifold is common in most tertiary care hospitals and often in the secondary care hospitals of the country. The liquid oxygen is manufactured by the cryogenic distillation process by an air separation unit through liquefaction of atmospheric air and separation of oxygen. The liquid oxygen so produced is transported through special vehicles to the hospitals, where it is transferred to the bulk storage tanks. The major advantage of liquid oxygen is that a large amount of oxygen can be stored in a relatively small space since each liter of liquid oxygen will yield 860 L of gaseous oxygen. Additionally, it is not dependent upon electricity and can work in areas with an unreliable power supply. The cost of infrastructure is high, and requires regular maintenance and is exhaustible if regular refilling is not done.

MECHANISM OF OXYGEN DELIVERY AT THE BEDSIDE

Oxygen is delivered at the patient's bedside through oxygen cylinders, centralized oxygen distribution system, and local cylinder bank.

Oxygen Cylinder

Oxygen cylinders contain compressed gas for oxygen delivery, as mentioned earlier. The cylinder is connected to the flow meter through the oxygen regulator. The flow meter is further connected to the patient oxygen administration tubing that delivers oxygen to the patient.

Centralized Oxygen Distribution System

This is the most efficient method of supplying oxygen in a modern hospital. The initial installation costs are high but are cost-effective in the long run. The centralized distribution of oxygen requires an adequately laid down supply manifold gas pipeline system. The significant factors while designing the pipeline distribution system are the flow required at each terminal unit, the flow required in branches of the distribution system, and the total flow required at any time point in the whole pipeline.

This pipeline originates from the gas source and goes up to the terminal unit. The supply pipes are usually made of copper. The pipeline joints are also made of copper and brazed by silver brazing filler material without the use of any flux. The pipeline must be supported at regular intervals to prevent sagging or distortion. It should be encased in sleeves when crossing through walls/slabs. To have a control mechanism, the pipeline has an evenly distributed valve system, area valve service units, and terminal units. The valves can be located at the entry of the pipeline into the building, exit from the building, and on the risers/branches within the building and should enable isolation of large parts of the pipeline. The area valve service unit isolates the upstream and downstream pipeline of the valve for service and repair and caters to limited areas. These valves should be visible, easily operable, and labeled to identify the area being supplied. Warning and alarm systems with pressure sensors are placed at the central monitoring point (central indicator panel) and at specific points on the pipeline to ensure safety and efficacy. The pipeline terminates in the color-coded wall outlets. The delivery points are located in bed head panels above the patient bed or the pendant, along with other medical supply assemblies. These outlet points are either diameter index safety type or one of the many other variants available in the market. The manifold gas pipeline system can have inadequate pressure, accidental valve shut down, leakage, kinking, or obstruction of the pipeline. Therefore, a regular maintenance contract must be in place to ensure uninterrupted supply to the terminal units.

Manifold Room

Healthcare facilities that have installed piped supply of medical gases, including oxygen, must have a central manifold room for continuous monitoring. The central supply will have a cylinder bank as primary and secondary supply if jumbo cylinders are being used as the oxygen source. Typically, J size cylinders with a usable supply of 6,540 liters (total 6,800 liters) at 137 bar or 1987 psi are used for cylinder manifold. Here, a row of cylinders is connected to the main header pipe of oxygen, which then branches out to the whole HCF for oxygen supply. The cylinders are connected in parallel so that gas is taken from each cylinder. Once the gas in the cylinders is consumed, the automatic switch shifts the supply to a secondary source/bank of cylinders. If this switchover is based on electrical power, an alternate power source must be in place in the event of a power failure. Meanwhile, the empty cylinders in the primary source are replenished. There is another bank of cylinders classified as an emergency bank used in case both the primary and secondary source fails due to some reason.

If HCFs have liquid oxygen or oxygen generator as the primary source of oxygen, there should be a secondary source of oxygen cylinders and an emergency bank. The manifold room should have a central alarm panel with visual and audible alarms to alert the staff about a drop in pressure and possible leakage from the pipeline. A similar alarm system will also be placed at strategic locations throughout the pipeline to alert the users about any change in pressure beyond permissible limits for taking corrective action.

Local Cylinder Bank

Large-sized cylinders are grouped at a central location and connected to the supply area through a copper pipeline. This setup is monitored by control panels and used in small hospitals. The area supplied through this system is limited. Empty cylinders are continuously replaced to maintain adequate pressure.

Cylinder Storage

A separate storage area for cylinders should be built near the manifold room for storing full and empty cylinders. There should be a clear demarcation between the full and empty cylinders to prevent any mixing of the two so that empty cylinders are not mistaken for full cylinders. The cylinder storage area should be built considering the relevant safety rules and guidelines. A few prominent ones are given below:

- The Ministry of Commerce and Industry regulates the manufacture, supply, and transportation of medical gases in India.
- The Drugs and Cosmetics Act 1940 regulates the manufacture, distribution, and sale of medical oxygen in India. The standards of identity, purity, and strength as per Indian pharmacopeia must be followed to manufacture medical oxygen.

- The Gas Cylinder Rules 2016, under section 18 of the Explosives Act 1884, apply to medical oxygen in cylinders or cryogenic containers and regulate the filling, possession, import, and transport of cylinders.
- The Static and Mobile Pressure Vessels (Unfired) Rules, 2016, required under sections 5 and 7 of the Explosives Act, 1884, regulates the construction, storage, transport, and licensing for cryogenic vessels.

SAFETY TIPS

- The cylinders are to be stored in a cool, dry, ventilated, clean area with ease of access. Exposure to direct sunlight should be avoided.
- The cylinders should be free of oil, grease, or other residues.
- Full and empty cylinders should be stored separately, even if kept in the same room. Cylinders with the oldest fill date must be used first, so storing must be done accordingly.
- Cylinders should be stocked in a manner to prevent accidental falling, which can have devastating consequences. Large cylinders must be kept secure by a chain or other restraining device, while smaller cylinders can be kept horizontally on metal racks. The cylinder banks should be fastened so that natural events like earthquakes do not cause their falling which can disrupt the supply of oxygen.
- Transportation of the cylinders must be done using a trolley/cart.
- The manifold room, liquid oxygen vessel/oxygen generator should be protected from any unauthorized access.
- All measures should be taken to ensure safety from fire accidents since oxygen is not inflammable per se but supports combustion. Signages depicting "no smoking", "no open flame" must be displayed prominently.
- Regular testing of the liquid oxygen tank and oxygen cylinders must be done, e.g., ultrasonic test, hydrostatic test, etc.
- The area around the manifold room should be free of vehicles for clear access to emergency vehicles and transport vehicles supplying liquid oxygen and cylinders.
- Standard operating protocols for exchanging cylinders, mounting, and dismounting of cylinders, and other procedures must be established.
- Finally, regular training of the employees must be performed to update them about the safe handling of oxygen.

SUGGESTED READING

1. Arlas G. A method to quickly estimate remaining time for an oxygen e-cylinder. Anesth Analg. 2004;98:1190.
2. Bland H. The supply of anesthetic and other medical gases. In Davey AJ, Diba A Editors. Ward's Anesthetic Equipment, 5th edition. London: Elsevier Saunders. 2005. pp. 23–49.
3. Das S, Chattopadhyay S, Bose P. The anaesthesia gas supply system. Indian J Anaesth. 2013;57(5):489–499.
4. Department of Health. Health Technical Memorandum 02.01. Medical Gas Pipeline Systems. Part B: Design, Installation, Validation and Verification 2006 London The Stationery Office.
5. Department of Health. Health Technical Memorandum 02-01. Medical Gas Pipeline Systems. Part A: Design, Installation, Validation and Verification 2006 London The Stationery Office.
6. Hardavella G, Karampinis I, Frille A, et al. Oxygen devices and delivery systems. Breathe. 2019;15:e108–e116.
7. Soni NN, Maheshwari DG. Current regulation of medical gases in India and future aspects. Int J Drug Reg Affairs. 2018;6(1):35–40.
8. Srivastava U. Anaesthesia gas supply: Gas cylinders. Indian J Anaesth. 2013;57(5):500–506.
9. WHO, UNICEF. WHO-UNICEF technical specifications and guidance for oxygen therapy devices. Geneva, Switzerland: World Health Organization (WHO); 2019.
10. Wyka KA, Mathews PJ, Rutkowski JA. Foundations of Respiratory Care, 2nd edition. Stamford, Connecticut, US: Cengage Learning; 2011.

Index

Page numbers followed by *b* refer to box, *f* refer to figure, and *t* refer to table.

C

D

H

R

S

T